ADULT NURSE PRACTITIONER CERTIFICATION REVIEW GUIDE

Fifth Edition

Edited by

Sally K. Miller
PhD, CRNP, ANP-BC, ACNP-BC, FNP-BC, GNP-BC, CNE, FAANP
Clinical Professor
Drexel University College of
Nursing and Health Professions
Philadelphia, Pennsylvania

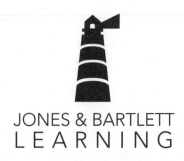

JONES & BARTLETT
LEARNING

World Headquarters
Jones & Bartlett Learning
5 Wall Street
Burlington, MA 01803
1-978-443-5000
info@jblearning.com
www.jblearning.com

Jones & Bartlett Learning books and products are available through most bookstores and online booksellers. To contact Jones & Bartlett Learning directly, call 1-800-832-0034, fax 1-978-443-8000, or visit our website, www.jblearning.com.

Substantial discounts on bulk quantities of Jones & Bartlett Learning publications are available to corporations, professional associations, and other qualified organizations. For details and specific discount information, contact the special sales department at Jones & Bartlett Learning via the above contact information or send an email to specialsales@jblearning.com.

Adult Nurse Practitioner Certification Review Guide is an independent publication and has not been authorized, sponsored, or otherwise approved by the owners of the trademarks or service marks referenced in this product.

The authors, editor, and publisher have made every effort to provide accurate information. However, they are not responsible for errors, omissions, or for any outcomes related to the use of the contents of this book and take no responsibility for the use of the products and procedures described. Treatments and side effects described in this book may not be applicable to all people; likewise, some people may require a dose or experience a side effect that is not described herein. Drugs and medical devices are discussed that may have limited availability controlled by the Food and Drug Administration (FDA) for use only in a research study or clinical trial. Research, clinical practice, and government regulations often change the accepted standard in this field. When consideration is being given to use of any drug in the clinical setting, the health care provider or reader is responsible for determining FDA status of the drug, reading the package insert, and reviewing prescribing information for the most up-to-date recommendations on dose, precautions, and contraindications, and determining the appropriate usage for the product. This is especially important in the case of drugs that are new or seldom used.

Production Credits
Publisher: Kevin Sullivan
Acquisitions Editor: Amanda Harvey
Editorial Assistant: Sara Bempkins
Production Editor: Amanda Clerkin
Associate Marketing Manager: Katie Hennessy
V.P., Manufacturing and Inventory Control: Therese Connell
Composition: Arlene Apone
Cover Design: Tim Dziewit
Cover Image: © Hocusfocus/Dreamstime.com
Printing and Binding: Courier Kendallville
Cover Printing: Courier Kendallville

To order this product, use ISBN: 978-1-4496-7046-7

Library of Congress Cataloging-in-Publication Data
Adult nurse practitioner certification review guide. -- 5th ed. / [edited by] Sally K. Miller.
    p. ; cm.
  Includes bibliographical references and index.
  ISBN-13: 978-0-7637-7535-3
  ISBN-10: 0-7637-7535-5
  I. Miller, Sally K.
  [DNLM: 1. Nurse Practitioners--Examination Questions. 2. Nurse Practitioners--Outlines. 3. Nursing Care--Examination Questions. 4. Nursing Care--Outlines. WY 18.2]
  610.7306'92--dc23
                    2011042568

6048

Printed in the United States of America
16 15 14 13 12   10 9 8 7 6 5 4 3 2 1

Dedication

This newest edition of the *Adult Nurse Practitioner Certification Review Guide* has been a labor of love and learning, and so many people in my life have contributed to the effort with their love, support, and tolerance. As always, hugs to my son Michael, now the 28-year-old version of the little boy to whom I dedicated my first book, to the teachers and mentors who brought me into the profession that I love, to the students who keep me on my toes and force me to be a life-long learner, and to my coworkers Ana and Linda who tolerate the unpredictable schedule and last-minute crises that characterize meeting a deadline.

Contents

Chapter 9

Endocrine Disorders 129

Sister Maria Salerno

Chapter 10

Genitourinary and Gynecological Disorders 147

Pamela A. Shuler
Mary D. Knudtson

Chapter 11

Pregnancy, Contraception, and Menopause 179

Beth M. Kelsey
Susan B. Moskosky

Chapter 12

Musculoskeletal Disorders 221

Madeline Turkeltaub

Chapter 13

Neurological Disorders   235

Sally K. Miller

Chapter 14

Psychosocial Disorders   249

Sister Maria Salerno

Chapter 15

Care of the Aging Adult   271

Debbie Gilbert Kramer

Chapter 16

Advanced Practice, Role Development, Current Trends, and Health Policy   289

Leanne C. Busby
Mary A. Baroni

Contributing Authors

Mary A. Baron, PhD, RN, CPNP
Professor
Nursing Program Director
University of Washington, Bothell
Bothell, Washington

Leanne C. Busby, DSN, RNC, FAANP
Dean and Professor
Jeanette Rudy School of Nursing
Cumberland University
Lebanon, Tennessee

Susan E. Chaney, EdD, APRN, BC, FNP-C
Professor
College of Nursing
Graduate Program Coordinator
Texas Woman's University
Family Nurse Practitioner
Homeless Outreach Medical Services
Parkland Health and Hospital System
Dallas, Texas

Sylvia Torres Fletcher, MS, RN, CS, FNP
Family Nurse Practitioner
Community Oriented Primary Care—
    Homeless Outreach Program
Parkland Health and Hospital System
Dallas, Texas

Nancy Dickenson-Hazard, MSN, CPNP, FAAN
Executive Officer
Sigma Theta Tau International
Indianapolis, Indiana

Beth M. Kelsey, MS, EdD(c), RNC, WHNP
Assistant Professor
Women's Health Nurse Practitioner
School of Nursing
Ball State University
Muncie, Indiana

Mary D. Knudtson, DNSc, NP-BC
Professor
Family Medicine
University of California, Irvine
Irvine, California

Debbie Gilbert Kramer, MS, RN, CS, CRNP
Gerontological/Adult Nurse Practitioner
Risk Management Department
Johns Hopkins Bayview Medical Center
Nurse Consultant
EHA Consulting Group, Inc.
Baltimore, Maryland

Sally K. Miller, PhD, CRNP, ANP-BC, ACNP-BC, FNP-BC, GNP-BC, CNE, FAANP
Clinical Professor
Drexel University College of Nursing and
    Health Professions
Philadelphia, Pennsylvania

Virginia L. Millonig, PhD, RN, CPNP
President
Health Leadership Associates, Inc.

Susan B. Moskosky, MS, RNC, WHCNP
Director, Office of Family Planning
Office of Population Affairs
U.S. Department of Health and
    Human Services
Washington, D.C.

Rosanne H. Pruitt, PhD, APRN-BC
Professor
School of Nursing
Clemson University
Clemson, South Carolina

Sister Maria Salerno, OSF, DNSc, APRN-BC
Associate Professor
Director Primary Care/Adult and Gerontological
    Nurse Practitioner Programs
Adult Nurse Practitioner, Gerontological
    Nurse Practitioner
Family Nurse Practitioner
Coordinator Adult CNS/Educator Program
School of Nursing
The Catholic University of America
Washington, D.C.

Pamela A. Shuler, DNSc, RN, CFNP
Family Nurse Practitioner
Great Smokies Medical Center
Asheville, North Carolina

Madeline Turkeltaub, PhD, CRNP
Nurse Practitioner
Greenbelt, Maryland

Margaret Hadro Venzke, MS, RN, CS, FNP
Instructor Nurse Practitioner Program
College of Nursing and Health Science
George Mason University
Fairfax, Virginia
Family Nurse Practitioner
Student Health Center
Georgetown University
Washington, D.C.

Preface

The fifth edition of this book has been developed especially for adult nurse practitioners preparing to take a national board certification examination. It is also an excellent tool for use in the clinical area for those who need an abbreviated, but comprehensive current clinical practice reference. All sections have been updated. The practice questions have been revised as appropriate and the chapter bibliographies updated and enhanced.

The purpose of the book is threefold. This book can be used by student nurse practitioners as they progress through their academic programs, it will assist new graduates and returning clinicians engaged in self-study preparation for certification examinations, and finally, the book can be used as a reference guide in the practice setting.

The book has been organized to provide the reader with test taking strategies first. This is followed by the chapter on health promotion. The next 13 chapters address common disorders and provide succinct summaries of definitions, etiology, signs and symptoms, physical findings, differential diagnoses, diagnostic evaluation, and clinical management. The final chapter addresses health policy, role, trends, and professional issues for the nurse practitioner in the healthcare industry at large.

Following each chapter are test questions, which are intended to help the reader assess recall and application of content and serve as an introduction to the testing arena. In addition, a bibliography is included for those who need a more in-depth discussion of the subject matter in each chapter. These references can serve as additional instructional material for the reader.

Many nurses preparing for certification examinations find that reviewing an extensive body of scientific knowledge requires a very difficult search of many sources that must be synthesized to provide a review base for the examination. This publication provides a succinct, yet comprehensive review of the core material.

The editor and contributing authors are certified nurse practitioners. They have designed this book to assist potential examinees to prepare for success in the certification examination process as well as enhance their clinical practice.

Certification is a process that is gaining recognition both within and outside the professional community. Most states, insurers, and employers require certification for licensure, hire, and reimbursement. For the professional, it is a means of gaining special recognition as a certified nurse practitioner, which not only demonstrates a level of competency, but may also enhance professional opportunities and advancement. For the consumer, it means that a certified practitioner has met certain predetermined standards set by the profession.

1

Test Taking Strategies and Techniques

Nancy A. Dickenson-Hazard

Virginia L. Millonig

We all respond to testing situations in different ways. What separates the successful test taker from the unsuccessful one is knowing how to prepare for and take a test. Preparing yourself to be a successful test taker is as important as studying for the test. Each person needs to assess and develop individual test taking strategies and skills. The primary goal of this chapter is to provide potential examinees with strategies that will help them develop studying and test taking skills. Of equal importance to this test preparation is a basic understanding of how certification examinations are developed. They are based upon a universal knowledge foundation. Test items are selected from generally recognized resources available to the examinee and specific to the specialty area.

◘ STRATEGY #1 KNOW YOURSELF

When faced with an examination, do you feel threatened, experience butterflies or sweaty palms, have trouble keeping your mind focused on studying or on test questions? These common symptoms of test anxiety plague many of us but can be used advantageously if understood and handled correctly. Over the years, each of us has developed certain test taking behaviors, some of which are beneficial, while others present obstacles to successful test taking. You can take control of the test taking situation by identifying undesirable behaviors, maintaining desirable ones, and developing skills to improve test performance.

Technique #1:

Find your personality type. Write down those characteristics that describe you even if they are from different personality types. Carefully review the pitfalls associated with your test taking personality characteristics. Write down the problems that are most troublesome. Then make a list of how you can remedy these problems from the improvement strategies list. Be sure to use these strategies as you prepare for and take examinations.

◘ STRATEGY #2 DEVELOP YOUR THINKING SKILLS

Understanding the Thought Process:

In order to improve your thinking skills and subsequent test performance, it is best to understand the types of thinking as well as the techniques to enhance the thought process.

Everyone has a personal learning style, but we all must proceed through the same process to think. Thinking occurs on six levels—from the basic levels of knowledge and comprehension to the more complex levels of application, analysis, synthesis, and evaluation (Bloom & Krathwohl, 1956). Knowledge is the ability to recall facts. Without adequate retrieval of facts, progression through the higher levels of thinking cannot occur easily. Comprehension is the ability to understand memorized facts. To be effective, comprehension skills must allow the person to translate recalled information from one context to another. Application, or the process of using information to know why something occurs, is a higher form of learning. Effective application relies on the use of understood, memorized facts to verify intended action. Analysis is the ability to use abstract or logical forms of thought to show relationships and to distinguish the cause and effect between the variables in a situation.

As related to testing situations, the thought process from memory to analysis occurs quite quickly. Some examination items are designed to test memory and comprehension while others test application and analysis. An example of a memory question is as follows:

Type 1 diabetes results from dysfunction of the:

a. Liver
b. *Pancreas*
c. Adrenal glands
d. Kidneys

To answer this question correctly, the individual has to retrieve a memorized fact. Understanding the fact, knowing why it is important, or analyzing what should be done in this situation is not needed. The following example is a question that tests comprehension:

You are taking a history on a 47-year-old white female during a routine health assessment visit. She reports that in the past month she has experienced increased thirst and needs to urinate frequently. She reports recurrent episodes of vaginitis and is concerned about an abrasion on her leg that will not heal. You note that her blood pressure is recorded at 150/90 mm Hg and that she is overweight at 5'1" and 195 lbs. Which of the following is the most likely cause of her symptoms?

a. Urinary tract infection
b. Hyperthyroidism
c. Type 1 diabetes mellitus
d. *Type 2 diabetes mellitus*

To answer this question correctly, an individual must retrieve facts about the physiology of diabetes mellitus in order to understand and differentiate the presenting symptoms.

In answering an examination question that requires a higher level of thought, an individual must be able to recall a fact, understand that fact in the context of the question, and apply this understanding to determine why one answer is correct, after analyzing possible answer choices as they relate to the situation (Sides & Korchek, 1994). The following example is an application analysis question:

A 48-year-old diabetic woman wants to enroll in a low-impact aerobics class. Her diabetes is well managed with twice-daily insulin injections. Your best advice is to suggest that she:

a. Increase daily doses of insulin
b. *Have an extra snack before exercise class*
c. Administer a dose of regular insulin after exercise is completed
d. Consider an activity that does not require physical exertion

To answer this question correctly, the individual must recall physiologic facts of insulin dependent diabetes, understand what is happening in this situation, consider each option and how it applies to the patient's condition, and analyze why each advice option works or doesn't work for this patient. Application/analysis questions require the examinee to use logical rationale based on a well-defined principle or fact. Problem solving ability becomes important as the examinee must think through each question option and determine its relevance and importance to the situation in the question.

Building Your Thinking Skills:

Effective memorization is the cornerstone to learning and building thinking skills (Olney, 1989). We have all experienced "memory power outages" at some time, due in part to trying to memorize too much, too fast. Developing skills to improve memorization is important for increasing the effectiveness of your thinking and subsequent test performance.

Technique #1:

Quantity is NOT quality, so concentrate on learning important content. For example, it is important to know the various pharmacologic agents appropriate for the management of chronic obstructive pulmonary disease (COPD), not the specific dosages for each medication.

Technique #2:

Memory from repetition, or saying something over and over again to remember it, usually fades. Developing memory skills that trigger retrieval of needed facts is more useful. Such skills include:

Acronyms: These are mental crutches that facilitate recall. Some are already established such as PERRLA (pupils equal, round, react to light, and accommodation), CHF (congestive heart failure), or TIA (transient ischemic attack). Developing your own acronyms can be particularly useful because they are your own word association arrangements in a singular word. Nonsense words or funny, unusual ones are often more useful since they attract your attention.

Acrostics: This mental tool arranges words into catchy phrases. The first letter of each word stands for something that is recalled as the phrase is spoken. Your own acrostics are most valuable in triggering recall of learned information because they are your individual situation associations. An example of an acrostic is as follows:

Sam **E**xercises **B**y **W**eight-lifting and **R**unning stands for the aspects of nondrug therapy/management for hypertension: **S**alt restriction, **E**xercise, **B**iofeedback, **W**eight reduction, and **R**elaxation techniques.

ABCs: This technique facilitates information retrieval by using the alphabet as a crutch. Each letter stands for a symptom, which when put together creates a picture of the clinical presentation of the disease. For example, the characteristics of peptic ulcer disease using the ABC technique are as follows:

Antacids relieve pain

Burning epigastric pain

Cycle of pain 2 hours after eating

Discomfort awakens at night

Experiences weight loss

Food sometimes aggravates pain

Imaging: This technique can be used in two ways. The first is to develop a nickname for a clinical problem that, when spoken, produces a mental picture. For example, "thin, barrel-chested, pink puffer" might be used to visualize a patient with emphysema who has a muscle-wasted body appearance, absent central cyanosis, hypertrophy of respiratory accessory muscles, and an AP chest diameter greater than the transverse chest. A second form of imaging is to visualize a specific patient while you are trying to understand or solve a clinical problem when studying or answering a question. For example, imagine a young woman who is experiencing an acute asthma attack. You are trying to analyze the situation and place her in a position that maximizes respiratory effort. In your mind you visualize her in various positions of sidelying, angular, and forward, imagining what will happen to the woman and her respiratory effort in each position.

Rhymes, music, and links: The absurd is easier to remember than the common. Rhymes, music, and links can add absurdity and humor to learning and remembering (Olney, 1989). These retrieval tools are developed by the individual for specific content. For example, making up a rhyme about diabetes may be helpful in remembering the predominant female incidence, origin of disease, primary symptoms, and management, as illustrated by:

There once was a woman
whose beta cells failed
She grew quite thirsty
and her glucose levels sailed
Her lack of insulin caused her to
increase her intake
And her increased urinary output
was certainly not fake
So she learned to watch her diet
and administer injections
That kept her healthy, growing,
and free of complications.

Setting content to music is sometimes useful to remembering. Melodies that are repetitious jog the memory by the ups and downs of the notes and the rhythm of the music. Links connect key words from the content by using them in a story. An example given by Olney (1989) for remembering the parts of an eye is IRIS watched a PUPIL through the LENS of a RED TIN telescope while eating CORN-EA on the cob.

Additional memory aids may also include the use of color or drawing for improving recall. Use different colored pens or paper to accentuate the material being learned. For example, highlight or make notes in blue for content about respiratory problems and in red for cardiovascular content. Drawing assists with visualizing content as well. This is particularly helpful for remembering the pathophysiology of the specific health problem.

> **The important thing to remember about remembering is to use good recall techniques.**

Technique #3:

Improving higher-level thinking skills involves exercising the application and analysis of memorized facts. Small-group review is particularly useful for enhancing these high-level skills. Small-group interaction allows verbalization of thought processes and receipt of input about content and thought process from others (Sides & Korchek, 1994). Individuals not only hear how they think, but how others think as well. This interaction allows individuals to identify flaws in their thought processes as well as strengthen their positive points.

Taking practice tests is also helpful in developing application/analysis thinking skills. Practice tests permit the individual to analyze thinking patterns as well as the cause-and-effect relationships between the question and its options. The problem solving skills needed to answer application/analysis questions are tested, giving the individual more experience through practice (Dickenson-Hazard, 1990b).

◻ STRATEGY #3 KNOW THE CONTENT

Your ability to study is directly influenced by organization and concentration (Dickenson-Hazard, 1990c). If effort is spent on both of these aspects of exam preparation, examination success can be increased.

Preparation for Studying: Getting Organized:

Study habits are developed early in our education experiences. Some of our habits enhance learning while others do not. To increase study effectiveness, organization of study materials and time is essential. Organization decreases frustration, allows for easy resumption of study, and increases concentrated study time.

Technique #1:

Create your own study space. Select a study area that is yours alone, free from distractions, comfortable, and well lighted. The ventilation and room temperature should be comfortable since a cold room makes it difficult to concentrate and a warm room may make you sleepy (Burkle & Marshak, 1989). All study materials should be left in a specific study space. The basic premise of a study space is that it facilitates a mind set that you are there to study. When study is interrupted, it is best to leave study materials just as they are. Don't close books or put away notes as they will have to be relocated, which will waste valuable time when study is resumed.

Technique #2:

Define and organize the content. Secure an outline or the content parameters that are to be examined from the examining body. If the outline is sketchy, develop a more detailed one for yourself using the recommended texts as a guideline. Next, identify available study resources: class notes, old exams, handouts, textbooks, review courses and books, home study programs, or study groups. For national standardized exams, such as initial licensing or certification, it is best to identify a few resources that cover the content being tested and stick to them. Attempting to review all available resources is not only mind boggling but increases anxiety and frustration as well. Make your selections and stay with them.

Technique #3:

Conduct a content assessment. Using a simple rating scale of:

1 = requires no review
2 = requires minimal review
3 = requires intensive review
4 = start from the beginning

Read through the content outline and rate each content area (Dickenson-Hazard, 1990a). **Table 1-1** provides a sample exam content assessment. Be honest in your assessment. It is far better to recognize your content weaknesses when you can study and remedy them rather than wishing during the exam that you had studied more. Likewise with content strengths: if you know the material, don't waste time studying it.

Technique #4:

Develop a study plan. Coordinate the content that needs to be studied with the time available (Sides & Korchek, 1994). Prioritize your study needs, starting with weak areas first. Allow for a general review at the end of the study plan. Finally, establish an overall goal

■ **Table 1-1** Sample Content Assessment

Exam Content: Gastrointestinal Health Problems of the Adult

Category: Provided by Examining Body	Rating: Provided by Examinee
I. Peptic Ulcer Disease	
A. Etiology	4
B. Pathophysiology	3
C. Symptomatology	3
D. Differential Diagnosis	4
E. Diagnostic Tests	3
F. Management/Treatment	4
II. Esophagitis	
A. Etiology	3
B. Pathophysiology	3
C. Symptomatology	2
D. Differential Diagnosis	3
E. Diagnostic Tests	2
F. Management/Treatment	4
III. Cholecystitis	
A. Etiology	2
B. Pathophysiology	2
C. Symptomatology	1
D. Differential Diagnosis	2
E. Diagnostic Tests	4
F. Management/Treatment	4
IV. Appendicitis	
A. Etiology	3
B. Pathophysiology	4
C. Symptomatology	3
D. Differential Diagnosis	2
E. Diagnostic Tests	3
F. Management/Treatment	4
V. Diverticulitis	
A. Etiology	3
B. Pathophysiology	4
C. Symptomatology	3
D. Differential Diagnosis	3
E. Diagnostic Tests	2
F. Management/Treatment	4
VI. Hepatitis	
A. Etiology	3
B. Pathophysiology	4
C. Symptomatology	4
D. Differential Diagnosis	4
E. Diagnostic Tests	2
F. Management/Treatment	4

■ **Table 1-1** Sample Content Assessment *(continued)*

Category: Provided by Examining Body	Rating: Provided by Examinee
VII. Acute Gastroenteritis	
A. Etiology	2
B. Pathophysiology	3
C. Symptomatology	2
D. Differential Diagnosis	3
E. Diagnostic Tests	4
F. Management/Treatment	3
VIII. Irritable Bowel Syndrome	
A. Etiology	3
B. Pathophysiology	3
C. Symptomatology	3
D. Differential Diagnosis	4
E. Diagnostic Tests	4
F. Management/Treatment	3

for yourself, something that will motivate you when brought to mind.

Table 1-2 illustrates a study plan developed on the basis of the exam content assessment in Table 1-1. Conducting an assessment and developing a study plan should require no more than 50 minutes. It is a wise investment of time with potential payoffs of reduced study stress and exam success.

Technique #5:

Begin now and use your time wisely. The smart test taker begins the study process early (Olney, 1989). Sit down, conduct the content assessment, and develop a study plan as soon as you know about the exam. DON'T PROCRASTINATE!

Getting Down to Business—the Actual Studying:

There is no better way to prepare for an examination than individual study (Dickenson-Hazard, 1989b). The

■ **Table 1-2** Sample Study Plan

Goal: Master Content on the Gastrointestinal Problems of the Adult Patient. Test Time Available: 2 Weeks		
Objective	**Activity**	**Date Accomplished**
Master content on diverticulitis.	Read Chapter 26. Take notes on chapter content according to outline.	Feb. 5 & 6, 1 hour
	Review class notes combined with chapter notes.	Feb. 6, 1 hour
	Review sample test questions.	Feb. 6, 1 hour
Understand content on peptic ulcer disease.	Read Chapter 25. Take notes on chapter content according to content outline.	Feb. 7, 2 hours
	Review class notes combined with chapter notes.	Feb. 8, 1½ hours
Master content on cholecystitis.	Read Chapter 24. Take notes on chapter content according to content outline.	Feb. 10, 2 hours
	Review class notes combined with chapter notes.	Feb. 11, ½ hour
	Review sample test questions.	Feb. 12, 1½ hours
Know material on irritable bowel syndrome.	Scan Chapter 27. Review class notes supplementing with text notes.	Feb. 14, 2 hours
Know material on esophagitis.	Scan Chapter 23. Review class notes supplementing with text notes.	Feb. 15, 2 hours
Know material on hepatitis.	Scan Chapter 28. Review highlights and important concepts.	Feb. 16, 2 hours
Know material on appendicitis and acute gastroenteritis.	Scan Chapter 29. Review highlights and important concepts.	Feb. 17, 2 hours
Demonstrate understanding of all material.	Review with another person.	Feb. 18, 2 hours
	Review all notes.	Feb. 19, 1½ hours
	Take sample test questions.	Feb. 19, 1½ hours
Think positively.	SMILE.	ONGOING
	Take frequent breaks.	
	Reward myself after each study session.	
	Keep my goal in mind.	

responsibility to achieve the goal you set for this exam lies with you alone. The means that you employ to achieve this goal will vary and should begin with identifying your peak study times and using techniques to maximize them.

Technique #1:

Study in short bursts. Each of us has our own biologic clock that dictates when we are at our peak during the day. If you are a morning person, you are generally active and alert early in the day, slowing down and becoming drowsy by evening. If you are an evening person, you don't completely wake up until late morning and hit your peak in the afternoon and evening. Each person generally has several peaks during the day. It is best to study during those times when your alertness is at its peak (Dickenson-Hazard, 1990d).

During our concentration peaks, there are mini peaks or bursts of alertness (Olney, 1989). These alertness ("mini") peaks occur during a concentration peak because levels of concentration are at their highest during the first part and last part of a study period. These bursts can vary from 10 minutes to 1 hour depending on the extent of concentration. If studying is sustained for 1 hour there are only two mini peaks; one at the beginning and one at the end. There are eight mini peaks if that same hour is divided into four, 10-minute intervals. Hence it is more helpful to study in short bursts (Olney, 1989). More can be learned in less time.

Technique #2:

Cramming can be useful. Since concentration ability is highly variable, some individuals can sustain their mini peaks for 15, 20, or even 30 minutes at a time. Pushing your concentration beyond its peak is fruitless and verges on cramming, which in general is a poor study technique. There are, however, times when cramming, a short-term memory tool, is useful. Short-term memory generally is at its best in the morning. A quick review or cram of content in the morning can be useful the day of the exam (Olney, 1989). Most studying, however, is best accomplished in the afternoon or evening when long-term memory functions at its peak.

Technique #3:

Give your brain breaks. Regular times during study to rest and absorb the content is needed by the brain. The best approach to breaks is to plan them and give yourself a conscious break (Dickenson-Hazard, 1990c). This approach eliminates the "day dreaming" or "wandering thought" approach to breaks that many of us use. It is better to get up, leave the study area, and do something unrelated to studying for longer breaks. For shorter breaks of 5 minutes or so, leave your desk, gaze out the window or do some stretching exercises. When your brain says to give it a rest, accommodate it! You'll learn more in time that is less stressful.

Technique #4:

Study the correct content. It is easy for all of us to become bogged down in the detail of the content we are studying. However, it is best to focus on the major concepts or the "state of the art" content. Leave the details, the suppositions, and the experience at the door of your study area. Concentrate on the major textbook facts and concepts that revolve around the subject matter being tested.

Technique #5:

Fit your studying to the test type. The best way to prepare for an objective test is to study facts, particularly anything printed in italics. Memory-enhancing techniques are particularly useful when preparing for an objective test. If preparing for an essay test, study generalities, examples, and concepts. Application techniques are helpful when studying for this type of an exam (Burkle & Marshak, 1989).

Technique #6:

Use your study plan wisely. Your study plan is meant to be a guide, not a rigid schedule. You should take your time with studying. Don't rush through the content just to remain on schedule. Occasionally study plans need revision. If you take more or less time than planned, readjust the plan for the time gained or lost. The plan can guide you, but you must go at your own pace.

Technique #7:

Actively study. Being an active participant in study rather than trying to absorb the printed word is also helpful. Ways to be active include taking notes on the content as you study, constructing questions and answering them, and taking practice tests and discussing the content with yourself. Also, using your individual study quirks is encouraged. Some people stand, others walk around, and some play background music. You should use whatever helps you to concentrate and study better.

Technique #8:

Use study aids. While there is no substitute for individual studying, several resources, if available, are useful in facilitating learning. Review courses are an excellent means for organizing or summarizing your individual study. They generally provide the content parameters and the major concepts of the content that you need to know. Review courses also provide an opportunity to clarify less-well-understood content as well as to review known material (Dickenson-Hazard, 1990a). Study guides, certification review books, and home study programs are useful for organizing study. They provide detail on the content that is important to the exam. Study groups are an excellent resource for summarizing and refining content. They provide an opportunity for thinking through your knowledge base, with the advantage of hearing another person's point of view. Each of these study aids increases understanding of content and, when used correctly, increases effectiveness of knowledge application.

Technique #9:

Know when to quit. It is best to stop studying when your concentration ebbs. It is unproductive and frustrating to force yourself to study. It is far better to rest or unwind, then resume at a later point in the day. Avoid studying outside your A.M. or P.M. concentration peaks and focus your study energy on your best time of day or evening.

◻ STRATEGY #4 BECOME TEST-WISE

Most advanced practice nursing certification examinations are composed of multiple choice questions (MCQ). This type of question requires the examinee to select the best response for a specific circumstance or condition. Successful test taking is dependent not only on content knowledge but on test taking skill as well. If you are unable to impart your knowledge through the vehicle used for its conveyance—for example, the MCQ—your test taking success is in jeopardy.

Computer-based examinations are offered by all certification organizations, with some continuing to offer pencil-and-paper alternatives. Computer-based testing has several advantages, such as flexibility in taking the examinations at your convenience and earlier notification of test results. Instructions will be provided prior to the examination and at the time of the examination. No computer experience is required, and tutorials or introductory lessons precede the computer-based testing to familiarize you with the process.

Technique #1:

Recognize the purpose of a test question. Most test questions are developed to examine knowledge at two separate levels: memory and comprehension or application and analysis. A memory question requires examinees to recall facts from their knowledge base while an application question requires examinees to use and apply the knowledge. Memory questions test recall while application questions test synthesis and problem solving skills. When taking a test, you need to be aware when you are being asked to recall a fact and when you are being asked to use that fact.

Technique #2:

Recognize the components of a test question. Multiple choice questions may include the basic components of a background statement, a stem, and a list of options. The background statement presents information that facilitates the examinee in answering the question. The stem asks or states the intent of the question. The options typically include four possible responses to the question. The correct option is called the keyed response, and all other options are called distracters (ABP, 1989). Knowing the components of a test question helps you sift through the information presented and focus on the question's intent (see **Table 1-3**).

Technique #3:

Identify the key word(s) in a test question. Don't jump to conclusions when you read the stem. Key words are generally included in the stem of a test question, whereas key concepts or conditions appear in the background statement. You should pay particular attention to the key words in the stem and their impact on the intent of the question. Never "read between the lines" of a question or make assumptions about the information given.

◼ **Table 1-3** Anatomy of a Test Question

Background Statement	A 32-year-old female is being seen for a complaint of sores in the vaginal area. She has been experiencing a low-grade fever, headache, and malaise over the past 5 days. Physical examination reveals inguinal lymphadenopathy, vaginal erythema, and multiple labial and vaginal vesicular lesions.
Stem	Which of the following causative organisms would you suspect?
Options	a. *Herpes simplex virus 2* b. Condylomata lata c. Herpes simplex virus 1 d. *Treponema pallidum*

Technique #4:

Recognize the item types. Basically two styles of MCQs are used for examinations. The more common type requires the examinee to select the one best answer; rarely, an exam will require selection of multiple correct answers. Among the one best answer styles are three types. The A type requires the selection of the best response among those offered. The B type requires the examinee to match the options with the appropriate statement. C-type items require the examinee to compare or contrast two related conditions. The X type asks the examinee to respond either true or false to each option (ABP, 1989). Many standardized tests such as those used for certification are composed of MCQ A-type questions.

Technique #5:

Read the directions to the questions carefully. Questions are sometimes answered incorrectly because the test taker did not carefully read the directions.

Technique #6:

Apply the basic rules of test taking. Examination candidates can avoid many problems associated with test taking if they give thought to the mechanics of sitting down, reading the question, and noting their answers. Timing yourself to avoid spending too much time on a question and not changing your answers are two techniques that can improve performance. Review these and apply them to the testing situation.

Technique #7:

Make educated guesses. An educated guess is the selection of an option (answer) when you are unsure of the correct answer. Elimination of all options except for two, followed by a reevaluation of these two options based on your knowledge base, allows you to make an educated guess.

The more common advanced practice nursing certification examinations will give credit when correct answers are selected and give no credit for incorrect answers. Directions for this type of examination may state that credit will be given for correct answers; therefore all questions should be answered and you will not be penalized for guessing.

Infrequently, examinations will only give credit for correct answers and subtract credit for incorrect answers. Directions for this type of examination will instruct you not to guess or will tell you that there is a penalty for guessing. However, even with this kind of an examination, it is still to your advantage to make an educated guess if you can reduce your possibilities to two options and then select the best of the two. WILD GUESSING should be avoided since it may not be to your advantage (Nugent & Vitale, 1997).

Technique #8:

Practice, practice, practice. Taking practice tests can improve performance. While they can assist in evaluation of your knowledge, *their primary benefit is to assist you with test taking skills*. You should use them to evaluate your thinking process; your ability to read, understand, and interpret questions, and your skills in completing the mechanics of the test.

Technique #9:

Be prepared for exam day. It is important to familiarize yourself with the test site, the building, the parking, and the travel route prior to the exam day. The night before the exam, go to bed at a reasonable hour and avoid excessive drinking or eating (Sides & Korchek, 1994). If you must travel, allow time for this familiarization. It is helpful to make a list of things you need on the exam day: pencils, admission card, watch, and a few pieces of hard candy as a quick energy source. On exam day allow yourself plenty of time to arrive at the site. Wear comfortable clothes and have a good breakfast that morning. The idea is to arrive on time at the test site as prepared and as rested as possible.

◻ STRATEGY #5 PSYCH YOURSELF UP: TAKING TESTS IS STRESSFUL

While a little stress can be productive, too much can incapacitate you in your studying and test taking (Divine & Kylen, 1979). Your attitude and approach to test taking and studying can influence your outcomes. Psyching yourself up can have a positive effect and help keep examinations from becoming anxiety-laden experiences (Dickenson-Hazard, 1990b). The following techniques are based on the principles of successful test taking as presented by Sides & Cailles (1989). Incorporation of these techniques can improve response and performance in examination situations.

Technique #1:

Adopt an "I can" attitude. Believing you can succeed is the key to success. Self-belief inspires and gives you the power to achieve your goals. Without a success attitude, the road to your goal is much harder. We all stand an equal chance of success in this world. It is those who believe they can who achieve it. This "I can" attitude must permeate all your efforts in test taking from studying to improving your skills to actually writing the test.

Technique #2:

Take control. By identifying your goal, deciding how to accomplish it, and developing a plan for achieving it, you take control. Do not leave your success or failure to chance; control it through action and attitude.

Technique #3:

Think positively. Examinations are generally based on a standard that is the same for all individuals. Everyone can potentially pass. Performance is influenced not only by knowledge and skill but attitude as well. Those individuals who regard an exam as an opportunity or challenge will be more successful.

Technique #4:

Project a positive self-fulfilling prophecy. While preparing for an examination, project thoughts of the positive outcomes you will experience when you succeed. Self-talk is self-fulfilling. Expect success, not failure, of yourself.

Technique #5:

Feel good about yourself. Without feeling a sense of positive self-worth, passing an examination is difficult. Recognize your professional contributions and give yourself credit for your accomplishments. Think "I will pass," not "I suppose I can."

Technique #6:

Know yourself. Focus exam preparation and test taking on your strengths. Try to alter your weaknesses instead of becoming hung up on them. If you tend to over-analyze, study and read test questions at face value. If you're a speed demon when taking a test, slow down and read more carefully.

Technique #7:

Failure is a possibility. We all have failed at something at some point in our lives. Rather than dwelling on the failure, making excuses, and believing you'll fail again, recognize your mistakes and remedy them. Failure is a time to begin again; use it as a motivator to do better. It is not the end of the world unless you allow it to be. It is best to deal with the failure and move on, otherwise it interferes with your success.

Technique #8:

Persevere, persevere, persevere! Endurance must underlie all your efforts. Call forth those reserve energies when you've had all you think you can take. Rely on yourself and your support systems to help you maintain a sense of direction and keep your goal in the forefront.

Technique #9:

Motivation is muscle. Most individuals are motivated by fear or desire. The fear in an exam situation may be one of failure, the unknown, or discovery of imperfection.

Put your fear into perspective; realize you are not the only one with fear and that all have an equal opportunity for success. Develop strategies to reduce fear and use fear to your advantage by improving the imperfections. Desire is a powerful motivator and you should keep the rewards of your desire foremost in your mind. Whatever motivates you, use it to be successful. Reward yourself during your exam preparation and after the exam has been completed. You alone hold the key to success; use what you have wisely.

Technique #10:

Overprepare. One of the best ways to reduce test anxiety is to overprepare. The more prepared you are the more confident you will be. Overpreparation requires you to study the same information over again even when you know the information. This activity will reinforce your learning and will build confidence and reduce anxiety when it comes time to take the examination.

Overpreparation cannot occur unless adequate time is allowed for this process. A last-minute cramming approach will not lead to an over-prepared test taker. Being over prepared definitely places an individual in control and in a position of power and confidence (Nugent & Vitale, 1997).

This chapter has provided concepts, strategies, and techniques for improving study and test taking skills. Your first task in improvement is to know yourself, how you study, and how you take a test. You should use your strengths and remedy the weaknesses. Next you need to develop your thinking skills. Work on techniques to improve memory and reasoning. Then you need to organize your study and concentrate on using these new skills to be successful. Create a study space, develop a plan of action, and then implement that plan during your periods of peak concentration. Before taking the exam be sure you understand the components of a test question, can identify key words and phrases, and have practiced. Apply the test taking rules during the exam process. Finally, believe in yourself, your knowledge, and your talent. Believing you can accomplish your goal makes it more likely that you will.

◻ BIBLIOGRAPHY

American Board of Pediatrics (ABP). (1989). *Developing questions and critiques.* Unpublished material.

Bloom, B. S., & Krathwohl D. R. (1956). *Taxonomy of educational objectives: The classification of educational goals, by a committee of college and university examiners. Handbook 1: Cognitive domain.* New York: Longman.

Burkle, C. A., & Marshak, D. (1989). *Study program: Level 1.* Reston, VA: National Association of Secondary School Principals.

Dickenson-Hazard, N. (1989a). Anatomy of a test question. *Pediatric Nursing, 15,* 395–399.

Dickenson-Hazard, N. (1989b). Making the grade as a test taker. *Pediatric Nursing, 15,* 302–304.

Dickenson-Hazard, N. (1990a). Develop your thinking skills for improved test taking. *Pediatric Nursing, 16,* 480–481.

Dickenson-Hazard, N. (1990b). The psychology of successful test taking. *Pediatric Nursing, 16,* 66–67.

Dickenson-Hazard, N. (1990c). Study smart. *Pediatric Nursing, 16,* 314–316.

Dickenson-Hazard, N. (1990d). Study effectiveness: Are you a 10 a.m. or p.m. scholar? *Pediatric Nursing, 16,* 419–420.

Divine, J. H., & Kylen, D. W. (1979). *How to beat test anxiety.* New York: Barrons Educational Series.

Millman, J., & Pauk, W. (1969). *How to take tests.* New York: McGraw-Hill.

Nugent, P. M., & Vitale, B. A. (1997). *Test success* (2nd ed.). Philadelphia: F. A. Davis.

Olney, C. W. (1989). *Where there's a will, there's an A.* NJ: Chesterbrook Educational Publishers.

Sides, M., & Cailles, N. B. (1989). *Nurse's guide to successful test taking.* Philadelphia: J. B. Lippincott.

Sides, M., & Korchek, N. (1994). *Nurse's guide to successful test taking* (2nd ed.). Philadelphia: J. B. Lippincott.

Health Promotion and Evaluation

Rosanne H. Pruitt

◻ THEORETICAL ASPECTS: HEALTH PROMOTION THEORIES AND MODELS

- High-Level Wellness—a *continuum* that demonstrates dynamic interaction of health and environment as one moves toward high-level wellness; health is dynamic with a continuing need for health-promoting activity to maintain and improve one's health

- Maslow's Hierarchy of Needs (Maslow, 1954)
  1. Survival needs—food, water, sleep
  2. Safety and security—protection from physical hazards
  3. Love and belonging—affection, companionship
  4. Self-esteem—sense of self-worth, recognition
  5. Self-actualization—achievement of personal potential

- Health Belief Model (Becker, 1972)—health is influenced by age, sex, race, ethnicity, and income
  1. Threats to health
     a. Perceived susceptibility
     b. Perceived seriousness of condition
  2. Outcome expectation of health action
     a. Perceived benefits of action
     b. Perceived barriers to taking action
     c. Efficacy expectations

- Self-Efficacy Theory (Bandura, 1986)—explains human behavior in terms of a dynamic, reciprocal interaction between behavior, personal factors, and environmental influences; key concepts include

  1. Personal factors, including the ability to symbolize behavior meaning, to foresee outcomes of given behavior, to learn by observing others, to self-determine and self regulate, and to reflect and analyze experience
  2. Reciprocal determinism refers to behavior as dynamic and dependent on environmental and personal constructs that influence each other simultaneously

- Health Promotion Model (Pender, 2002)—health-promoting behaviors are motivated by multiple cognitive-perceptual factors such as the importance of health and perceived benefits, and the perceived control of health and self-efficacy, and are modified by factors such as demographics and interpersonal influences

- Erikson's Stages of Psychosocial Development (Erikson, 1963)—degree of success in accomplishing developmental tasks influences the accomplishment of tasks of older adults
  1. Trust versus mistrust—trust of self and others
  2. Autonomy versus shame and doubt—self-expression and cooperation with others
  3. Initiative versus guilt—focus on purposeful behavior
  4. Industry versus inferiority—belief in one's ability
  5. Identity versus role confusion—clear sense of self
  6. Intimacy versus role confusion—capacity for reciprocal love relationships

7. Generativity versus stagnation—creativity and productivity
8. Ego identity versus despair—acceptance of one's life as worthwhile and unique

- Health Behavior Change Models
  1. PRECEDE Model (Green & Kreuter, 1991)—involves identifying and assessing the learner's quality of life; identifying health problems and risk factors; the acronym PRECEDE stands for Predisposing, Reinforcing, and Enabling Causes in Educational Diagnosis and Evaluation: Predisposing factors (perception, knowledge, and attitudes), Reinforcing factors (significant others), and Enabling factors (environmental factors of accessibility and costs) are used to develop educational interventions for change and policies to support change
  2. Change Theory (Lewin, 1951)—advanced practice environments are dynamic; planned change involves unfreezing of current approach, implementing change, refreezing or creating, and acceptance and regular use of new approach
  3. Transtheoretical Model (Prochaska & Velicer, 1997)—temporal model of behavioral change; model emerged from comparative analysis of over 300 theories
     a. Precontemplation—no intention to take action within next 6 months; not ready and often resistant to health promotion change efforts; appropriate to use consciousness-raising education
     b. Contemplation—intention to take action within next 6 months; not ready and ambivalent toward change; appropriate to use consciousness-raising education
     c. Preparation—intends to take action within 30 days and has taken some behavioral steps in this direction; individuals at this stage should be recruited for action toward behavior change
     d. Action—individual has changed behavior for less than 6 months
     e. Maintenance—individual has changed overt behavior for more than 6 months; support and encouragement of continued behavior change

- Systems Theories
  1. General Systems Theory (von Bertalanffy, 1968)—views world in terms of sets of integrated reactions in an effort to see parts in relation to the whole; key concepts include
     a. System—goal directed unit with interdependent, interacting parts that also interact with environment
     b. Boundaries regulate exchange of energy, information, and matter between systems; may be open or closed depending on interaction with surrounding environment
     c. Input, output, and feedback loop provide for an exchange of energy, information, and matter
  2. Neuman's Systems Model (Neuman & Fawcett, 2002)—uses a systems format and includes levels of prevention as well as multiple dimensions of health promotion (physical, psychological, spiritual, and social); health promotion efforts are used to strengthen line barriers of defense

◻ RELATED CONCEPTS

- Levels of prevention from public health science are used by most authorities when differentiating health promotion activities from other interventions. *Healthy People 2020* and other federal documents use a broader interpretation, including health protection with specific screenings and safety factors, which are also included in this chapter
  1. Primary prevention includes measures to promote optimum health prior to the onset of any problems—health promotion and care intended to minimize risk factors and subsequent disease (e.g., promoting a healthy diet, exercise, stress management, safety, avoiding harmful substances)
  2. Secondary prevention focuses on early identification and treatment of existing health problems (e.g., screening for disease, pap smear, mammogram)
  3. Tertiary prevention is care intended to improve the course of a disease; the rehabilitation and restoration to health (e.g., cardiac rehabilitation)

- Cultural influence must be considered with any healthcare encounter. Cultural beliefs of disease causation influence health practices (e.g., magic or evil spirits—Latino); violation of a natural law (American Indian); imbalance between "hot" and "cold" forces (Asian, Latino). Varied beliefs affect the acceptance of practices such as hand washing and immunizations. There are differences between and among cultural groups. Certain beliefs are common among cultural groups
  1. Native Americans—harmony with nature and supernatural forces are important factors in health beliefs; social networking is also important; note taking is often considered taboo; silence is a sign of respect
  2. Hispanic Americans—extended family is important in decision making; illness may be

related to imbalance of hot and cold; sustaining eye contact is considered rude (*mal ojo*); higher risk of vitamin A, iron, and calcium deficiency due to dietary habits

3. Asian Americans—naturalistic beliefs are common; saying no is considered rude and is avoided; eye contact may be avoided out of respect; a need to balance hot and cold through food and medication is prevalent; use of acupuncture therapy is widespread

4. African-Americans—diverse group with beliefs that include "health is harmony with nature" and "life is a process, not a state"; maternal grandmother is often important in decision making

◻ LIFESTYLE/HEALTH BEHAVIORS

- Stress Management—stress is an imbalance between environmental demands and one's individual and social resources required to cope with those demands

  1. Types of stressors
     a. Major life events—discrete events that disrupt normal functioning (e.g., marriage, divorce, death of family member)
     b. Daily hassles—minor daily events perceived as frustrating
     c. Chronic strains—challenges, hardships, and problems
     d. Cataclysmic events—sudden disasters that require major adaptive responses (e.g., natural disasters)
     e. Ambient stressors—continuous and often unchanging conditions in physical environment, such as chronic pollution or noise

  2. Theoretical basis of stress
     a. General Adaptation Syndrome—Selye's (1974) continuum demonstrates how small amounts of stress are motivating and improve the quality of life (eustress or good stress); however, beyond a certain point the stress becomes psychologically and physically debilitating (distress)
     b. Physical indicators of stress
        (1) Gastrointestinal symptoms—upset stomach, change of appetite
        (2) Headache, muscle tension, elevated blood pressure (BP)
        (3) Restlessness
        (4) Cold, sweaty palms
     c. Emotional indicators of stress
        (1) Irritability, emotional outbursts, crying
        (2) Depression, withdrawal
        (3) Hostility, tendency to blame others
        (4) Anxiety, suspiciousness
     d. Behavioral indicators of stress
        (1) Lethargy, loss of interest
        (2) Poor concentration, forgetfulness
        (3) Decreased productivity, absenteeism
        (4) Sleep disturbance
     e. Related terminology—*Karoshi* (Japanese), which means death by overwork; associated with long hours and stressful working conditions

  3. Stress management intervention techniques
     a. Stress reduction techniques
        (1) Time management—determine goals and priorities, set time priorities, and learn to say no to non-goal-related activities
        (2) Time blocking—set aside time to adapt to change and incorporate it into daily routine
        (3) Change avoidance—during periods of high life change, avoid unnecessary change to prevent need to make multiple adjustments simultaneously
        (4) Habituation—incorporate routine into daily activities during stressful situation (e.g., park in same place to avoid having to look for car upon return)
        (5) Environmental modification—identify experiences and/or personalities that are abrasive or stress producing and minimize contact as much as possible
        (6) Involvement with activities of interest—doing something for others and helping with activities of interest to decrease focus on self
     b. Behavioral aspects to build stress resistance
        (1) Increase self-esteem—focus on own strengths and attributes
        (2) Increase assertiveness—substitute positive assertive behavior for negative passive actions
        (3) Meditation/prayer (includes Zen and yoga)
     c. Counter-conditioning to lower stress response
        (1) Autogenic training—repetition of autogenic suggestions such as "my hands are warm"
        (2) Imagery—image visualization used to relax or assist with past frightening experiences
        (3) Tension-relaxation exercises—tense muscles for 8–10 seconds, then relax; longer training sessions are usually required initially to enhance benefits (may be contraindicated in individuals with severe heart disease or hypertension)

(4) Biofeedback—awareness and control to influence response that is not ordinarily under voluntary control
   (a) Electromyography—measures the amount of electrical discharge in muscle fibers (usually forearm and forehead)
   (b) Skin temperature feedback—peripheral temperature measurement by vasomotor control found in bio-dots, mood rings, etc.
(5) Exercise—produces physiological changes that counteract effects of stress

d. Contraindications for stress management
   (1) Severe depression
   (2) Hallucinations or delusions
   (3) Temporary hypotensive or hypoglycemic states
   (4) Severe pain

- Social Support—strong relationship between social support and health (Bomar, 2004)
  1. Four types of supporting behaviors
     a. Emotional support—provision of empathy, love, trust, and caring (strongest, most consistent relationship to positive health status)
     b. Instrumental support, such as direct assistance or services, including money and time
     c. Informational support, such as advice, suggestions, and information
     d. Appraisal support or provision of information useful for self-evaluation purposes (feedback, affirmation)
  2. Related research
     a. Research evidence suggests that quality of supportive relationships rather than quantity is a better predictor of health—relationships are thought to provide buffering effects to protect people from the negative consequences of stressful situations
     b. The importance of social support has been demonstrated in multiple studies related to recovery from illness, disaster, success with weight loss, and other positive life changes; support groups can provide encouragement for those without a strong positive social network (Pender, 2002)

- Nutrition
  1. Healthy diet guidelines
     a. Eat a variety of foods with more fruit, vegetables, whole grains, poultry, and fish (herbs/spices can enhance diminished taste associated with normal aging)
     b. Calorie breakdown—55–60% carbohydrates, < 30% fat with remainder protein (0.8–1.0 g/kg)
     c. Limit total fat to less than 30% of total calories and saturated fat to less than 10% of total calories (low in saturated fat and cholesterol, moderate in total fat)
     d. Limit cholesterol intake to 300 mg/day
     e. Use sugar, salt, and sodium in moderation; choose and prepare foods with less salt and moderate sugar content
     f. The food guide pyramid (U.S. Department of Agriculture, 2011) includes the following daily recommendations
        (1) Bread, cereal, rice—6–11 servings; variety daily, especially whole grain
        (2) Vegetables—4–5 servings; fruits—3–4 servings
        (3) Milk, yogurt, and cheese—2–3 servings
        (4) Meat, poultry, fish, dry beans, eggs, and nuts—2– 3 servings for a total of 6–7 oz
        (5) Oils, sweets, and fats used sparingly
     g. Multivitamins with folic acid (0.4 mg/day) are recommended for all women of child-bearing age
     h. Vitamin D is needed for proper calcium absorption—400–800 IU/day
     i. Calcium (see **Table 2-1**)
  2. Assessment for weight loss
     a. Symptoms indicative of underlying pathology (associated with and/or aggravated by excessive weight)
        (1) Polyuria/polyphagia/polydipsia (diabetes)
        (2) Joint pain or marked swelling (osteoarthritis or gout)
        (3) Angina/palpitations/dyspnea (cardiovascular disease)
        (4) Edema/cold intolerance (hypothyroidism)
        (5) Recent weight gain with edema, pruritus (renal disease

■ Table 2-1 Recommended Calcium Intakes

	Amount mg/day
Adolescents (13–18 years); Pregnant/lactating women	1,300
Men, women, pregnant women (19–50 years)	1,000
Men 51–70 years	1,000
Women 51–70 years	1,200
Men and women 71+ years	1,200

Food sources of calcium: yogurt, milk, cheese, calcium-fortified juices and cereal, turnip and mustard greens, collards, kale, broccoli, sardines and salmon with bones

b. Contraindications for weight loss
(1) Pregnancy
(2) Chemotherapy due to already compromised nutritional status and potential impact on therapy
3. Body mass determinations—useful in determining both under- and over-nutrition or weight-for-frame size; calculate the body mass using the body mass formula in **Table 2-2** or the body mass index chart in **Table 2-3**; body mass index is weight (in kilograms) divided by the squared height (in meters)
4. Guidelines for healthy weight loss should include
a. A diet characterized by a reduction in calories, not nutrients, with a focus on diet composition/preparation methods
b. A balanced diet (food guide pyramid); should not depend on vitamins, weight loss pills, prepared liquids, "fad diets"

■ **Table 2-2** Body Mass Formula

1. To convert weight to kilograms, divide pounds (without clothes) by 2.2

2. To convert to meters, divide height in inches (without shoes) by 39.4, then square it

3. Divide weight in kilograms (#1) by meters squared (#2)

c. A diet that supplies all essential vitamins and minerals
d. Adequate fiber for proper GI functioning
e. Adequate fluid for renal functioning
f. Enough fat to supply essential fatty acid linoleic acid
g. Consumption of a variety of highly nutritious foods
h. A goal of up to 3 lbs/wk (gradual) weight loss

■ **Table 2-3** Body Mass Index Chart

Weight (lbs)	5'0"	5'2"	5'4"	5'6"	5'8"	5'10"	6'0"	6'2"
125	24	23	22	20	19	18	17	16
130	25	24	22	21	20	19	18	17
135	26	25	23	22	21	19	18	17
140	27	26	24	23	21	20	19	18
145	28	27	25	23	22	21	20	19
150	29	27	26	24	23	22	20	19
155	30	28	27	25	24	22	21	20
160	31	29	28	26	24	23	22	21
165	32	30	28	27	25	24	22	21
170	33	31	29	28	26	24	23	22
175	34	32	30	28	27	25	24	23
180	35	33	31	29	27	26	25	23
185	36	34	32	30	28	27	25	24
190	37	35	33	31	29	27	26	24
195	38	36	34	32	30	28	27	25
200	39	37	34	32	30	29	27	26
205	40	38	35	33	31	29	28	26
210	41	38	36	34	32	30	29	27
215	42	39	37	35	33	31	29	28
220	43	40	38	36	34	32	30	28
225	44	41	39	36	34	32	31	29
230	45	42	40	37	35	33	31	30

BMI
Underweight ≤ 18.5
Normal weight 18.6–24.9
Overweight 25–29.9
Obese 30 and above

From: NHLBI, June 17, 1998

i. A focus on eating regular meals, avoiding snacks, and modifying bad eating habits
j. Follow tips on healthy behavior changes that consider cultural needs
k. A plan to keep weight off after loss

5. Weight control strategies
   a. Regular physical activity increases caloric use, aids and sustains weight loss, preserves lean body mass and metabolism
   b. Social support by family, friends, colleagues, and support groups
   c. Focus on internal motivation for loss (e.g., control, personal goals, self-monitoring) and positive health benefits
   d. Smaller, more frequent meals to maintain blood sugar levels and avoid feeling hungry
   e. Control home environment (e.g., limit eating to one room, sit down at table without watching television)
   f. Control eating environment (e.g., avoid serving bowls at the table, use smaller plates and glasses, and eat slowly)
   g. Limit snacks (e.g., keep ready-to-eat, low-calorie snacks available)
   h. Control work environment (e.g., eat away from your desk, store food away from work area, and take exercise breaks)
   i. Use a shopping list; do not shop when hungry
   j. Keep a food diary (thoughts and feelings regarding eating patterns for 2 weeks) to guide intervention strategies

6. Health effects of severe dieting (metabolic response to starvation)
   a. Lower metabolic rate
   b. Hypertension as a result of norepinephrine release
   c. Overcompensation, gain beyond pre-diet weight
   d. Loss of fat and protein; regain fat
   e. Fat cells multiply as protective response against starvation

7. Weight loss prognostic factors
   a. Stability of present weight—number of years at present weight
   b. Motivation to change; conditions making weight loss a high priority
   c. Realistic expectations

8. Nutritional risk factors for older adults—three or more factors indicate a moderate nutritional risk (Hudgens & Langkamp-Henken, 2004)
   a. Illness or condition with potential impact on appetite, ability to eat, alertness, and memory
   b. Tooth loss or mouth pain
   c. Eating poorly, low variety, skipping meals, or more than two alcoholic beverages daily
   d. Inadequate finances for food (economic hardship)
   e. Physically unable to shop, cook, or feed self (needs assistance in self-care)
   f. Multiple medications related to influence on appetite and GI response
   g. Unintentional loss or gain of 10 pounds in past 6 months
   h. Elder years beyond 80
   i. Three or more different medications taken daily
   j. Reduced social contact

- Physical Activity for Health—any physical activity performed regularly is beneficial; current guidelines emphasize benefits of an exercise plan with optimal health benefits derived when that activity is in accordance with certain minimums. Health derived benefits include
  1. Physical fitness
     a. Psychological benefits
        (1) Increased alertness
        (2) Improved self-esteem, feeling better
        (3) Decreased depression
        (4) Lower stress
     b. Physical benefits
        (1) Heart—increases efficiency, lowers heart rate, lowers BP, increases oxygen capacity
        (2) Decreases LDL, increases HDL
        (3) Muscles—improves strength and endurance
        (4) Improves flexibility
        (5) Increases basal metabolic rate (BMR) during and after exercise
        (6) Weight loss of fat, not muscle
        (7) Body composition—lowers fat percentage
        (8) Antiaging effect
     c. Components of effective exercise
        (1) Moderate intensity aerobic activity (brisk walking or equivalent) for 30 minutes 5 days weekly or
        (2) Vigorous activity (jogging or equivalent) for 20 minutes 2 days weekly
        (3) Approaches may be combined
        (4) All adults should also perform resistance training 2 days weekly
        (5) Enjoyable for participant
        (6) Rhythmic movement with alternating relaxation and contraction of large muscle groups
     d. Components of an exercise plan
        (1) Warm up (increases blood flow, loosens and strengthens muscles), e.g., brisk walk and deep breathing
        (2) Stretch (maintains and increases flexibility), e.g., stretch slowly and hold

position several seconds to point of tightness, not pain; do not bounce

    (3) Endurance—select a variety of activities to work different muscle groups; start slow and build up gradually

    (4) Cool down period allows body temperature and heart rate to decrease slowly, prevents pooling of blood in extremities and decreases muscle soreness, e.g., walk, deep breathe, and loosely shake extremities

  e. Exercise counseling

    (1) Exercises to avoid

      (a) Bouncing with stretch (strains involved joints)

      (b) Sit ups with legs straight or double leg lifts (strains lower back)

      (c) Duck or bent knee walk (stresses knees)

      (d) Toe touching (stresses hamstrings)

      (e) Leg splits and leg thrusts in kneeling position (stresses legs and groin area, also creates potential hip strain)

    (2) Exercise self-care

      (a) Appropriate clothing with layers in winter

      (b) Caps for cold weather and summer heat

      (c) Appropriate footwear, snug socks

      (d) Plenty of fluids before, during, and after exercise

      (e) Alternate exercise program during weather extremes, e.g., stationary bike, treadmills, steppers, etc.

    (3) Tolerance barometer—refers to potentially dangerous physical symptoms or early signs of injury

      (a) Breathlessness (inability to talk while exercising)

      (b) Excessive fatigue—fatigue for more than 1 hour after exercise

      (c) Chest discomfort, dizziness, faintness, exertional dyspnea, nausea, or vomiting

      (d) Stiffness in joints with slight loss of motion

      (e) Swelling and localized pain

  f. Exercise prescription components

    (1) Specify duration, intensity, and frequency

    (2) Progression of physical activity—gradual onset, increasing in intensity/duration, e.g., begin walking, then gradually replace with jogging

    (3) Individualized to client capabilities

    (4) Client motivation, goals, and interest (motivators)—adolescent females— weight control, improved appearance; adolescent males—increased skills, strength, competition; women—weight control, appearance, stress reduction; men—pleasure, fun, and challenge abilities

    (5) Based on available time, equipment, and facilities

    (6) Refer individuals with abnormal exercise stress tests (bicycle ergometer or treadmill), chronic/recent heart or lung pathology, or any positive cardiac risk factors to the appropriate health-care provider

  g. Physical fitness evaluation

    (1) Baseline—resting heart rate, blood pressure, and weight (calculate BMI)

    (2) Skinfold test or other determination of body fat composition

    (3) Back flexibility is tested with sit and reach test; joints should be evaluated with range of motion

    (4) Muscle strength—tested by determining maximum amount of weight that can be lifted comfortably, a single time, by four different muscle groups; test is usually conducted following completion of approximately 6 weeks of training

    (5) Aerobic capacity with bicycle ergometer or treadmill, heart is stressed to level of steady state

  h. Nutrition for athletic performance

    (1) Drink 17 ounces of fluid approximately 2 hours prior to exercise to promote hydration; allow time for excretion of excess ingested fluid; drink approximately 2 cups of fluid for every pound of weight loss during extended athletic activities

    (2) Maintain well-balanced diet—adequate carbohydrates to optimize respiratory metabolism, adequate protein to preserve lean body mass, adequate minerals to maximize oxygen delivery, and calcium to develop high-density bones (Kenney, 1996)

- Safety and Environment
  1. General
     a. Fire safety (smoke alarms, fire extinguishers)
     b. Home safety (secure locks on doors and windows, secure firearms)
     c. Automobile (use of safety belts, harnesses, defensive driving)
     d. Helmets and safety pads (bikes, motorcycles, roller blades); mouth guards appropriate for sport

e. Personal safety (avoid risk-taking behaviors; always be alert to danger)

2. Safety for aging adult
   a. Home safety
      (1) Adequate lighting especially around stairs; light switches near doorways and accessible from bed
      (2) Home should be surveyed for risk factors that may create walking hazards (loose rugs, furniture placement, electrical cords); maintain traffic lanes in each room free of hazards
      (3) Nightlight or flashlight by bed is recommended to avoid falls or disorientation in the dark
      (4) Avoid housekeeping hazards by cleaning up spills as they occur and avoiding clutter on floors/stairways
      (5) Bathroom—nonslip mat in tub/shower, secure "grab bar"
      (6) Stairwell—secure handrail, steps in good repair with contrasting color/surface at edge of steps
   b. Personal safety
      (1) Avoid dangers of hypothermia with adequate heat and caloric intake
      (2) Set up daily surveillance system with others
      (3) Assess ability to take medications correctly
   c. Physical deficit concerns
      (1) Gait and balance problems
         (a) Slippery or irregular surfaces
         (b) Clutter or obstructions
         (c) Stairs steep or without rails
         (d) Lack of space to maneuver assistive device (e.g., walker)
         (e) Bathtub without secure rail or slip guards
      (2) Decreased vision
         (a) Inadequate lighting
         (b) Poorly marked stairs
      (3) Decreased sensitivity to pain/heat
         (a) Hot water bottle/heating pad
         (b) Hot bath water
      (4) Potential driving/traffic hazards
         (a) Decreased visual acuity and hearing
         (b) Decreased reaction time
         (c) Difficulty moving head due to arthritis or disc problems
         (d) Ambulation too slow for traffic signals

3. Four categories of environmental hazards
   a. Biological (e.g., viruses, microorganisms)
   b. Chemical (e.g., lead, asbestos)
   c. Physical (e.g., natural disasters)
   d. Sociological and psychological hazards (e.g., overcrowding, lack of resources)

4. Components of an environmental assessment
   a. Home hazards—fire safety, pest control, inadequate heat or toilet facilities
   b. Work site hazards and protection—noise, inhalants, lifting, hazardous materials; related exposures
   c. Neighborhood hazards—noise, air/water pollution, inadequate police protection, overcrowding or isolation from neighbors
   d. Community hazards—lack of availability of grocery stores, drugstores, public transportation

◘ HEALTH EVALUATION ACROSS THE LIFESPAN

- Health History—important in identifying risk behaviors and need for health education
  1. Demographics and biographical data
  2. History of present illness
     a. Symptom analysis (OPQRST)

       O—Onset
       P—Provocative/Palliative (better or worse)
       Q—Quality/Quantity
       R—Region/Radiation
       S—Setting
       T—Timing

     b. Reason for seeking health care or chief complaint—signs/symptoms and duration; preferably in client's own words
  3. Past medical history
     a. General state of health (client's perception)
     b. Past illnesses (hospitalizations)
     c. Past injuries, surgery (dates, treatment, and follow-up)
     d. Emotional health (past problems including assistance, history of domestic violence)
     e. Sexual health (obstetric and contraceptive history, number of partners, sexual preference, sexual problems, disease prevention efforts)
     f. Food or drug allergies (specify reaction and treatment, if any)
     g. Medications (prescription, over the counter, herbal, folk remedies)
     h. Immunizations (type and date)
     i. Sleep patterns (approximate hours, difficulties, e.g., difficulty falling asleep [DFA], early morning awakening [EMA], nightmares)
     j. Last examinations (physical, dental, vision, hearing, radiography, electrocardiogram [ECG], cancer screenings)
  4. Personal habits
     a. Tobacco use—cigarettes, pipe, cigars, smokeless; record number of cigarettes per day, number of years used, if stopped,

how long ago; approach adolescents with declarative statements related to drugs at school, drugs in common use at school, drugs used by friends, and by individuals; inquire about tobacco use in terms of number of packs smoked daily

b. Alcohol and drug use (type, amount)

c. Use of caffeine (coffee, colas, etc.)

d. Diet (24-hour intake, including nutritional supplements)

e. Exercise (type, frequency)

f. Leisure activities (type, frequency)

g. Sexual practices and activities (disease prevention, contraception, number of partners, and sexual preferences)

h. Sports (type, frequency)

i. Information required regarding sports participation, especially contact sports includes (Armado & Thomas, 2002)

   (1) Family history of heart disease, high blood pressure, or Marfan's syndrome

   (2) Prior limitation from sports

   (3) Exertional dyspnea or chest pain

   (4) Seizure, concussion, or history of unconsciousness

   (5) Ability to run ½ mile or more

   (6) Missing kidney

5. Psychosocial history

a. Living situation at present

b. Education—for adolescents ask, if in school, grades, positive or negative attitudes toward school

c. Religious beliefs in relation to health and treatment

d. Positive or negative perspective of the future

e. Perception of "typical day"

f. Stress, stress management

g. Depression or anxiety, suicide ideation (adolescents and young adults require direct questioning, e.g., have you ever thought of killing yourself)

h. Support systems

6. Family history—include age, health status, or cause of death of parents, siblings, children in a genogram (diabetes, heart disease, cancer, hypertension, lung disease, alcoholism, blood disorders, birth defects, and any other illnesses that seem to run in the family)

7. Occupational and environmental history

a. Type of work, former occupation(s)

b. Hazardous exposures at home or work

c. Military service, wartime employment, if any

d. Location of home, length of time

e. Home location adjacent to factories, shipyards, or other potentially hazardous facilities

f. Hobbies, potential exposures

8. Adolescent interviewing guidelines

a. Adolescent is primary historian, interviewed alone

b. Explain ground rules—unless serious problem emerges threatening life or health, interview is confidential

c. Home, Education, Activities, Drugs, Sex, Suicide (HEADSS) interview format is widely suggested—see age-related anticipatory guidance

• Risk Factor Identification—virtually every disease and condition has risk factors; select conditions are presented related to prevalence, in addition to protective factors

1. Research over the past 20 years has identified factors associated with physical health and longer, healthier life (Pender, 2002)

a. Exercise—regular (see exercise, this chapter)

b. Nonsmoker, recently extended to smoke-free environment

c. Seven to eight hours of sleep

d. Moderate or no alcohol

e. Regular and moderate eating (including breakfast)

f. Weight control

2. Cardiac risk factors

a. Age—male 40+, female 50+ or premature menopause

b. Family history of premature heart disease, myocardial infarction, or death of father/first degree male relative < 55, mother/female relative < 65

c. Cigarette smoking

d. Hypertension ≥ 140/90 mm Hg, or on antihypertensive medication

e. Low HDL cholesterol < 40 mg/dL (> 60 mg/dL negative risk)

f. LDL > 100 mg/dL

g. Diabetes mellitus

3. Obesity (20% above desirable weight)—mortality rates increase with weights 10% above desirable weights; obesity is associated with multiple attendant health risks (USPS Task Force, 2007)

a. Three times more prevalent in hypertensives and Type 2 diabetes

b. Increased risk of high cholesterol and coronary artery disease

c. Increased risk of cancer (colon, rectal, prostate, gallbladder, biliary tract, breast, cervical, endometrial, and ovarian)

d. Abdominal adiposity associated with increased risk of stroke and death from all causes

4. Suicide risk factors

a. Family history of psychiatric disorders (especially depression or suicide)

b. Previous suicide attempts
c. Family violence (verbal, physical, or sexual abuse)
d. Family instability (frequent separation from, or loss, of loved one)
e. Alcohol or substance abuse
f. Availability and accessibility of firearms in the home

- Age-Related Health Monitoring (if asymptomatic)—specific health screenings are part of secondary prevention, see **Table 2-4**
1. Screening guidelines
   a. Generalized screening indicated for diseases of high prevalence in the population and diseases with profound morbidity/ mortality if not diagnosed
   b. Screening tests must be reliable with acceptable technical process; must include appropriate follow-up
   c. Tests should be sensitive (those with disease screen positive); may need confirmatory testing with high-specificity testing (those who are positive have the disease for which they are tested)
2. Adolescence (12–19 years of age)—American Medical Association (AMA) recommends three visit intervals, 11–14 years, 15–17 years, and 18–21 years, unless more frequent examinations are indicated; information available on AMA website, "Guidelines for Adolescent Preventative Services (GAPS)"
   a. Complete physical examination including
      (1) Height/weight (use anthropometric chart)
         (a) Screen for eating disorders if indicated
         (b) Assess perception of food, weight
      (2) Complete skin examination
      (3) Assessment for gingivitis, caries, and malalignment
      (4) Assessment for signs of abuse or neglect
      (5) Hearing assessment (if exposed to excessive noise) and vision assessment
   b. Blood pressure (BP) every 2 years, normal 120/80 mm Hg or below
   c. Tuberculin skin test (PPD) every 2 years with any exposure or if at risk
   d. Female
      (1) Teach self-breast examination (SBE)
      (2) Determine Tanner stage
         (a) Stage I— prepubertal, average age for girls 10 years
         (b) Stage II—breast bud, sparse pubic hair
         (c) Stage III—breast mound development, pubic hair becomes coarser, growth spurt

         (d) Stage IV—menarche
         (e) Stage V—mature stage
      (3) If sexually active or 18 years old— Papanicolaou (pap) smear
   e. Male
      (1) Teach self-testicular examination (STE)
      (2) Determine Tanner stage
         (a) Stage I—prepubertal, average age for boys 9 years
         (b) Stage II—scrotum skin thins, reddens, testicular volume increases
         (c) Stage III—growth spurt, penis lengthens
         (d) Stage IV—male organ enlargement in length and width
         (e) Stage V—mature stage
   f. If high risk, counseling and test for human immunodeficiency virus (HIV) and venereal disease research laboratory (VDRL); assess knowledge of contraceptives and protective barriers
   g. Immunization
      (1) Tetanus-diphtheria booster (Td)
      (2) Others if needed; see immunization guidelines, this chapter
   h. Remain alert for depressive symptoms, any suicide risk factors
   i. Dental checkup with cleaning annually
3. Young adult (20–39 years of age) (see Table 2- 4)
   a. Complete physical examination (age 20, then every 5–6 years)
   b. BP every 2 years; normal systolic 110–130 mm Hg, diastolic 60–80 mm Hg
   c. Fractionated cholesterol screening every 5 years (may substitute nonfasting total cholesterol screen in low-risk individuals)
   d. Female
      (1) Pap and pelvic examination every 3 years, gonorrhea (GC) and chlamydia tests
      (2) Clinical breast examination (by health professional) every 3 years
   e. Male—clinical testicular examination every 3 years
   f. PPD if exposed to tuberculosis
   g. Immunizations—Td every 10 years; substitute 1 Tdap
   h. Self-skin examination
   i. Dental checkup with cleaning annually
4. Middle-aged adult (40–59 years of age) (see Table 2-4)
   a. Complete physical examination (every 5–6 years)
   b. BP every 2 years; normal systolic 110–130 mm Hg, diastolic 60–80 mm Hg; goal <120/80 with diabetes or chronic renal disease (NHLBI, 2003)

c. Cholesterol screening every 5 years; low-risk screening option not indicated over age 40

d. ECG, age 40+ with cardiac risk factors

e. Female
  (1) Clinical breast exam yearly (performed by a health professional)

  (2) Mammogram annually (ACS), every 1–2 years (USPSTF)
  (3) Pap and pelvic examination every 3 years if no risk factors

f. Male—prostate screening age 50 and annually (high-risk begin age 45) (ACS)

g. Colorectal screen (fecal occult or sigmoidoscopy)—age 50 annually

■ **Table 2-4** Adult Screening Guidelines (U.S. Preventive Services Task Force, American Cancer Society, NCEP ATP-III, NHLBI JNC VII)

Service	Who Needs	Frequency*	Risk Factors
Blood pressure	All adults	Every 2 years	male, blk, fam hx
Cholesterol	All adults	Every 5 years	male, tob, htn, fam hx
Dental	All adults	Annual	
ECG	Adults 40+	Annual (only with cardiac risk factors)	
Pap smear	Women 3 years after onset of intercourse but no later than age 21	Recommended every 3 years after two normal exams for women without risk factors**	
Self-breast exam	No recommendation for or against (ACS)		
Clinical breast exam	Women 40+	Annual (age 20–39 every 3 years)	
Mammogram (ACS)	Women 40+	Annual (ACS) (USPSTF every 1–2 years)	
Colorectal screen (fecal occult annually or colonoscopy every 10 years)	Adults 50+	Annual	
Prostate specific antigen (PSA)****	Men 50+	Annual (ACS)	blk, fam hx
Glaucoma screen****	Adults 40+	Annual (with risk factors)***	
Hearing	Only w/excessive noise exposure		
Chest x-ray	Not recommended		
Thyroid palpation****	Adults 20–39 Adults 40+	Every 3 years Annual	
Urinalysis	Controversy		Yes, w/sx, pregnancy, dm
Hgb/Hct	Controversy		Yes, w/sx, pregnancy
Health education/promotion (nutrition, exercise, stress management, substance abuse, safety, safe sex, and cancer prevention)	All adults	Every encounter	

*Increased frequency in the presence of risk factors
**Risk factors for cervical cancer—history of STD, multiple partners, tobacco use (tob), first intercourse before age 18
***Risk factors for glaucoma—myopia, diabetes mellitus (dm), family history, African-American (blk) > 40
****Insufficient evidence to recommend for or against screening
The term *controversy* indicates that the U.S. Preventive Services Task Force recommends against routine screening.

Adapted from: *Guide to Clinical Preventive Services 2007*, by U.S. Preventive Services Task Force, American Cancer Society, National Cholesterol Education Program ATP-III, and National Heart Lung and Blood Institute JNC VII (2003). Consult full reports for details.

h. Glaucoma screen, annually

i. Dental examination with cleaning every 6–12 months

j. Cancer screening yearly

k. Immunizations—tetanus every 10 years

5. Elderly adult (60+ years of age) (see Table 2-4)

a. Complete physical examination every 2 years with laboratory assessments

b. BP every 2 years, normal systolic 110–120 mm Hg, diastolic 60–80 mm Hg

c. Fractionated cholesterol every 5 years

d. ECG annually with cardiac risk factors

e. Female

(1) Mammogram—annual (ACS); every 1–2 years (USPSTF)

(2) Pap and pelvic examination every 3 years

f. Male—clinical testicular examination annually

g. Colorectal screen (fecal occult or sigmoidoscopy) age 50—annually

h. Glaucoma screen—annually

i. Dental examination with cleaning every 6–12 months

j. Immunizations—tetanus every 10 years, pneumococcal vaccine once, annual influenza vaccine, varicella zoster vaccine

- Age-Related Anticipatory Guidance (Allender, 2002)

1. Adolescence (12–19 years of age)

a. Leading causes of death—motor vehicle accidents (MVA), suicide, other accidents, homicide, cardiovascular disease, congenital disease

b. Normal growth and development

(1) Physical changes with puberty

(2) Need for increased self-responsibilities for own health—nutrition, exercise, adequate sleep and safety habits

c. Nutrition

(1) Variety of foods, including breakfast

(2) Nutritious snacks, limit sweets and fast food

d. Skin care/skin protection

e. Dental care (brushing and flossing)

(1) Fluoride supplementation

(2) Dental visits with cleaning every 6–12 months

f. Injury prevention

(1) Athletics, safety helmets, pads, mouthguards

(2) Safety belts

(3) Firearm safety

(4) Defensive driving, driver education

(5) Violent behavior/gangs

g. Physical activity

(1) Need for regular physical activity

(2) Encourage team activities, peer interaction

(3) Encourage participation in after school and/or church activities

h. Substance abuse

(1) Tobacco use avoidance or cessation emphasizing unattractive cosmetic effects (stained teeth and fingernails, foul-smelling breath and clothes) and athletic consequences (decreased endurance, shortness of breath)

(2) Smokeless tobacco is not safer, can be addicting/life-threatening

(3) Alcohol and other drugs

i. Sexuality

(1) Dating

(2) Responsible sexual behaviors, abstinence, contraception

(3) Risks, sexually transmitted diseases, unwanted pregnancy

2. Young adult (20–39 years of age)

a. Leading causes of death—motor vehicle accidents, homicide, suicide, injuries, heart disease

b. Nutrition and exercise

(1) Weight management with changing basal metabolic rate

(2) Selection of exercise program

c. Dental care

d. Sexuality

(1) Family planning, contraception

(2) Sexually transmitted diseases

e. Cancer warning signs, skin protection

f. Substance use/abuse

(1) Tobacco cessation, primary prevention

(2) Alcohol and other drugs

g. Injury prevention

(1) Athletics

(2) Safety belts, safety helmets

(3) Firearm safety

(4) Defensive driving

(5) Violent behavior

h. Lifestyle choices

(1) Family and parenting skills

(2) Stress management

i. Safety and environmental health

3. Middle-aged adult (40–59 years of age)

a. Leading causes of death—heart and vascular disease; lung, breast, prostate, and colorectal cancer

b. Nutrition and exercise

(1) Weight management with changing basal metabolic rate

(2) Selection of exercise program

    c.   Dental care

    d.   Sexuality

        (1)   Menopause

        (2)   Sexual changes due to aging

        (3)   Sexually transmitted diseases

    e.   Cancer warning signs, skin protection

    f.   Substance use/abuse

        (1)   Tobacco cessation, primary prevention

        (2)   Alcohol and other drugs

    g.   Injury prevention

        (1)   Athletics

        (2)   Safety belts, safety helmets

        (3)   Firearm safety

        (4)   Defensive driving

        (5)   Violent behavior

    h.   Midlife changes

        (1)   Empty nest syndrome, grandparenting

        (2)   Planning for retirement

        (3)   Stress management

    i.   Safety and environmental health

4.   Elderly adult (age 60+ years of age)

    a.   Leading causes of death—heart and vascular disease, cancers as described for 40–59 age group, and influenza and pneumonia

    b.   Nutrition and exercise

        (1)   Weight management with changing basal metabolic rate

        (2)   Selection of exercise program

    c.   Dental care

    d.   Sexuality

        (1)   Sexual changes due to aging

        (2)   Sexually transmitted diseases

    e.   Cancer warning signs, skin protection

    f.   Substance use/abuse

        (1)   Tobacco cessation, primary prevention

        (2)   Alcohol and other drugs

    g.   Injury prevention

        (1)   Athletics

        (2)   Safety belts, safety helmets

        (3)   Firearm safety

        (4)   Defensive driving

        (5)   Violent behavior

    h.   Life changes

        (1)   Retirement

        (2)   Loss of spouse, friends

        (3)   Physical changes (vision, hearing, reaction time, alterations of bowel and bladder habits)

    i.   Safety and environmental health

        (1)   Home safety

        (2)   Personal safety

- Immunization Guidelines (Centers for Disease Control and Prevention [CDC], 2004)

1.   Tetanus-diphtheria vaccine (Td)—primary series is recommended if not completed during childhood with two doses at least 4 weeks apart and a third dose 6–12 months after the second; Td booster is recommended every 10 years; adolescents 14–16 years of age should receive booster if no dose in past 5 years

2.   Measles-Mumps-Rubella vaccine (MMR)—recommended for adolescents who have not received two doses at or after 12 months of age; second dose is now given routinely as part of preschool immunizations or at age 12–14 years, or prior to postsecondary education or military service; adults without documentation of disease or immunization need only one dose; adults born prior to 1956 are considered immune due to prevalence of diseases before that time

3.   Varicella vaccine—recommended for individuals who have never had chicken pox; adolescents and adults need two doses 4–8 weeks apart

4.   Influenza vaccine—recommended annually for all adults

    a.   Groups that can transmit influenza to high-risk persons should be prioritized for immunization (e.g., healthcare workers and household members)

    b.   Optimal time for immunization (mid-October through mid-November)

    c.   Contraindications—history of anaphylactic hypersensitivity to eggs or other components; refer to physician for appropriate therapy and possible allergy evaluation

5.   Pneumococcal vaccine—recommended for any person over 2 years of age who is at increased risk of complications due to chronic illness (e.g., heart or lung disease and diabetes, alcoholism, Hodgkin's disease, cirrhosis, sickle cell disease) and individuals who work or live with high-risk individuals); anyone over age 65 and persons without a spleen; revaccination after 5 or more years is recommended for those at highest risk of antibody decline, e.g., those with renal disease or who have undergone organ transplant and persons vaccinated before age 65

6.   Hepatitis B vaccine (HBV)—three-dose regimen now recommended for all individuals at time 0, 1–2 months, and 4–6 months. Adults who are at increased risk of infection include healthcare workers, individuals at high risk of exposure to blood and blood products, and individuals at increased risk of exposure due to sexual practices. The timing and need for periodic boosters is determined by serologic testing. Immunization series is now recommended for all adolescents who were not previously immunized.

7. Zostavax vaccine is a live, attenuated virus indicated for the prevention of herpes zoster (shingles) in adults > age 60. It is given as a single dose 0.65 cc subcutaneous injection. Should not be given to those who are immunocompromised or who have a history of allergic response to gelatin or neomycin.

8. Hepatitis A vaccine (HAV)—two doses at time 0 and 6–12 months are recommended for individuals working in or traveling to countries with high levels of HAV infection; men who have sex with men, parenteral drug users, persons exposed to nonhuman primates, persons with chronic liver disease

9. Polio—inactivated poliovirus vaccine-enhanced potency (IVP-e) is indicated for unimmunized adults who are traveling outside the United Sates and healthcare workers; partially immunized or unimmunized adults with close contact with children receiving OPV; the second dose is given 1 month after the first with a third dose 6 months later

10. Lyme disease—people age 15+ working in endemic geographic areas may be at risk and should receive Lyme disease vaccine

11. Catch-up schedule, contraindications and precautions
    a. For individuals with uncertain immunization histories (lacking documentation)
       (1) First visit—Td, IPV, MMR, HBV, HAV, varicella, influenza, pneumococcal are optional depending upon risk factors
       (2) Second visit (4–6 weeks after first visit)—Td, IPV, HBV, with second dose of HAV, varicella, if given initially
       (3) Third visit (6 months after second visit)—Td, IPV, HBV, with third dose of HAV for adolescents
    b. Contraindications
       (1) Anaphylactic reaction to known component
          (a) MMR and influenza (eggs)
          (b) Hepatitis (baker's yeast)
          (c) IPV (streptomycin, polymyxin B or neomycin)
          (d) Varicella (gelatin or neomycin)
       (2) Moderate to severe illness (fever > 100.4°F)
       (3) Immunocompromised individuals (no live virus)
    c. Precaution with MMR—delay pregnancy for 3 months following immunization

12. Immunization schedule synopsis for adolescents and adults with documentation of immunizations during childhood
    a. Adolescents and adults
       (1) Hepatitis B series
       (2) Td booster, repeat every 10 years
       (3) Varicella, if needed, two doses 4–8 weeks apart
       (4) MMR if born after 1956
    b. Adults over 65, chronic disease (heart, lung, or diabetes; those who work or live with high-risk individuals)
       (1) Influenza vaccine each fall
       (2) Pneumococcal vaccine

◘ RESOURCES

Agency for Healthcare Research and Quality (AHRQ)
AHRQ Publications Clearinghouse
540 Gaither Road, Suite 2000
Rockville, MD 20850
www.ahrq.gov/
1-800-358-9295   FAX 1-301-594-2800
Automated instructions available 24 hours/day (Pocket guide on smoking cessation, etc.)

American Association for Retired Persons (AARP)
601 E. Street NW
Washington, DC 20049
www.aarp.org
1-888-687-2277 M–F 7:00 A.M.–12 :00 A.M.
Services for age 50 and older include lobby for senior citizens, mail-order pharmacy, bimonthly magazine, support group for widowed persons

Office of Cancer Communications National Cancer Institute
Building 31, Room 10A16
9000 Rockville Pike
Bethesda, MD 20892
www.cancer.gov/aboutnci/cis
1-800-4-CANCER   1-800-422-6237
Pamphlets on breast examination, pap smear, colorectal screening

National Institute on Aging Information Center
National Institute on Aging
Building 31, Room 5C-27 31 Center Drive, MSC 2292
Bethesda, MD 20892
www.nih.gov/nia/health
1-301-496-1752
Self-care and self-help groups for the elderly (directory)

Office of Disease Prevention and Health Promotion
200 Independence Ave. SW Room 738G
Washington, DC 20201
www.health.gov
1-202-205-8611   Fax 1-202-205-9478
Check the telephone directory for local chapters

American Cancer Society Cancer Response System
2525 Ridge Point Dr., Suite 100
Austin, TX 78754
www.cancer.org
1-800-227-2345

American Heart Association
7272 Greenville Avenue
Dallas, TX 75231
www.americanheart.org
1-800-AHA-USA1   1-800-242-8721

American Lung Association
61 Broadway, 6th floor
New York, NY 10006
www.lungusa.org/
1-212-315-8700

◼ ADDITIONAL INTERNET RESOURCES FOR HEALTH PROMOTION

American College of Nurse Practitioners
www.acnpweb.org/i4a/pages/index.cfm?pageid=1

American Dietetic Association
www.eatright.org

American Health Line
www.americanhealthline.com

American Journal of Nursing
www.ajn.org

American Nurses Association
www.nursingworld.org

American Red Cross
www.redcross.org

Centers for Disease Control and Prevention
www.cdc.gov

Consumer Health Information
www.healthfinder.gov

Food and Drug Administration
www.fda.gov/

Food and Nutrition Information
www.fns.usda.gov/fns

Healthgate
www.healthgate.com

Healthy People 2020
www.health.gov/healthypeople

Modern Healthcare
www.modernhealthcare.com

National Health Information Center
www.health.gov/nhic/

National Heart, Lung, and Blood Institute Information Center
www.nhlbi.nih.gov

New England Medical Journal Online
www.nejm.org

National Institute for Occupational Safety and Health
http://www.cdc.gov/NIOSH/

National Institute on Alcohol Abuse and Alcoholism
www.niaaa.nih.gov

◼ QUESTIONS

Select the best answer.

1. Using the Health Belief Model, determine which of the following individuals would be most motivated for behavior change:

    a. 42-year-old married female with excess weight for over 20 years
    b. 16-year-old female with poorly controlled sugar levels and poor dietary habits consistent with her friends
    c. 50-year-old male with recent myocardial infarction, whose prognosis is good with positive changes in diet and weight loss
    d. 40-year-old male who reports spouse wants him to lose weight

2. Which of the following activities would prepare an individual planning retirement to successfully resolve the final developmental tasks proposed by Erickson?

    a. Plan to simultaneously complete any community obligations
    b. Become involved with community activities
    c. Plan several extended trips early in retirement while able
    d. Avoid any commitments initially; wait for opportunities to present themselves

3. Screening for breast cancer is which level of prevention?

    a. Primary
    b. Secondary
    c. Tertiary
    d. Preliminary

4. Client (age 70) comes into your clinic the first week of November for health screening. Her last immunization, Td (tetanus), was 10 years ago. Which immunization(s) will you recommend?

    a. Td, influenza, and pneumococcal vaccine
    b. Influenza and pneumococcal vaccine and schedule Td within 3 months
    c. Td and influenza
    d. Td only

5. A temporary certificate for school attendance is given following initial immunizations for a 14-year-old boy. When should the adolescent return for more immunizations?

    a. 6 months
    b. 4–6 weeks
    c. 1 year
    d. 4 months

6. A woman, age 19, will be entering college in January. She is not pregnant. Without evidence of recent immunization, she should receive which of the following today?

   a. Second MMR, Td, and polio boosters
   b. Hemophilus influenza (HIB) and a tetanus booster
   c. Second MMR and Td
   d. Immunization for rubella, tetanus, and influenza

7. Joe, age 15, has just moved to your community and is staying in a temporary foster home. He has no record of any immunizations. Which of the following does Joe need today?

   a. MMR, Td, and varicella
   b. IPV, MMR, HBV, and Td
   c. Td only
   d. MMR and Td

8. According to research, which type of social support has the strongest relationship with health status?

   a. Emotional
   b. Instrumental
   c. Informational
   d. Appraisal

9. According to research, how much sleep is associated with a longer, healthier life?

   a. 5–6 hours
   b. 6–7 hours
   c. 7–8 hours
   d. 8–9 hours

10. Josh, age 32, is ready to start exercising and wants to jog. Guidelines should include which of the following?

    a. Jog 1 mile initially, then add distance daily until goal is reached
    b. Jog at least once a week for 30 minutes to condition his heart and lungs
    c. Begin with brisk walking and gradually replace with jogging for at least 20 minutes 2 times weekly
    d. Warm-up exercises before or after jogging

11. Several cups of coffee immediately prior to the clinic visit would likely elevate which of the following?

    a. Heart rate
    b. Respiratory rate
    c. Cholesterol
    d. Blood sugar

12. Jim asks why cooling down is necessary for an exercise plan. You tell him cooling down will:

    a. Allow the body temperature and heart rate to decrease slowly
    b. Loosen and strengthen muscles
    c. Maintain and increase flexibility
    d. Sustain heart rate for a longer period of time

13. According to the Transtheoretical Model, intervention at which level is most likely to result in behavior change?

    a. Maintenance
    b. Contemplation
    c. Precontemplation
    d. Preparation

14. Which stress management technique would be most appropriate for a newly diagnosed diabetic?

    a. Change avoidance
    b. Habituation
    c. Time blocking
    d. Imagery

15. According to the U.S. Preventive Services Task Force Recommendations, a woman age 21 needs which of the following annually?

    a. Blood pressure and cholesterol screen
    b. Clinical breast exam
    c. Pap and pelvic exam
    d. Dental screen

16. Your female client, age 49, has had a normal baseline mammogram. She asks when she should get her next mammogram. You advise:

    a. Annually or every 1–2 years
    b. Every other year from age 50 to 59, then yearly
    c. Every 3 years until age 60
    d. Every 5 years for the rest of her life

Answers

1. **c**	9. **c**
2. **b**	10. **c**
3. **b**	11. **a**
4. **a**	12. **a**
5. **b**	13. **d**
6. **c**	14. **c**
7. **b**	15. **d**
8. **a**	16. **a**

◻ BIBLIOGRAPHY

Allender, M. (2002). Adolescent. In C. Edelman & C. Mandie (Eds.). *Health promotion throughout the lifespan* (5th ed.). Baltimore: Mosby.

Armado, J., & Thomas, D. (2002). Early recognition of Marfan's syndrome. *JAANP, 14*(5), 201–204.

Bandura, A. (1986). *Social foundations of thought and action*. Englewood Cliffs, NJ: Prentice-Hall.

Becker, M. (1972). The health belief model and personal health behavior. *Health Education Monographs* 2, 326–327.

Bomar, P. (2004). *Promotion health in families, applying research and theory*. Philadelphia: Saunders.

Centers for Disease Control and Prevention. (2009). Adult immunization schedule. Retrieved from http://www.cdc.gov/vaccines/recs/schedules/Adult-schedule.htm

Clark, M. (2003). *Nursing in the community* (4th ed.). Norwalk, CT: Appleton & Lange.

Erikson, E. (1963). *Childhood and society* (2nd ed.). New York: Norton.

Friedman, M., Bowden, V., & Jones, S. (2003). *Family nursing: Research, theory, and practice* (5th ed.). Upper Saddle River, NJ: Prentice-Hall.

Green L, & Kreuter M. (1991). *Health promotion planning: An educational and environmental approach*. Mountain View, CA: Mayfield Publishing.

Haskell, W. L., Min-Lee, I., Pate, R. R., Powell, K. E., Blair, S. N., Franklin, B. A., et al. (2007). Physical activity and public health: Recommendations for adults from the American College of Sports Medicine and the American Heart Association. *Circulation, 116*, 1081–1093.

Hudgens, J. & Langkamp-Henken, B. (2004). The Mini Nutritional Assessment as an Assessment Tool in Elders in Long-Term Care, *Nutrition in Clinical Practice, 19*(5): 463–470.

Keller, C., Oveland, D., & Hudson, S. (1997). Strategies for weight control success in adults. *Nurse Practitioner, 22*(3), 33–54.

Kenney, W. (1996). *American college of sports medicine fitness book*. Champaign, IL: Human Kinetics.

Lewin, K. (1951) *Field theory in social science; selected theoretical papers*. D. Cartwright (ed.). New York: Harper & Row.

Maslow, A. (1954). *Motivation and personality*. New York: Harper & Row.

Neuman, B., & Fawcett, J. (2002). *The Neuman systems model*. Upper Saddle River, NJ: Prentice-Hall.

National Heart, Lung, & Blood Institute (NHLBI) (2003). 7th Report Joint National Committee on Prevention, Detection, Evaluation, and Treatment of High Blood Pressure (JNC 7). *JAMA, 289*, 2573–2574.

Pender, N. (2002). *Health promotion in nursing practice* (4th ed.). Upper Saddle River, NJ: Prentice-Hall.

Prochaska, J., & Velicir, W. (1997). The transtheoretical model of health behavior change. *American Journal of Health Promotion, 12*(I).

Selye, H. (1974). *Stress without distress*. Philadelphia: Lippincott Co.

Smith, R. A., Cokkinides, V., Eyre, H. (2006). American Cancer Society guidelines for the early detection of cancer, 2006. *CA: A Cancer Journal for Clinicians, 56*, 11–25.

U.S. Department of Agriculture (USDA). (2011). Food Guide Pyramid. Retrieved November 5, 2011 from http://www.nal.usda.gov/fnic/Fpyr/pmap.htm

U.S. Department of Health and Human Services. (2011). *Healthy people 2020* Washington, DC: Government Printing Office.

U.S. Department of Health and Human Services (2006). *Dietary guidelines for Americans*. Washington, DC: Government Printing Office.

U.S. Preventive Services Task Force. (2007). *The guide to clinical preventive services: Recommendations of the United States Preventive Services Task Force*. Retrieved from http://www.ahrq.gov/clinic/pocketgd.htm

Selye, H. (1974). *Stress without distress*. New York: J. B. Lippincott.

Swartz, M. (2009). *Textbook of physical diagnosis* (4th ed.). Philadelphia: W. B. Saunders.

von Bertalanffy (1968). *General systems theory*. New York: George Braziller.

3

Dermatological Disorders

Sylvia Torres Fletcher

Susan E. Chaney

◘ ACNE VULGARIS

- Definition—self-limited or chronic disorder characterized by development of open comedones (black heads) and closed comedones (white heads) due to an increase in sebum release by the sebaceous glands after puberty; if further inflammation is present, pustules, cysts, and nodules on erythematous bases may be present

- Etiology/Incidence
  1. Four primary pathogenic factors
     a. *Propionibacterium acnes*
     b. Increased sebum production
     c. Abnormal follicular keratinization
     d. Chemotactic factors
  2. Factors that predispose to comedone formation
     a. Cosmetics and hair products
     b. Coal tar and insoluble oils
     c. Corticosteroids (topical and systemic), oral contraceptives, lithium, dilantin
  3. Contributing host factors
     a. Heredity
     b. Environment
     c. Stress
  4. May occur as a result of polycystic ovarian disease
  5. May be worse in fall and winter seasons
  6. Seen primarily in adolescents and young adults; may persist to fifth decade
  7. More common in males than females
  8. Circumstances characterized by increased androgen production increase risk

- Signs and Symptoms
  1. Lesions are nonpruritic, may be erythematous and tender
  2. Females may notice an increase in symptoms prior to menses

- Differential Diagnosis
  1. Acne rosacea
  2. Eosinophilic folliculitis (seen in HIV patients)
  3. Drug-induced folliculitis
  4. Pyogenic folliculitis

- Physical Findings
  1. Morphology
     a. Closed comedones, "white heads," are pustular lesions found in hair follicles due to blockage of sebum and keratinous materials
     b. Open comedones, "black heads," are dilated follicular orifices with easily expressed darkened oily debris
     c. Inflamed comedones, pustules, cysts, and nodules
  2. Distribution
     a. Forehead
     b. Cheek, nose, and chin
     c. Chest, upper arms, back, and buttocks

- Diagnostic Tests/Findings—culture for causative agent rarely necessary

- Management/Treatment
  1. For mild or episodic cases
     a. Mild skin cleansing twice daily
     b. Benzoyl peroxide 2.5–10%—apply to affected area daily

c. Topical benzoyl peroxide/antibiotic combinations (Benzaclin, Benzamycin)

d. For moderate cases
(1) Oral antibiotic therapy for at least 2 months (options include tetracycline 250–500 mg, initially 1 g/day, may increase to 2–3 g/day; minocycline 50–100 mg b.i.d.
(2) Females—combination oral contraceptives with high estrogen component

2. Prevent development of comedone with comedolytic agent
a. Retinoic acid cream 0.025% or retinoic acid gel 0.1%
b. Caution patient about photosensitivity
c. Erythromycin/benzoyl peroxide gel in morning and topical retinoid at night 3 times a week most effective regimen

3. Severe nodulocystic acne may require aggressive treatment to decrease sebum production—13-cis-retinoic acid 0.5–2.0 mg/kg/day for 16–20 weeks (typically prescribed by dermatologists or professionals who have completed manufacturer education)
a. Teratogenic—use with extreme caution in females of child-bearing age
b. Multiple systemic side effects
c. Monitor liver function tests (LFT), CBC, triglyceride levels
d. Associated increase in suicide; monitor mood and suicide risk

4. Patient education
a. Noticeable improvement may not be apparent for 6 weeks
b. Reassure patient, advise on stress reduction
c. Skin care including mild skin cleansing twice daily; advise patient to not squeeze or pick lesions
d. Be alert to changes in mood; seek help immediately if suicidal thoughts occur

❑ ALOPECIA

- Definition—the complete or partial loss of hair from areas where it normally is present; may be total, diffuse, patchy, or localized

- Etiology/Incidence
1. Hair loss involving hair matrix or follicle destruction due to chemical agents, physical agents, or both, and by infectious or immunologically mediated inflammation; may also result from a slowing of hair growth due to metabolic diseases
2. Cicatricial alopecia—scarring
a. Destruction of hair follicles from inflammatory processes with healing resulting in scarring
b. Permanent and irreversible

3. Noncicatricial alopecia—nonscarring alopecia
a. 95% of alopecia seen in primary care
b. Most common is male or female baldness, which is genetic or developmental
c. Considered an autoimmune disease
d. Other causes include vitiligo, thyroid disease, familial autoimmune polyendocrinopathy syndrome

4. Androgenetic alopecia
a. Males after puberty, females after age 60
b. Cause is combined effects of androgen on genetically predisposed hair follicles

- Signs and Symptoms
1. Usually the client is symptom free but verbalizes distress over hair loss
2. Hair loss resulting from physical agents or infectious disease such as tinea capitis may cause pain or pruritus

- Differential Diagnosis
1. Secondary syphilis
2. Traction alopecia
3. Early chronic systemic lupus erythematosus (SLE)
4. Dermatomyositis

- Physical Findings
1. Genetic pattern baldness of
a. Males—frontotemporal hairline recession with various amounts of hair loss at scalp vertex
b. Females—diffuse or vertex hair loss
2. Traumatic alopecia findings are patchy hair loss and breakage of hairs
3. Infectious alopecia—patches of partial hair loss
4. Alopecia areata (immunologic)—smooth, salmon-colored patches

- Diagnostic Tests
1. Usually a clinical diagnosis
2. Hair pull test of 10–20 grouped hairs; if over 40% of shafts are removed, disease is more advanced
3. KOH preparation—negative for fungus
4. ANA to rule out SLE
5. RPR to rule out secondary syphilis

- Management/Treatment
1. Treatment for scarring alopecia areata—hair transplant
2. Treatment for nonscarring alopecia areata
a. Intralesional injection with triamcinolone acetate 3.5 mg/mL
b. Systemic glucocorticoids
c. Systemic cyclosporine

3. Treatment of androgenetic alopecia
   a. Topical minoxidil 5% solution for 4–12 months
   b. Oral finasteride 1 mg daily for 6–12 months
   c. Antiandrogens for women (spironolactone, cimetadine)
4. Patient education
   a. About 40% of clients have moderate hair growth within 1 year
   b. Discontinuation of treatment will result in regression to pretreatment levels of baldness within 2–3 months

◻ BACTERIAL INFECTIONS/ PYODERMAS

- Definitions
  1. Impetigo—contagious and autoinoculable bacterial infection of skin; the two types are small vesicle and bullous
  2. Folliculitis—infection surrounding hair follicle caused by occlusion of ostium
  3. Furunculosis—deep-seated, autoinoculable infection involving entire hair follicle and adjacent subcutaneous tissue
  4. Carbuncle—several furuncles developing in adjoining hair follicles and coalescing to form deep mass with multiple drainage points
  5. Hidradenitis suppurativa—chronic suppurative disease of the apocrine gland-bearing areas of the skin
  6. Cellulitis—spreading infection of epidermis, subcutaneous tissue, and superficial lymphatic system

- Etiology/Incidence
  1. Impetigo
     a. Most frequent causative organisms—*Staphylococcus aureus* (*S. aureus*), group A beta hemolytic *Streptococcus pyogenes* (GAS)
     b. Seen primarily in children, bullous in children and young adults
     c. Predisposing factors
        (1) Humid, warm climate
        (2) Preexisting skin disease, especially atopic
        (3) Prior antibiotic therapy
        (4) Poor hygiene, crowded living conditions
        (5) Chronic staph carrier (nose, axilla, perineum, bowel)
  2. Folliculitis, furunculosis, carbuncle
     a. Most frequent causative organism—*S. aureus*
     b. Predisposing factors
        (1) Shaving hairy areas such as beard, axillae, legs
        (2) Occlusion of hair-bearing areas (plastic, clothing, positioning)
        (3) Topical glucocorticoid steroids, systemic antibiotics
        (4) Diabetes
  3. Hidradenitis suppurativa
     a. Pathogenesis unknown, mechanism plugging apocrine duct with subsequent ulceration, fibrosis, and sinus tract formation
     b. Males—anogenital involvement; females— axillary involvement
     c. Predisposing factors
        (1) Obesity
        (2) Family history of nodulocystic acne, hidradenitis suppurativa
  4. Cellulitis
     a. Most frequent causative organisms *S. aureus* and GAS
     b. Less common—*H. influenzae*, group B streptococci (GBS), pneumococci
     c. Diabetic/immunocompromised—*E. coli*, *Proteus mirabilis*, *Acinetobacter*, *Enterobacter*, *Pseudomonas aeruginosa*
     d. Predisposing factors
        (1) Multiple dermatoses—tinea, inflammatory, bullous, ulceration, pyodermas
        (2) Trauma
        (3) Surgical wounds
        (4) Infections
     e. Risk factors
        (1) Immunocompromised, cancer, and diabetes
        (2) Alcohol and drug abuse
        (3) Cancer, cancer chemotherapy

- Signs and Symptoms
  1. Localized pain, redness, swelling, or heat
  2. More severe infections (e.g., cellulitis)—systemic symptoms such as malaise, fever, chills

- Differential Diagnosis
  1. Contact dermatitis
  2. Allergic dermatitis
  3. Fungal dermatitis
  4. Herpes dermatitis

- Physical Findings
  1. Severe infections
     a. Regional lymphadenopathy
     b. Fever
     c. Skin tracking
  2. Morphology
     a. Impetigo—small vesicle caused by streptococcus
        (1) Small, red macules that progress to water-filled vesicles
        (2) Ruptured vesicles leave characteristic honey-colored crusted area
     b. Bullous impetigo caused by *S. aureus*
        (1) Large flaccid blister
        (2) Cloudy to purulent contents

c. Folliculitis, furuncle, carbuncle,
(1) Abscess—tender, fluctuant nodule
(2) Furuncle—firm, tender nodule with central necrotic plug
(3) Carbuncle—multiple abscess/furuncles with sieve-like openings draining purulent material
d. Hidradenitis suppurativa
(1) Initial—inflamed nodule/abscess with serous/purulent drainage and sinus tracks; open, black comedones when active nodules are absent
(2) Late phase—fibrous "bridge" scarring and contractures
e. Cellulitis
(1) Bright red plateau, erythema with indistinct margins
(2) Lymphangitis (red streaking from the area of cellulitis toward proximal lymph nodes) may be present
3. Distribution
a. Impetigo—anywhere
b. Folliculitis, furuncle, carbuncle
(1) Hair-bearing area—beard, axilla, occipital scalp, back of neck
(2) Any non-weight-bearing area, buttock, upper trunk, puncture wound site
c. Hidradenitis suppurativa—regions rich with apocrine glands
(1) Axilla
(2) Inguinal area
(3) Anogenital area
(4) Buttocks, scalp
d. Cellulitis
(1) Any area where normal lymphatic drainage has been disrupted
(2) Recent venous and lymphatic surgical sites
(3) Previous cellulitis sites
(4) Cheek or cheek bone and lower extremities

• Diagnostic Tests/Findings
1. Gram's stain— may be positive for cocci
2. Culture and sensitivity of exudate especially on immunocompromised patient
3. KOH—negative
4. Wood's lamp—no fluorescence
5. Tzanck test—negative

• Management/Treatment
1. GAS—small vesicular impetigo
a. Small, localized affected area may be treated with topical Bactroban
b. Larger surface involvement requires systemic antistreptococcal treatment
(1) Penicillin (PCN) VK 250 mg q.i.d. for 10 days

(2) Benzethine penicillin 1.2 million units
(3) Cephalexin 250–500 mg q.i.d. for 10 days
2. *S. aureus*—bullous impetigo
a. Small, localized affected area may be treated with topical Bactroban
b. Dicloxacillin 250–500 mg q.i.d. for 10 days (adults)
c. Cephalexin 250–500 q.i.d. for 10 days
3. PCN allergy for GAS and *S. aureus*
a. Erythromycin ethylsuccinate 500 mg q.i.d.
b. Clarithromycin 500 mg b.i.d. for 10 days
4. MRSA (treat for at least 10 days)
a. Minocycline 100 mg b.i.d.
b. Trimethoprim-sulfamethoxazole DS b.i.d.
c. Rifampin 300 mg b.i.d. for 5 days may be added to above regimens
d. Linezolid 300 mg p.o. b.i.d. for five days in resistant cases
5. Folliculitis, furuncle, carbuncle, and hidradenitis suppurativa
a. Mild folliculitis
(1) See impetigo
(2) Terbinafine 250 mg daily for 14 days—fungal folliculitis
b. Moderate infection
(1) Warm moist compresses to promote spontaneous drainage
(2) Incision and drainage (I & D) usually required
(3) Culture recurrent abscesses
(4) See impetigo
c. Hidradenitis suppurativa—additional measures to reduce inflammation
(1) Intralesional triamcinolone 3–5 mg/mL diluted with lidocaine
(2) Prednisone 70 mg tapered over 14 days
6. Cellulitis
a. Facial involvement—consult with physician for possible inpatient management
b. I & D may be required
c. See impetigo
d. Rest, immobilization, elevation, moist heat, analgesia
e. Reevaluate in 48 hours

◘ DERMATITIS

• Definition—group of inflammatory pruritic skin diseases that have different etiologies but share common symptoms and clinical manifestations
1. Atopic dermatitis—acute, subacute, but usually chronic, pruritic inflammation of the epidermis and dermis; term often used synonymously with eczema, IgE dermatitis
2. Contact dermatitis—acute or chronic inflammatory reactions to substances that come in contact with the skin

3. Stasis dermatitis—inflammatory response to extravasated blood in dermis and subcutaneous tissue resulting from stasis
4. Seborrheic dermatitis—chronic dermatosis characterized by redness and scaling reaction where sebaceous glands are most active

- Etiology/Incidence
  1. Atopic dermatitis
     a. Thought to have genetic basis; often seen as part of an "atopy" triad; dermatitis, asthma, and allergic rhinitis
     b. Two-thirds of patients have personal or family history of respiratory atopy
     c. Seen in all populations and geographic locations
     d. More common in males than in females
     e. Highest incidence in childhood, usually resolves by third decade
     f. More prevalent in urban areas and developed countries
     g. Exacerbated by allergies, skin dehydration, emotional stress, hormonal changes, and infection
  2. Contact dermatitis
     a. Irritant contact dermatitis
        (1) More common than allergic contact dermatitis
        (2) Most irritants used daily in work and home environments
        (3) Accounts for high percentage of work-related skin disorders
            (a) Low-caustic irritants—soapy water, cleansers, rubbing alcohol, kerosene
            (b) High-caustic irritants—bleach, strong acids, alkalines
        (4) Higher incidence in those with compromised skin integrity
     b. Allergic contact dermatitis
        (1) Delayed (type IV) cell-mediated hypersensitivity to a substance
            (a) Substance (antigen) binds with epidermal protein
            (b) Antigen-protein complex presented to T-helper cells causing release of mediators
            (c) T-helper cell expansion occurs in regional lymph nodes producing T-effector lymphocytes
            (d) T-effector lymphocytes circulate in bloodstream and produce the epidermal response
            (e) Entire process occurs in 5–21 days
            (f) Reexposure—dermatologic response in 12–48 hours
        (2) Most common sensitizer in United States is oleoresin of Rhus family of plants—poison oak, poison ivy, and poison sumac
        (3) Other common sensitizers are nickel in jewelry, fragrances, and preservatives in topical preparations
  3. Stasis dermatitis
     a. Occurs as a result of chronic venous insufficiency
     b. Complicated by low-grade tissue ischemia associated with stasis at capillary level
     c. History of varicosities, thrombophlebitis, or postphlebitic syndrome
     d. Often complicated by allergic contact dermatitis and chronic infection
  4. Seborrheic dermatitis
     a. Etiology unknown, thought to have a genetic basis
     b. Overgrowth of naturally occurring yeast, *Pityrosporum ovale*
     c. Often begins in early adulthood, aggravated by stress
     d. Can be an early cutaneous sign of HIV infection
     e. Often severe in patients with chronic neurological diseases
     f. Seen in patients with severe acne
     g. More common in males

- Signs and Symptoms—pruritic scaly rash

- Differential Diagnosis
  1. Scabies
  2. Tinea
  3. Atopic/eczema dermatitis
  4. Contact dermatitis
  5. Nummular dermatitis
  6. Psoriasis (seborrheic dermatitis)
  7. Cellulitis (stasis dermatitis)

- Physical Findings
  1. Common clinical findings for all types of dermatitis
     a. Initial stage—erythema, papules, microvesicles, and excoriation
     b. Chronic stage—lichenification
  2. Atopic dermatitis
     a. Papules, erythema, excoriations, and lichenification
     b. Pustules represent secondary infections with staphylococci
     c. Distribution—flexural areas of neck, antecubital fossae, and popliteal fossae
     d. Other locations—face, wrist, and forearm
  3. Irritant contact dermatitis
     a. Mild irritants—erythema, chapped skin, dryness, and fissuring
     b. Severe cases—edema, serous oozing, tender, crusting, scaling

    c. Painful bullae may develop with potent irritant

    d. Distribution—hands most common, also face and eyes

  4. Allergic contact dermatitis

    a. Erythema, edema, papules, vesicles, serous oozing, crusting, scaling

    b. Distribution—corresponds to exposed area

    c. Lesions outline site of irritant, often linear pattern with plant exposure

  5. Stasis dermatitis

    a. Early stage—mottled pigmentation and slight erythema

    b. Evidence of varicosities, ankle edema

    c. Mild tenderness with deep palpation; pulses normal

    d. Chronic stage—subcutaneous tissue becomes thick, fibrous

    e. Distribution—lower legs

  6. Seborrheic dermatitis

    a. Ill-defined, greasy yellow scales overlying erythematous patches

    b. Distribution—scalp, within external ear, postauricular area, eyebrows, nasolabial folds, central chest, and at times axilla, groin, submammary folds

- Diagnostic Tests/Findings

  1. Serum IgE—levels elevated in patients with atopy

  2. KOH—negative for spores/hyphae

  3. Skin scrapings—negative for burrows

- Management/Treatment

  1. Three goals of therapy

    a. Treatment of inflamed skin

    b. Control of pruritus

    c. Control of exacerbating factors

  2. Treatment of inflamed skin

    a. Mild disease—low-potency steroid cream

      (1) Hydrocortisone 1–2.5% cream 2–4 times daily

      (2) Desonide 0.05% b.i.d. (face or areas resistant to hydrocortisone)

    b. Severe disease—medium potency steroid cream (2–4 weeks)

      (1) Triamcinolone acetonide 0.1% cream 2–4 times daily

      (2) Fluocinolone acetonide 0.025% cream b.i.d.

    c. Topical corticosteroid with occlusion may be helpful

      (1) Treat area with steroid cream and cover with plastic wrap

      (2) Leave on overnight and remove plastic wrap in morning

    d. Lesions resistant to medium potency steroids use ultra-high potency—betamethasone dipropionate 0.05% b.i.d., with or without occlusion

    e. Pimecrolimus 1%—apply twice daily for steroid-resistant cases or for cases requiring steroid cessation

    f. Acute flares may require short-term oral glucocorticoids

      (1) Prednisone 40–60 mg tapered over 14–21 days

      (2) Solu-Medrol dose pak

    g. Ultraviolet light therapy and oral glucocorticoids for most severe cases

    h. Wet to dry compresses with water or aluminum acetate (Burow's solution) to dry vesicular lesions

    i. Bullous lesions—may be drained; do not remove top thin skin

  3. Control of pruritus

    a. Antihistamines

      (1) Cetirizine 10 mg q.d./b.i.d. prn

      (2) Desloratadine 5 mg q.d./b.i.d. prn

      (3) Hydroxyzine 25 mg t.i.d./q.i.d. prn

      (4) Diphenhydramine 25–50 mg every 4–6 hours prn

      (5) Doxepin 10–25 mg b.i.d./t.i.d. prn

    b. Tepid baths to cool and hydrate skin

    c. Mild soaps, avoid dry scaly areas

    d. Emollients

    e. Control of exacerbating factors

      (1) Treat secondary bacterial infections, usually staphylococcus

      (2) Maintain good hydration and integrity of skin

      (3) Gently towel dry skin, no brisk rubbing

      (4) Continued use of emollients to prevent skin drying

      (5) Wear gloves to avoid contact irritants

      (6) Identify and avoid offending irritants

      (7) Stasis dermatitis—special measures

        (a) Elevate legs; support stockings

        (b) Exercise daily to help reduce venous pressure and edema

      (8) Seborrheic dermatitis—special measures

        (a) Daily use of shampoos containing tar, sulfur, salicylic acid, or selenium

        (b) Ketoconazole 2% cream and shampoo (twice weekly) is an alternative to topical steroids

        (c) Low-potency topical steroid, hydrocortisone 1%

      (9) Educate patient on stress reduction to avoid exacerbation

      (10) Follow-up in 1–2 weeks

◘ FUNGAL AND YEAST INFECTIONS

- Definitions
  1. Tinea (dermatophytosis)—fungal infection of skin, nails, and hair; characteristic lesions varies by site
  2. Tinea (pityriasis) versicolor—chronic, asymptomatic, scaly dermatitis
  3. Candidiasis—yeast-like fungal infection of skin and mucous membrane

- Etiology/Incidence
  1. Tinea
     a. Causative organisms—*Trichophyton*, *Microsporum*, and *Epidermophyton*
     b. Transmitted by people through fomites, animals (pets), and, to a lesser extent, soil
  2. Tinea versicolor
     a. Causative organism—nondermatophyte fungus *Pityrosporum orbiculare*; normal inhabitant of skin
     b. Most common in young adults when sebum production is high
  3. Candidiasis
     a. Causative organism usually *Candida albicans*; normal saprophytic inhabitant of GI tract; overgrowth often due to antibiotic use
     b. Occurs in intertriginous, moist, cutaneous areas
  4. Contributing factors
     a. Warm, moist environments for fungal infections
     b. Obesity
     c. Altered immunity
        (1) HIV
        (2) Diabetes
        (3) Pregnancy
        (4) Inhaled or oral steroids
     d. Oral contraceptives
     e. Antibiotic therapy

- Signs and Symptoms (depends upon area of involvement)
  1. Mild pruritus
  2. Inflamed, tender rash
  3. Thickened nails
  4. Hair loss

- Differential Diagnosis
  1. Seborrheic dermatitis
  2. Psoriasis
  3. Alopecia
  4. Atopic dermatitis
  5. Contact dermatitis
  6. Pityriasis rosea
  7. Bacterial infection

- Physical Findings
  1. Morphology
     a. Tinea (dermatophytosis)—characteristic lesion varies by site
        (1) Tinea capitis—well-defined or irregular, diffuse areas of scaling and hair loss on scalp
        (2) Tinea corporis—annular appearance (ringworm), deep inflammatory nodules, or granulomas
        (3) Tinea cruris—sharply demarcated, erythematous, scaly patches
        (4) Tinea pedis—erythema/edema, scaling, and occasional vesiculation; fissured toe webs
        (5) Tinea unguium—opacified thickened nails with subungual debris
        (6) Immunocompromised patient—may see abscess or granulomas
     b. Tinea (pityriasis) versicolor—oval scaly hyper- or hypopigmented macules
     c. Candidiasis
        (1) Skin (intertrigo)—erythematous macerated areas with satellite pustules
        (2) Mucous membranes—white friable patches on mucous membranes
  2. Distribution
     a. Tinea
        (1) Capitis—scalp
        (2) Corporis—non-hair-bearing skin
        (3) Cruris—(males) groin and upper thigh sparing scrotum
        (4) Pedis—feet, usually between 4th and 5th toes
        (5) Unguium—nails, usually 1st and 2nd toenails
     b. Tinea versicolor
        (1) "Shawl like" back, chest, and shoulders
        (2) Less common—groin, thigh, genitalia
     c. Candidiasis
        (1) Body folds—axillae, submammary, groin, intergluteal, webspaces of fingers and toes
        (2) Oral and vaginal mucous membranes

- Diagnostic Tests/Findings
  1. Direct microscopy of skin, hair, or nail samples
  2. Wood's lamp (tinea versicolor)—golden fluorescence
  3. KOH—positive for hyphae, pseudohyphae, and/or spores
  4. Fungal culture—may be useful for inflammatory tinea corporis and tinea capitis

- Management/Treatment
  1. Tinea
     a. Scalp
        (1) Prevention—ketoconazole or selenium sulfide shampoo, may eradicate carrier state
        (2) Terbinafine 250 mg daily 4–8 weeks

(3) Itraconazole 200 mg daily 6–8 weeks

(4) Griseofulvin microsized 250 mg daily 4–8 weeks

(5) Fluconazole 200 mg daily 2 weeks

(6) Ketoconazole 200–400 mg daily

(7) Advise hair regrowth will be slow

  b. Body/feet

(1) Prevention—apply powder containing miconazole to fungus-prone areas after bathing

(2) Multiple topical imidazoles and triazoles applied b.i.d. until 1–2 weeks after clinical clearing

(3) Terbinafine 1% cream b.i.d. 1–2 weeks after clinical clearing

(4) If topical antifungals fail, use oral agents (see tinea capitis)

(5) Avoid occlusive footwear for tinea pedis

  c. Nails

(1) Itraconazole 200 mg daily or terbinafine 250 mg daily

    (a) Fingernails—6 weeks

    (b) Toenails—12 weeks

(2) Poor results with topical agents; usually reserved for maintenance after successful systemic treatment

  d. Follow up in 2 weeks to reevaluate treatment

2. Tinea versicolor (pityriasis versicolor)

  a. Selenium sulfide lotion 2.5%—apply and leave on for 10–15 minutes, then rinse, for 1 week

  b. Ketoconazole shampoo (same as selenium sulfide)

  c. Terbinafine 1% solution b.i.d. for 7 days

  d. Imidazole or triazole creams b.i.d. for 1 week

  e. Retreat if no improvement in 1 month

  f. Recurrence common as organism is normal inhabitant of skin

3. Candidiasis

  a. Nystatin cream or powder b.i.d. 2–4 weeks

  b. Ketoconazole cream daily for 2–4 weeks

  c. Fluconazole 150 mg orally once

  d. Dry intertriginous area—wet Burow's compresses 3–4 times daily

  e. Rule out HIV or diabetes in patients with multiple recurrences

◘ PAPULOSQUAMOUS DISORDERS

- Definition—group of disorders with unique scales due to abnormal keratinization process; these lesions are sharply delineated, which distinguishes them from scaling lesions of eczematous diseases

1. Psoriasis vulgaris—genetically determined, chronic, epidermal proliferate disease of unpredictable course

2. Pityriasis rosea—self-limited, mild, inflammatory skin disease lasting 3–8 weeks

- Etiology/Incidence

1. Psoriasis

  a. Genetic predisposition, although not totally understood

  b. Autoimmune component

  c. Affects 2% of population in United States, Caucasians > African-Americans

  d. Type 1, early onset, occurring in 2nd decade

  e. Type 2, late onset, occurring in 6th to 8th decades

  f. Approximately 5% of patients will develop psoriatic arthritis affecting primarily distal interphalangeal (DIP) joints

  g. Abrupt onset seen with early HIV infection

  h. Trigger factors

    (1) Physical trauma

    (2) Infection

    (3) Stress

    (4) Drugs—corticosteroids, lithium, antimalarial, interferon, beta-blockers

2. Pityriasis rosea

  a. Etiology unknown; herpes 7 is suspected

  b. Seen primarily in the spring and fall seasons

  c. Patients frequently report recent upper respiratory infection

  d. Equal incidence in males and females

- Signs and Symptoms

1. Psoriasis

  a. Frequently asymptomatic, indolent lesion may be present for months

  b. Severe pruritus in body fold eruptions

  c. Constitutional symptoms, joint pain, acute fever, and chills

2. Pityriasis rosea

  a. Mild pruritus, 50%

  b. Initial lesion precedes general eruption by 1–2 weeks

  c. Self-limiting—heals without scarring in 4–8 weeks

- Differential Diagnosis

1. Psoriasis

  a. Seborrheic dermatitis

  b. Candidiasis

  c. Psoriasiform dry eruptions (beta-blockers, methyldopa)

  d. Tinea corporis

2. Pityriasis rosea

  a. Secondary syphilis

  b. Tinea infections

  c. Drug eruptions, e.g., captopril, barbiturates

- Physical Findings
  1. Psoriasis
     a. Cutaneous lesions reveal four prominent features
        (1) Sharply demarcated lesions with clear-cut borders
        (2) Erythematous plaque base
        (3) Overlapping silvery scales
        (4) Auspitz sign—removal of scales results in small blood droplets
     b. Fingers/nails
        (1) Stippling or pitting of nail plate
        (2) Yellow or brown-red staining of oncholytic patches with accumulation of yellow debris under nails
        (3) Swelling, redness, and scaling of paronychial margins
  2. Pityriasis rosea—classic disease pattern
     a. A single lesion termed *herald patch* precedes generalized eruption by 7–10 days
     b. Herald patch is found usually on neck or lower trunk; oval, slightly erythematous, rose or fawn-colored
     c. Oval patches seen in general eruption have an unusual fine, white scale located near the border of the plaques, forming a collarette
     d. Lesions follow skin cleavage lines in a "Christmas tree" pattern

- Diagnostic Tests/Findings
  1. Psoriasis
     a. Diagnosis generally based on clinical presentation
     b. Biopsy may be necessary
     c. HIV serology
     d. Serum uric acid
  2. Pityriasis rosea
     a. Diagnosis generally based on clinical presentation
     b. KOH—negative for spores/hyphae
     c. Throat culture or rapid strep test—negative for scarlatina
     d. RPR—negative for syphilis

- Management/Treatment
  1. Psoriasis—localized to palm/soles/scalp < 5% involvement
     a. Strong potency topical corticosteroid—adjunctive therapy for 2–3 weeks
        (1) Topical fluorinated high-potency glucocorticoids
        (2) Occlusion with plastic wrap
        (3) More effective if scales removed prior to application
     b. Tar-based preparations are useful adjuncts
     c. Anthralin cream 0.1–1% at bedtime
     d. Calcipotriene ointment or cream twice daily

     e. Goeckerman regimen—phototherapy ultraviolet B radiation, sun (UVB) exposure 4–6 hours daily for 4 weeks
     f. Ingram regimen—phototherapy ultraviolet B radiation (UVB) used in combination with anthralin 0.1–0.5% applied daily
  2. Psoriasis—generalized (> 30% body surface affected)
     a. Referral to dermatologist
     b. May include some combination of UVB, PUVA (psoralen with UVA), etretinate, methotrexate, cyclosporine, acitretin, immunomodulators
     c. Patient education for localized and generalized psoriasis—family issues, emotional support, stress reduction, National Psoriasis Foundation
  3. Pityriasis rosea
     a. Treatment often not necessary
     b. UVB light treatments for 1 week
     c. Topical corticosteroids and antihistamines for control of pruritus

◘ SCABIES

- Definition—common highly pruritic transmissable ectoparasite infection

- Etiology/Incidence
  1. Caused by itch mite, *Sarcoptes scabiei*
  2. Adult female mite burrows into skin shortly after contact; lives for 4–6 weeks
  3. Incubation period 4 weeks from initial contact; generalized hypersensitivity eruption 1–2 weeks later
  4. Transmitted primarily by person-to-person or sexual contact
  5. Transmission via clothing, bedding less common—mite typically cannot survive more than 24–48 hours without host
  6. May affect entire families
  7. Frequently seen in institutionalized persons, such as homeless shelters, nursing homes, correctional facilities

- Signs and Symptoms
  1. Pruritus always present; most intense when individual is in bed or after a hot shower
  2. Pruritus frequently less intense in the HIV client

- Differential Diagnosis
  1. Atopic dermatitis
  2. Contact or irritant dermatitis
  3. Adverse cutaneous drug reaction
  4. Pediculosis

- Physical Findings
  1. Burrows, small pruritic vesicles, or wavy dark lines a few millimeters to 1 cm in length with papule at open end

2. May be difficult to visualize since client scratching destroys burrows
3. Lesions are believed to be due to a hypersensitivity reaction to the excreta deposited by mite
4. Generalized excoriations surrounding vesicles and pustules on fingers, palms, wrists, elbows, axillae, feet, nipples in females, scrotum or penis in males, buttocks
5. Usually spares the head and neck, except in the elderly or patients with AIDS—in the client with HIV, hyperkeratotic plaques may be located on any area of the body

- Diagnostic Tests/Findings—microscopic examination of skin scraping in oil immersion detects presence of mite, eggs, or fecal pellets

- Management/Treatment
  1. Treatment of choice is 5% permethrin cream applied to all areas of the body from the neck down; left on for 8–14 hours and then removed with soap and water; may be repeated in 1 week
  2. Alternative is 1% lindane (no longer the drug of choice)
     a. Lotion or cream applied from neck down to all areas of the body and removed with soap and water after 8 hours
     b. Not recommended for pregnant or lactating women, patients with extensive dermatitis, or infants
  3. Alternative is 10% crotamiton cream applied to the body from the neck down for 2 consecutive nights and then removed with soap and water 48 hours after the last application
  4. All household members and sexual partners should be evaluated and treated if necessary to prevent reinfection
  5. For persistent pruritus, triamcinolone 0.1% cream to affected areas b.i.d.
  6. Secondary pyoderma is generally due to staphylococcus; treat with topical mupirocin or oral erythromycin
  7. Patient education
     a. Launder all bedding and clothing in hot water and on hot dryer cycle
     b. Place clothing that cannot be laundered in plastic storage bags for at least 4 days—mites will not survive off the host longer than 4 days
     c. Advise client that pruritus may continue for several weeks

◘ SKIN CANCER

- Definition
  1. Basal cell carcinoma (BCC)—slow-growing locally destructive carcinoma of basal cell layer of epidermis; metastasis rarely seen but can occur
  2. Squamous cell carcinoma (SCC)—malignant, nodular, tumor arising from squamous cells in epithelium; hyperkeratotic growth
  3. Malignant melanoma (MM)—cancer that arises in melanocytes; accounts for 5% of all skin cancers; two most common types are superficial spreading melanoma (SSM) and nodular melanoma (NM)
  4. Kaposi's sarcoma (KS)—multisystem vascular neoplasm characterized by mucocutaneous and violet lesions and edema; involves nearly all body organs

- Etiology/Incidence
  1. Basal cell carcinoma
     a. Cause is multifactorial; cumulative sunlight exposure (UVB) is most significant factor
     b. Primarily affects fair-skinned persons with tendency to sunburn easily
     c. Most common form of human cancer
     d. Over 400,000 new cases in United States per year; mostly persons in 4th decade
     e. Additional risk factors
        (1) Extensive sun exposure as a youth
        (2) History of treatment with x-ray for facial acne
  2. Squamous cell carcinoma
     a. Causal/contributing factors
        (1) UVB light
        (2) Human papillomaviruses (HPV) have also been implicated
        (3) Immunocompromised
        (4) Chemical carcinogens—topical nitrogen mustard; oral PUVA (psoralens with UVA [used to treat psoriasis]); industrial carcinogens
        (5) Increased risk of oral and lip SCC in cigarette and cigar smokers
     b. Mainly seen on sun-damaged areas of fair-skinned persons, but can appear anywhere on the body
     c. Also found in brown- and black-skinned person on plantar surface of foot
     d. Frequency of metastasis is by location; SCC of the cutaneous tissue has an overall metastatic rate of 3–4%; invasive SCC arising from chronic osteomyelitis sinus tracts, burn scars, and sites of radiation dermatitis have metastatic rates of 31%, 20%, and 18% respectively
  3. Malignant melanoma
     a. All causes not known
     b. Brief, intense exposure to long-wave ultraviolet radiation contributes to development
     c. Predisposing/risk factors
        (1) Presence of precursor lesions, e.g., Clark's dysplastic melanocytic nevus, congenital melanocytic nevus

(2) Family history of melanoma

(3) Fair complexion; red or blonde hair; freckles; tendency to sunburn easily

(4) Excessive sun exposure

d. Peak age distribution 30–50 years

e. SSM more common in women, NM equal in women and men

f. Incidence has increased 300% in 40 years

4. Kaposi's sarcoma

a. Human herpesvirus 8 present in all forms

b. Epidemic clusters in United States predominantly found in HIV-infected individuals—incidence has decreased from 40% to 18% of HIV population

c. Occurs when CD4$^+$ count < 500

d. Non-HIV-related forms are less common but do occur

(1) African-endemic—accounts for 8–12% of malignancies in Zaire

(2) Classic (European)—occurs predominantly in elderly white males, rarely fatal

(3) Iatrogenic immunosuppressive drug associated—occurs infrequently in patients on immunosuppressive or cytotoxic chemotherapy; resolves when drug withdrawn

- Signs and Symptoms

1. BCC/SCC—painless sore that will not heal, especially on sun-damaged skin, lower lip, or on radiodermatitis

2. Malignant melanoma—6 signs (ABCDEE)

a. **A**symmetry in shape

b. **B**order is irregular

c. **C**olor is mottled

d. **D**iameter is usually large (> 6.0 mm)

e. **E**levation is almost always present

f. **E**nlargement or a history of an increase in size is perhaps the most important sign

3. Kaposi's sarcoma—small reddish-purple to brown macule

- Differential Diagnosis

1. BCC/SCC

a. Seborrheic keratosis

b. Malignant melanoma

c. Actinic keratosis

d. Psoriasis

e. Nummular eczema

2. Malignant melanoma

a. Melanoma in situ

b. Solar lentigo

c. Dysplastic melanocytic nevus with marked atypia

d. Recurring melanocyte nevus

e. Hemangioma

f. Pyogenic granuloma

g. Pigmented BCC

3. Kaposi's sarcoma

a. Sclerosing hemangioma

b. Ecchymosis

c. Stasis dermatitis

- Physical Findings

1. Basal cell carcinoma

a. Most commonly found on face and head

b. Types—nodular, ulcerated, sclerosing pigmented and superficial lesions

c. Pearly appearance with telangiectatic vessels is most diagnostic (nodular)

d. Lesions may have a central crust or erosion (sclerosing)

2. Squamous cell carcinoma

a. In situ (Bowen's disease)

(1) Sharply demarcated, scaling, or hyperkeratotic macule, papule, or patch

(2) Red, sharply demarcated, glistening macule or plaque-like on genital and perineum

b. Invasive squamous cell carcinoma

(1) Highly differentiated SCC

(a) Keratinization within or on surface of tumor

(b) Firm or hard upon palpation

(2) Poorly differentiated SCC

(a) Shows no sign of keratinization

(b) Fleshy, granulomatous; soft on palpation

3. Malignant melanoma

a. SSM

(1) Pigment variation of dark brown, black, pink, or gray; starts as flattened papule, progressing to plaques, and then nodules

(2) Asymmetrical to 12 mm (early), to 25 mm (late)

(3) Isolated single lesions found primarily on sun-exposed areas—back (men), legs (women)

(4) Regional lymphadenopathy (later stages)

b. NM

(1) Dark blue, black uniformly elevated "blueberry-like" nodule ranging in size from 1 to 3 cm; oval or round with smooth sharply defined borders

(2) Distribution and regional lymphadenopathy same as SSM

4. Kaposi's sarcoma

a. Red, purple, or dark color palpable plaques or nodules on cutaneous or mucosal surfaces

b. Oral lesions are often initial manifestation

c. Lymph node involvement in 50% of patient's with HIV-associated KS

d. May also involve the lung, gastrointestinal tract, lymphatic system, or urogenital system

- Diagnostic Tests/Findings—total excisional biopsy with narrow margins for SSM and NM

- Management/Treatment
  1. Basal cell carcinoma
     a. Simple excision—5–10% recurrence
     b. Referral to oncology for therapy
        (1) Three cycles of curettage and electro-dessication
        (2) Radiotherapy with 4,000–5,000 rads in 6–10 doses (cure 95%)
        (3) Mohs surgery—removal of tumor; 98% cure rate
  2. Squamous cell carcinoma
     a. Referral to oncologist for therapy
     b. Surgical excision, Mohs surgery, radiotherapy (invasion SCC)
     c. Cryotherapy, 5-fluorouracil chemotherapy
  3. Malignant melanoma
     a. Refer to oncologist for therapy—Initial excision to establish diagnosis
        (1) Total excisional biopsy with narrow margins where possible
        (2) If total excision not possible, punch biopsy followed by extensive surgery
     b. Close follow-up for evidence of recurrence of metastasis
  4. Kaposi's sarcoma
     a. Referral for cryotherapy, radiation, or laser surgery—treatment depends upon underlying condition and location of sarcoma
     b. Supportive care, counseling for HIV-progressive disease

❑ VIRAL DERMATOSES

- Definitions
  1. Herpes simplex I (HS-I) ("fever blister")—recurrent cutaneous viral infection characterized by single or multiple clusters of small vesicles on an erythematous base; lesions appear on the lips, in the mouth, or in the pharynx
  2. Herpes (varicella) zoster ("shingles")—an acute CNS cutaneous viral infection characterized by vesicular eruptions and neurologic pain; involves primarily the dorsal root ganglia
  3. Human papillomavirus —cutaneous infections (HPV-CI), common contagious epithelial tumors; usually benign

- Etiology/Incidence
  1. Herpes simplex
     a. Caused by herpes simplex virus (HSV-I)
     b. Usually follows a minor infection, trauma, stress, or sun exposure
     c. 90% of adults have serologic evidence of virus
     d. Incubation period 2–20 days

  2. Herpes (varicella) zoster
     a. Reactivation of varicella zoster virus (VZV) in chickenpox
     b. Proposed that VZV is dormant in dorsal root ganglia
     c. May occur at any age, but most common after age 50
     d. May precede marked immunosuppression in patients with HIV or Hodgkin's disease
     e. Post-transplant patients on immunosuppression medication are also at risk
  3. HPV (cutaneous infections)
     a. Caused by any of more than 150 human papillomaviruses
     b. Squamous cell carcinoma associated with HPV infections in anogenital region
     c. Common in young adults, but uncommon in the aged

- Signs and Symptoms
  1. HS-I
     a. Small umbilicated vesicles appear after a short prodrome of tingling, burning, or itching
     b. Vesicles dry to a yellow crust within a few days
  2. Herpes zoster
     a. Pain along nerve root precedes eruption by 2–3 weeks
     b. Characteristic crops of vesicles then appear in 3–5 days
  3. HPV (cutaneous infections)—generally asymptomatic
  4. Post-herpetic neuralgia months to years

- Differential Diagnosis
  1. HS-I
     a. Aphthous stomatitis
     b. Hand, foot, and mouth disease
     c. Herpangina
  2. Herpes zoster (local lesion and pre-eruptive pain)
     a. Contact dermatitis
     b. Herpes simplex
     c. Migraine
     d. Myocardial infarction
     e. Acute abdomen
  3. HPV (cutaneous infection)
     a. Squamous cell carcinoma
     b. Hypertrophic actinic keratosis
     c. Molluscum contagiosum
     d. Seborrheic keratosis

- Physical Findings
  1. Regional lymphadenopathy may be seen with herpetic diseases
  2. HS-I
     a. Small, grouped vesicles on an erythematous base that progress to crusted erosion

b. Duration 5–7 days

c. Distribution lips, mouth, pharynx

3. Herpes zoster

   a. Prodrome (2–3 weeks); papules (24 hours); vesicles-bullae (48 hours); pustules (96 hours); crust (7–10 days)

   b. Painful unilateral vesicular eruptions with crust formation within a dermatome lasting 3–5 days

   c. Duration 2–3 weeks

   d. Distribution—face and trunk

   e. Regional lymph glands may be tender or edematous

   f. Complication of post-herpetic neuralgia involving trigeminal region

4. Warts

   a. Common wart (verruca vulgaris)

     (1) Solitary flesh-colored papule with scaly irregular surface 2–10 mm in diameter

     (2) Appear most often on fingers, around nail plate, elbows, knees (site of trauma)

   b. Flat wart (verruca plantaris)

     (1) Groups of smooth flat-topped, flesh-colored lesions

     (2) Distribution—face and extremities (site of trauma)

   c. Plantar warts

     (1) Endophytic (growing inward) with thick keratin surface

     (2) Common on sole of foot, toes

     (3) May be exquisitely painful

- Diagnostic Tests/Findings

1. HS-I and zoster

   a. Direct immunofluorescent antibody (ELISA)—positive

   b. Tzanck smear—multinucleated cells (least sensitive)

   c. Viral culture—positive (not highly sensitive)

   d. Consider testing for HIV or Hodgkin's if recurrence of herpes

2. Warts

   a. Acetic acid 5%—lesions turn white

   b. Biopsy—rule out squamous cell carcinoma

- Management/Treatment

1. HS-I

   a. Immunocompetent patient

     (1) Initial episode—7–10 days

       (a) Acyclovir 400 mg 3 times/day for 7–10 days

       (b) Valacyclovir 1,000 mg b.i.d. for 7 days

       (c) Famciclovir 250 mg t.i.d. for 5–10 days

     (2) Recurrent episodes—5 days

       (a) Acyclovir 400 mg 3 times/day for 5 days

       (b) Valacyclovir 1,000 mg b.i.d. for 5 days

       (c) Famciclovir 125 mg b.i.d. for 5 days

     (3) Topical acyclovir not recommended, minimally effective

   b. Immunosuppressed patient

     (1) Initial episode

       (a) Acyclovir 200 mg 5 times/day for 7–10 days

       (b) Acyclovir 5 mg/kg/IV every 8 hours for severe cases

     (2) To prevent reactivation (i.e., immediate post-transplant)—acyclovir 400 mg 3–5 times/day

   c. Caution family—virus may remain on fomites for several hours

2. Herpes zoster

   a. Immunocompetent

     (1) Immunization for those > 60 years old with Zostavax—not intended to treat existing disease

     (2) Acyclovir 800 mg 4 times/day for 7–10 days started within 48–72 hours

     (3) Famciclovir 500 mg t.i.d. for 7 days started within 48–72 hours

     (4) Valacyclovir 1,000 mg t.i.d. for 7 days started within 48–72 hours

     (5) Good hydration essential

     (6) Nerve block for analgesia may be necessary

     (7) Acute pain—prednisone 60 mg/day for 3 weeks

     (8) Monitor renal function in patient with renal disease

   b. Immunosuppressed patient

     (1) Consult with physician

     (2) Antiviral therapy as with immunocompetent except of longer duration until lesions have completely crusted

   c. Post-zoster neuralgia

     (1) Capsaicin ointment 0.025–0.075% every 4 hours

     (2) Chronic regional nerve blockade

     (3) Antiepileptic or antidepressant medications (e.g., pregabalin, amitriptyline)

   d. HPV (cutaneous infection)

     (1) Most are unresponsive to all therapeutic modalities

     (2) Most will resolve spontaneously in 1–2 years

     (3) Multiple keratolytic agents—salicylic acid or salicylic acid and lactic acid combination

     (4) Imiquimod cream—apply, leave on for 6–10 hours, then wash, 3 times a week

     (5) Plantar warts—hyperthermia with hot water ½ to ¾ hour 3 times a week

◻ QUESTIONS

Select the best answer.

1. Mrs. Trevino is a 35-year-old patient with patchy hair loss as a result of chronic systemic lupus erythematosus. You have determined that she has scarring or cicatricial alopecia. What is the most effective treatment you can offer?

    a. Topical minoxidil
    b. Intralesional corticosteroids
    c. Topical estrogen
    d. Referral for hair transplants

2. Mr. Johnson is a 45-year-old patient with diabetes who is homeless. He presents with tender fluctuant nodules on the skin around his beard. He has been previously treated with benzoyl peroxide 5% with minimal response. You order warm moist compresses and:

    a. Dicloxacillin 500 mg q.i.d. for 10 days
    b. Trimethoprim/sulfamethoxazole every day for 5 days
    c. Acyclovir topical
    d. Clotrimazole 1% b.i.d. for 10 days

3. Mr. Johnson returns to your office with his friend. His friend presents with multiple abscesses and "boils" on the back of his neck that have coalesced and developed sieve-like openings draining pus. Your diagnosis is:

    a. Scabies
    b. Folliculitis
    c. Carbuncle
    d. Contact dermatitis

4. To reduce inflammation in a hidradentitis suppurativa lesion, immediately prior to incision and drainage you would:

    a. Apply cold packs to axilla
    b. Order Solu-Medrol Dosepak
    c. Apply tretinoin topically
    d. Inject intralesional triamcinolone 3–5 mg/mL diluted with lidocaine

5. What is the most common sensitizer in the United States responsible for allergic contact dermatitis?

    a. Oleoresin
    b. Tinea
    c. Rubbing alcohol
    d. Bleach

6. Mrs. Waterman is a 64-year-old with a history of varicosities and a single episode of thrombophlebitis. On inspection of both lower extremities you note mottled pigmentation, erythema, varicosities, and ankle edema. What is your initial impression?

    a. Cellulitis
    b. Stasis dermatitis
    c. Atopic dermatitis
    d. Contact dermatitis

7. What is the most effective antifungal agent used in the treatment of tinea capitis?

    a. Terbinafine orally
    b. Clotrimazole 1% cream
    c. Triamcinolone 0.025% cream
    d. Nystatin cream

8. Janet is a 22-year-old white female who presents for evaluation of lesions on the palm of her right hand. The lesions consist of silvery scales on an erythematous base and are isolated by a sharply demarcated border. You remove the scales and minute drops of blood appear giving a positive Auspitz sign. Your diagnosis is:

    a. Pityriasis rosea
    b. Squamous cell carcinoma
    c. Psoriasis
    d. Eczema

9. Common mode(s) of transmission of scabies include:

    a. Moist fomites
    b. Person to person
    c. Household pets
    d. Soil

10. A 24-year-old presents to clinic with a 5-cm purple, palpable plaque on the upper right posterior chest. He admits to unprotected homosexual activity for the past 10 years. On further exam you note axillary and inguinal lymphadenopathy. You suspect this patient may have:

    a. Squamous cell carcinoma
    b. Malignant melanoma
    c. Basal cell carcinoma
    d. Kaposi's sarcoma

11. Initial laboratory evaluation(s) for this patient in question 10 should include:

    a. HIV antibody screening
    b. Complete blood count
    c. GC/chlamydia cultures
    d. Liver function tests

12. The common wart, verruca vulgaris, is characterized as:

    a. Solitary flesh-colored papule with scaly irregular surface
    b. Group of flat-topped flesh colored papules
    c. Thick, endophylitic papules or plaques
    d. Papular, nodular, ulcerated sclerosing pigmented lesion

13. Joan is a 15-year-old with multiple closed comedones and a few pustules on her face and upper back. She has been on tretinoin for her face but is distressed at the progression of acne to her back. What would you would prescribe?

    a. 13-cis-retinoic acid (Accutane)
    b. Erythromycin 500 mg b.i.d. for 10 days
    c. Benzoyl peroxide cleansing soap
    d. Amoxil 250 mg t.i.d. for 10 days

14. Janice is an 18-year-old who presents to your clinic with a scaly, pruritic rash on the dorsal aspect of her toes. This rash has occurred each winter for the past 8 years. Her family history is unremarkable except for her father who has asthma. What is the most likely diagnosis?

    a. Psoriasis
    b. Candidiasis
    c. Contact dermatitis
    d. Atopic dermatitis

15. Overgrowth of *Pityrosporum orbiculare* in the young adult results in:

    a. Tinea corporis
    b. Tinea versicolor
    c. Tinea capitis
    d. Tinea pedis

16. A 30-year-old male presents with multiple, scattered, discrete vesicular lesions on the right leg for 5 days. There are honey-colored "stuck-on" crusts and erosions in some of these lesions. The culture yields *Staphylococcus aureus.* What is the most likely diagnosis?

    a. Herpes simplex
    b. Herpes zoster
    c. Stasis dermatitis
    d. Impetigo

17. A 19-year-old female presents with small grouped vesicles on an erythematous base on her lower lip. The lesion is painful. She has had this before and it has always gone away in a week or so. You suspect herpes simplex 1. You would confirm your diagnosis with which of the following laboratory tests?

    a. Direct immunofluorescent antibody (ELISA)
    b. KOH test
    c. Culture and sensitivity
    d. Wood's lamp

18. Mr. Smith, age 46, presents to the adult nurse practitioner (ANP) with fever, malaise, and a painful, linear vesicular rash on just one side of his trunk. What is the most likely diagnosis?

    a. Tinea corporis
    b. Carbuncle
    c. Herpes simplex
    d. Herpes zoster

19. Mr. Thompson has chronic eczema. He presents with pruritic, dry, leathery patches with accentuated skin markings on his forearm. What is the most appropriate treatment?

    a. Amoxicillin orally
    b. Clotrimazole 1% cream
    c. Desonide 0.05%
    d. UVB with coal tar

20. Melissa, age 22, presents to the ANP's office with a slightly pruritic red rash on her trunk and breast following the line of skin cleavage giving a "Christmas tree" configuration. She states that the rash started as a single red patch on her abdomen. Medical history is unremarkable, except for a recent upper respiratory infection. What is your initial diagnosis?

    a. Tinea versicolor
    b. Folliculitis
    c. Pityriasis rosea
    d. Seborrheic dermatitis

21. Mr. Kirk is a 45-year-old African-American who presents with a sore on his lip that will not heal. Medical history includes psoriasis treated with oral PUVA. Upon inspection you note an erythematous plaque, slightly raised with sharp borders, and no sign of infiltration or telangiectatic vessels. You make a referral to the dermatologist for further evaluation of what you suspect is:

    a. Basal cell carcinoma
    b. Squamous cell carcinoma
    c. Kaposi's sarcoma
    d. Psoriasis refractory to treatment

22. Mrs. Summers presents to the ANP with a complaint of red rash and large blister after wearing a new prosthetic leg for 3 days. This prosthesis has a new polyurethane material she did not have with her old prosthesis. Her leg was amputated below the right knee secondary to an accident as a child. Upon inspection you note a tender, erythematous, scaly, maculopapular rash. It is warm and edematous with a large bullous lesion on the posterior popliteal fossae. What is your initial diagnosis?

    a. Eczema
    b. Severe irritant contact dermatitis
    c. Herpes zoster
    d. Carbuncle

23. Your management of Mrs. Summers includes oral glucocorticoids steroids, UVB (sunlight exposure) and:

    a. Reducing bullae with sterile needle and syringe
    b. Leaving bullae alone and let rupture spontaneously
    c. Advising continued use of new prosthesis
    d. Removing top of bullae and applying high-potency steroid cream

24. Which of the following medications has no severe teratogenic properties and is safe for use in the sexually active young female with acne?

    a. Erythromycin
    b. Tretinoin
    c. Accutane
    d. Tetracycline

25. Mrs. Lopez is a 45-year-old who presents with a tender, mildly pruritic rash under both breasts and on her abdomen. She is a diabetic with poor control due to poor medication compliance and is at 160% ideal body weight (IBW). Upon inspection you note moist erythematous macerated areas with satellite pustules under both breasts. What is your initial impression?

    a. Candidiasis intertrigo
    b. Tinea corporis
    c. Herpes zoster
    d. Pityriasis rosea

26. Along with better control of Mrs. Lopez's diabetes and continued effort at weight modification, you would prescribe which of the following:

    a. Nystatin cream or powder
    b. Selenium sulfide lotion 2.5%
    c. Terbinafine 1% cream
    d. Hydrocortisone 1% cream

27. What is the most appropriate treatment for tinea versicolor?

    a. To apply selenium sulfide lotion 2.5% to the body and leave on for 10–15 minutes, then rinse, for 1 week
    b. To apply topical steroids t.i.d. to the rash for 7 days
    c. To apply coal tar preparations such as estar gel
    d. To use psoralen with UV light

Answers

1.	**d**	15.	**b**
2.	**a**	16.	**d**
3.	**c**	17.	**a**
4.	**d**	18.	**d**
5.	**a**	19.	**c**
6.	**b**	20.	**c**
7.	**a**	21.	**b**
8.	**c**	22.	**b**
9.	**b**	23.	**a**
10.	**d**	24.	**a**
11.	**a**	25.	**a**
12.	**a**	26.	**a**
13.	**b**	27.	**a**
14.	**d**		

◘ BIBLIOGRAPHY

Braunwald, E. (Ed.). (2008). *Harrison's principles of internal medicine* (17th ed.). New York: McGraw-Hill.

Brodell, R. T., & Elewski, B. (2000). Antifungal drug interactions. *Postgraduate Medicine, 107* (1). Retrieved from http://www.postgradmed.com/issues/2000/01_00/brodell.htm

DiPiro, J. T., Talbert, R. L., Yee, G. C., Matzke, G. R., Wells, B. G., & Posey, L. M. (Eds.). (2008). *Pharmacotherapy: A pathophysiologic approach* (7th ed.). New York: Lange Medical Books/McGraw-Hill.

Edmunds, M. V., & Mayhew, M. S. (2003). *Procedures for primary care practitioners.* St. Louis: Mosby.

Hay, W. W., Levin, M. J., Deterding, R., & Sondheimer, J. M. (2008). *Current pediatric diagnosis and treatment* (19th ed.). New York: McGraw-Hill.

McPhee, S. J., & Papadakis, M. A., & Rabow, M. W. (Eds.). (2011). *Current medical diagnosis and treatment* (51st ed.). New York: McGraw-Hill.

Ozgediz, D., Smith, E.B., Zheng, J., Otero, J., Tabatabi, Z. L., & Corvera, C. U. (2008). Basal cell carcinoma does metastasize. *Dermatology Online Journal, 14*(8), 5. Retrieved from http://dermatology.cdlib.org/148/case_reports/bcc/corvera.html

Uphold, C. R., & Graham, M. V. (2003). *Clinical guidelines in family practice* (4th ed.). Gainesville, FL: Barmarrae Books.

Wolff, K., & Johnson, R. A. Polano (2009). *Fitzpatrick's color atlas and synopsis of clinical dermatology common and serious diseases* (6th ed.). New York: McGraw-Hill.

4

Eye, Ear, Nose, and Throat Disorders

Margaret Hadro Venzke

◻ CONJUNCTIVITIS

- Definition—inflammation of palpebral and/or bulbar conjunctiva; classic description is "pink eye"

- Etiology/Incidence
  1. Bacterial
     a. *Staphylococcus aureus*
     b. *Streptococcus pneumoniae*
     c. *Haemophilus influenzae*
     d. *Neisseria gonorrhoeae*
     e. Proteus species
  2. Viral
     a. Adenoviruses (most common)
        (1) Adenopharyngeal conjunctivitis (APC) —"swimming pool"
        (2) Epidemic keratoconjunctivitis (EKC) —highly contagious, corneal involvement
     b. Herpes simplex
     c. Herpes zoster
  3. Allergic
     a. Seasonal allergies—pollen, grass, trees
     b. Hypersensitivity
     c. Chemical irritants
  4. Chlamydia/trachoma
  5. Other
     a. Trauma
     b. Contact lens wearer—more susceptible than general population
     c. Foreign body
     d. Drug induced—preservative in eye drops, antimicrobials
     e. Systemic illness
        (1) Measles
        (2) Varicella
        (3) Rocky Mountain spotted fever
        (4) Reiter's syndrome
     f. Contaminated contact lens solution
     g. Mascara/eyeliner, makeup
  6. Mode of transmission—direct contact with contagion or allergen
  7. Most common eye disease in primary care; usually benign, self-limiting disorder

- Signs and Symptoms
  1. Mild to moderate redness and irritation
  2. No change in visual acuity
  3. Absence of photophobia and eye pain
  4. Mild discomfort, often associated with itching, burning sensation or excessive tearing
  5. Discharge may be watery, stringy, purulent; scant to copious
  6. Bacterial conjunctivitis
     a. Mucopurulent discharge (profuse exudate suggests *Neisseria gonorrhoeae*)
     b. Thick purulent crust of material on eyelids after night's sleep
     c. Unilateral (initially)
     d. Self-limiting—10–14 days without treatment, resolves in 2–4 days with treatment
  7. Viral conjunctivitis
     a. Redness, general discomfort, profuse watery discharge
     b. Preauricular adenopathy common
     c. Association with upper respiratory illness, fever, pharyngitis

d. Unilateral (initially)

e. Symptoms last 2–3 weeks (contagious, viral shedding in tears for approximately 2 weeks)

8. Allergic

a. Moderate to severe bilateral itching

b. Clear to stringy mucoid discharge

c. Chronic hypersensitivity—vernal conjunctivitis associated with corneal ulceration

9. Chlamydial conjunctivitis

a. More often unilateral than bilateral

b. Moderate exudate

c. Enlarged, tender preauricular nodes

d. Symptoms persist 3–9 months without treatment

• Differential Diagnosis

1. Urgent ophthalmic conditions—prompt referral to avoid compromised eyesight. See **Table 4-1**.

a. Acute uveitis/iritis

b. Acute glaucoma

c. Corneal trauma/infection

d. Orbital cellulitis

• Physical Findings

1. Injected conjunctiva

2. Discharge (see signs and symptoms)

3. Cornea—clear

4. Pupillary response—equal and reactive to light

5. Visual acuity (Snellen)—no acute change

6. Preauricular adenopathy—often viral etiology

• Diagnostic Tests/Findings

1. Typically none indicated; uncomplicated cases diagnosed based upon clinical examination

2. Fluorescein uptake staining—dye uptake suggests corneal involvement

3. Culture—only if chronic problem or gonococcal conjunctivitis suspected

4. Gram stain of discharge/scrapings—rarely done unless gonococcal conjunctivitis suspected

5. Giemsa stain of scrapings—for *Chlamydia trachomatis* infection

• Management/Treatment

1. Pharmacologic

a. Bacterial conjunctivitis

(1) Sodium sulfacetamide 10% ophthalmic solution, 1–2 drops every 4 hours while awake or q.i.d. for 5–7 days

(2) Bacitracin/polymyxin ophthalmic ointment, apply thin layer in lower conjunctival sac b.i.d. for 7 days

(3) Erythromycin ophthalmic ointment, apply thin layer in lower conjunctival sac q.i.d. for 5–7 days

(4) Tobramycin 0.3% or gentamycin 0.3% ophthalmic solution, 1–2 drops q.i.d. for 7 days

b. Gonococcal conjunctivitis—refer to ophthalmologist immediately

(1) Topical antibiotics—erythromycin

(2) Intravenous (IV) antibiotics

(a) Ceftriaxone

(b) Aqueous penicillin

(3) Culture discharge

(4) Report to health department

c. Chlamydia conjunctivitis

(1) Doxycycline 100 mg orally b.i.d. for 21 days

(2) Erythromycin 250 mg 6 times/day for 21 days

d. Viral conjunctivitis

(1) Self-limiting

(2) Topical antibiotics—to prevent secondary bacterial infection

(3) Corticosteroids contraindicated

e. Allergic conjunctivitis

(1) Topical vasoconstrictors/antihistamines

(a) Naphazoline HCL/pheniramine maleate—1–2 drops q.i.d.

(b) Ketotifen 1–2 drops every 12 hours

■ **Table 4-1** Characteristics of the Common Ophthalmic Conditions

	Conjunctivitis	Iritis	Acute Glaucoma
Pain	mild	moderate	severe
Vision	normal	slightly blurred	blurred
Discharge	clear, stringy, or mucopurulent	clear	clear
Cornea	clear	clear	cloudy
Pupil	normal	small irregular	mid-dilated and nonreactive
Light response	normal	poor	none
Conjunctival injection	diffuse toward fornices	circumcorneal	corneal/conjunctival hyperemia

       (2) Oral antihistamines

       (3) Allergen avoidance

       (4) Topical antihistamine mast cell stabilizer

          (a) Azelastine 0.05% 1 drop b.i.d.

          (b) Olopatadine 0.1% 1 drop b.i.d.

       (5) NSAID-ophthalmic (for ocular pruritus)—ketorolac tromethamine 0.5% 1 drop q.i.d.

2. General measures

   a. Cool/warm compresses

   b. Frequent gentle eye wash to remove discharge

   c. Artificial tears

   d. Strict hand washing

   e. Use separate towels; avoid handshaking

   f. Contact lens care—clean contacts or change disposable lens, use new solutions, avoid "homemade" tap water solutions

   g. Avoid eye cosmetics during infection; change eye products frequently

   h. Refer if no improvement in 48 hours or if vision is impaired

◘ BLEPHARITIS

- Definition—inflammation of eyelid margins and eyelashes

- Etiology/Incidence
  1. Commonly affects elderly persons
  2. Associated with seborrheic dermatitis and acne rosacea
  3. Often a chronic condition
  4. Seborrheic blepharitis
     a. Erythematous lid margins
     b. Dry flakes, oily secretions
     c. Cosmetics and chemicals aggravate the condition
  5. Staphylococcal (ulcerative) blepharitis
     a. Acute/chronic inflammation of glands of lid margins
     b. *Staphylococcus aureus* and *Staphylococcus epidermidis* are causative organisms
     c. Mild ulceration of lid margin
     d. Loss of lashes
  6. Mixed blepharitis—most common (seborrheic with secondary staphylococcal infection)
  7. Infestation of eyelashes with lice

- Signs and Symptoms
  1. Gritty, burning sensation
  2. Crusted material on eyelids upon awakening
  3. Redness
  4. Swelling of lid margins
  5. Irritation and itching common
  6. Dry or greasy scales on lashes

7. Mild conjunctival irritation and erythema

8. Discomfort typically less than expected given appearance

- Differential Diagnosis
  1. Conjunctivitis
  2. Chronic chalazia
  3. Sebaceous cell carcinoma (rare)
  4. Keratitis

- Physical Findings
  1. Erythematous eyelid margins bilaterally
  2. Scaly lesions on lashes
  3. Sclera—white
  4. Conjunctivae—usually clear
  5. Masses on lids/lid margins (palpate with gloves)
  6. Preauricular adenopathy
  7. No change in visual acuity

- Diagnostic Tests/Findings—none indicated

- Management/Treatment
  1. Warm water compresses
  2. Eyelid margin gentle scrubs 2–4 times a day
     a. Use washcloth or cotton tip applicator, moisten with dilute solution of water and baby shampoo or commercial lid cleaner
     b. Rinse well
  3. Antibiotic ointment q.i.d. to lid margins for 7 days (erythromycin, sulfacetamide sodium)
  4. Systemic antibiotics for severe infection—doxycycline 100 mg b.i.d. for 6 weeks
  5. Coexisting seborrhea of face/scalp—treat with selenium sulfide shampoo
  6. Maintain hygiene (lid washes) to prevent recurrence of seborrheic and mixed blepharitis
  7. Infestation of lice
     a. 1% permethrin cream rinse, following shampoo of head, which kills both lice and eggs; requires one application whereas others require more than one
     b. Apply thick petrolatum to eyelashes b.i.d.
     c. Remove nits from lashes and hair

◘ FOREIGN BODY IN EYE

- Description—object or debris in eye causing irritation

- Etiology/Incidence
  1. Most common ocular injury in primary care
  2. Foreign body (FOB) often lodges in conjunctiva or cornea

- Signs and Symptoms
  1. Unilateral, acute onset
  2. Sensation of "something in the eye"

3. Photophobia
4. Redness
5. Mild pain
6. Mild decrease in visual acuity

- Differential Diagnosis
  1. Intraocular foreign body (penetrates eye globe)
  2. Corneal laceration
  3. Corneal abrasion
  4. "Contact lens wearer" keratitis

- Physical Findings
  1. Diagnosis based on physical findings
  2. Visual acuity may be normal
  3. Cornea—examine under magnification and bright light, FOB may show up as a dark speck
  4. Ring-shaped orange stain—embedded iron or steel body
  5. Observe for laceration, hyphema, irregular pupil, or absent red reflex—immediate ophthalmic referral
  6. Conjunctiva—instruct patient to look down, grasp lashes, evert eyelid, inspect upper eye and lid

- Diagnostic Tests/Findings—fluorescein stain highlights presence of foreign body and corneal abrasion

- Management/Treatment
  1. Remove simple (nonpenetrating) foreign body with moistened cotton applicator with water or sterile normal saline; reevaluate visual acuity
  2. Irrigation of eye—use only for chemical splash to eyes
  3. Antibiotic ophthalmic ointment
  4. Eye pad
  5. Follow up in 24 hours to evaluate
  6. Patient education
     a. Caution—no rubbing of eye
     b. Advise protective eye wear
  7. Refer
     a. Intraocular foreign body
     b. Change in visual acuity
     c. Acute ocular pain
     d. Large corneal abrasion

◘ CORNEAL ABRASION

- Definition—disruption in the epithelial surface of the cornea by mechanical or chemical factors

- Etiology/Incidence
  1. Common eye injury
  2. Direct trauma to eye; most commonly a scratch from contact lens, fingernail, or piece of paper
  3. Chemical splash
  4. Chronic dry eye

- Signs and Symptoms
  1. Unilateral severe eye pain, progresses over period of hours
  2. Redness
  3. Tearing
  4. Photophobia
  5. Scratchy sensation that worsens with blinking
  6. Decreased visual acuity
  7. Difficulty keeping eye open

- Differential Diagnosis
  1. Keratitis (viral, bacterial, or acanthamoeba)
  2. Foreign body
  3. Corneal laceration

- Physical Findings
  1. Document visual acuity—often decreased
  2. Visualization of corneal lesion following fluorescein stain illuminated with cobalt blue light

- Diagnostic Tests/Findings
  1. Fluorescein dye; abraded or ulcerated areas will become stained and fluoresce yellow-green color
  2. Magnetic resonance imaging (MRI) of orbit if high-velocity injury or suspect embedded foreign body

- Management/Treatment
  1. Antibiotic ointment or sulfonamide drops to affected eye
  2. Ophthalmic nonsteroidal anti-inflammatory agent, e.g., ketorolac
  3. Oral analgesics or short-acting cycloplegic agent for pain relief
  4. Pain should be markedly improved in 48 hours; typically much better in 24 hours; if not, refer to ophthalmology
  5. Topical antibiotics q.i.d. for 24–48 hours
  6. Avoid topical anesthetic drops after initial examination; retard healing and mask symptom progression
  7. Topical steroids contraindicated; retard healing and increase risk of infection
  8. If chemical or thermal injury to eye, refer immediately to ophthalmology

◘ GLAUCOMA

- Definition—increased intraocular eye pressure resulting in atrophy of optic nerve, loss of visual fields and acuity; may be acute or chronic

- Etiology/Incidence
  1. Inadequate drainage of aqueous fluid in the anterior chamber of the eye
  2. Most common type is chronic open angle (wide angle)
  3. Acute closed angle (angle closure, narrow angle) occurs in patients with an anatomically narrow angle

4. Chronic open angle
   a. Accounts for 90% of all cases
   b. Predominately seen over age 40
   c. African-Americans are affected more frequently
   d. Positive first-degree family history
   e. Diabetes mellitus and steroid use are risk factors
5. Primary angle closure (closed angle or narrow angle)
   a. Positive family history
   b. African-Americans and Asians more affected than Caucasians
   c. Predominately age 55–75 years
   d. Females more than males
   e. Less common than open angle but more severe in presentation
   f. May be precipitated by stress, anxiety, darkness, increased fluid intake or medications—anticholinergic medications are common triggers
6. Congenital glaucoma (developmental) in young children
7. Approximately 0.5% of total population

- Signs and Symptoms
  1. Chronic open angle glaucoma—obstruction to aqueous outflow
     a. Asymptomatic at onset
     b. Mid-peripheral vision affected in early stages
     c. Frequent change of glasses
     d. Central vision loss is a late sign
     e. Gradual, painless visual loss and ultimate blindness
  2. Primary angle closure—mechanical obstruction of flow of aqueous humor; iris may obstruct the trabecular meshwork at canal of Schlemm resulting in elevated intraocular pressure
     a. Acute ocular pain
     b. Nausea, vomiting
     c. Photophobia
     d. Blurred vision
     e. Halos around lights at night
     f. Unilateral frontal headache
     g. Tearing
     h. Erythema

- Differential Diagnosis
  1. Uveitis
  2. Conjunctivitis
  3. Ocular trauma
  4. Neurological disease

- Physical Findings
  1. Visual acuity—decreased
  2. Cornea is clear
  3. Change in peripheral vision as measured by direct confrontation

4. Chronic open angle glaucoma
   a. Cupping of optic disc
   b. Elevated intraocular pressure (IOP)
5. Primary angle closure
   a. Lid edema
   b. Injected conjunctiva
   c. Fixed mid-dilated pupil
   d. Shallow anterior chamber, often cloudy
   e. Markedly elevated IOP
   f. Firm eye globe

- Diagnostic Tests/Findings
  1. Tonometry (normal range 10–20 mm Hg)
  2. Pressure reading 20 mm Hg or greater requires further evaluation
  3. U.S. Preventive Services Task Force reports insufficient evidence to recommend glaucoma screening; no consensus on frequency of screening
  4. May screen certain at-risk populations (African-Americans, diabetes mellitus, or severe myopia)

- Management/Treatment
  1. Refer all patients with
     a. Elevated IOP
     b. Decreased visual acuity
     c. Visual field loss
     d. Nonreactive pupil
  2. Goal of therapy to stabilize IOP to prevent optic nerve damage and visual loss
  3. Pharmacological—chronic open angle glaucoma
     a. Parasympathomimetics—topical miotics (pilocarpine) facilitates aqueous outflow
     b. Beta blockers decrease aqueous (timolol, betaxolol) production
     c. Carbonic anhydrase inhibitors (acetazolamide)—reduces aqueous production
     d. Hyperosmotics—reduces formation of fluid (mannitol)
     e. Alpha agonists—decrease aqueous production, increase outflow
  4. Pharmacological—primary angle closure
     a. Emergency treatment with IV acetazolamide, mannitol, and oral glycerol
     b. Maintenance therapy with additional miotic agents and corticosteroids
  5. Laser and surgical intervention are indicated for all patients with acute glaucoma after initial stabilization; may be indicated for chronic glaucoma after maximizing medication therapy
  6. General measures
     a. Encourage frequent follow-up with ophthalmology
     b. Monitor side effects of medications
     c. Avoid over-the-counter cold preparations that may exacerbate glaucoma

◘ CATARACTS

- Definition—clouding/opacity of crystalline lens, causing disruption of visual acuity

- Etiology/Incidence
  1. Single largest cause of blindness
  2. 90% of cataracts due to aging process (senile cataract)
  3. Congenital cataract (rubella)
  4. Systemic disease (diabetes and thyroid)
  5. Drug induced, especially steroid use
  6. Ocular trauma
  7. Chronic uveitis
  8. Ultraviolet B light exposure

- Signs and Symptoms
  1. Painless
  2. Cloudy, fuzzy, blurred vision
  3. Change in refractive error
  4. Glare associated with bright lights (night driving)
  5. Alteration in color perception
  6. Unilateral or bilateral development

- Differential Diagnosis
  1. Senile macular degeneration (loss of central vision)
  2. Retinal detachment
  3. Diabetic retinopathy
  4. Ocular tumor

- Physical Findings
  1. Lens opacity
  2. Disruption of red reflex
  3. Visual acuity decreased
  4. Reduced color discrimination

- Diagnostic Tests/Findings—refer to ophthalmology

- Management/Treatment
  1. Refer to ophthalmologist
  2. Surgical intervention—lens implant is preferred treatment
  3. Follow up postoperatively to observe for hemorrhage or infection
  4. Nonsurgical treatment—frequent changes in glasses, bifocals, or contacts
  5. Optimize the environment of the inoperable patient with increased light sources, decreased glare; reorganize living space to prevent accidents/falls
  6. Prevention with protective eyewear to filter ultraviolet B exposure

◘ IMPAIRED VISION

- Definition—decreased/blurred visual acuity

- Etiology/Incidence
  1. Associated with lens opacity, damage to photoreceptor cells, damage to optic nerve, visual cortex or refractory error
  2. Legal blindness—20/200 or less in best eye with correction
  3. Presbyopia—loss of accommodative capacity of lens with age; inability to focus on objects at normal reading distance

- Signs and Symptoms
  1. Decreased vision
     a. Sudden or gradual
     b. Unilateral or bilateral
  2. Pain
  3. Floaters
  4. Peripheral vision loss
  5. Association with systemic symptoms

- Differential Diagnosis
  1. Refractive error
  2. Cataract
  3. Macular degeneration
  4. Glaucoma
  5. Retinal vascular occlusion/detachment
  6. Temporal arteritis
  7. Optic neuritis—often first sign of multiple sclerosis
  8. Cerebrovascular accident (CVA) or tumor

- Physical Findings—vary according to etiology
  1. Decreased visual acuity
  2. Unilateral visual loss, often seen in retinal detachment, temporal arteritis, or optic neuritis
  3. Conjunctiva—clear or injected (glaucoma)
  4. Cornea—clear or cloudy (cataracts)
  5. Visual field deficit—associated with glaucoma, cerebrovascular disease, or tumor
  6. Pupils—small, irregular size, with poor response to light; common in iritis or glaucoma
  7. Extraocular movements—nystagmus associated with neurological disease
  8. Funduscopic examination may reveal
     a. Absent red reflex (cataracts)
     b. Hemorrhages, exudates (diabetes)
     c. Optic disc swelling/cupping (glaucoma, papilledema)

- Diagnostic Tests
  1. Tonometry
  2. Slit lamp

- Management/Treatment—based upon cause of visual loss
  1. Refer to ophthalmologist
     a. Sudden loss of vision—requires emergency consultation
     b. Abnormal physical examination findings
     c. Complaints of flashing lights
     d. Visual loss associated with systemic disease
     e. Diabetics

2. Prevention
   a. Visual disorders in the elderly often lead to trauma from falls and motor vehicle accidents
   b. U.S. Preventive Services Task Force recommends screening for glaucoma after age 65; no consensus on routine visual acuity screening—generally recommended at each health maintenance examination

◘ ACUTE OTITIS MEDIA (AOM)

- Definition—inflammation of middle ear

- Etiology/Incidence
  1. Eustachian tube dysfunction (ETD) or obstruction secondary to viral nasal pharyngitis—major pathogenic factors causing ineffective drainage of middle ear
  2. Bacterial pathogens
     a. *Streptococcus pneumoniae* (most common)
     b. *Haemophilus influenzae*
     c. *Moraxella catarrhalis*
     d. Occasional *Staphylococcus aureus*
  3. More frequent in young children (under age 7) than adults
  4. Risk factors include
     a. Recent URI
     b. Congenital disorders—cleft palate, Down syndrome
     c. Active or passive smoking
     d. Native American/Eskimo heritage

- Signs and Symptoms
  1. Otalgia
  2. Fever
  3. Hearing loss (conductive)
  4. Otorrhea (if perforated eardrum)
  5. Intense pain, followed by popping sound; acute relief indicative of perforated tympanic membrane (TM)
  6. Vertigo

- Differential Diagnosis
  1. Otitis externa
  2. Referred pain from jaw/teeth
  3. Dental abscess
  4. Mastoiditis
  5. Ear canal furuncle

- Physical Findings
  1. Bulging tympanic membrane uncommon; suggests imminent rupture
  2. Distorted light reflex/obscured landmarks
  3. Pneumatic otoscopy may show decreased TM mobility
  4. Erythema

5. Bullae may form on TM—associated with *Mycoplasma pneumoniae* organism
6. Postauricular or cervical adenopathy

- Diagnostic Tests/Findings
  1. Usually no tests ordered
  2. Needle aspiration of middle ear fluid for culture—only in immunosuppressed patients and severe mastoiditis
  3. Tympanometry—indicator of fluid posterior to TM
  4. CBC with differential—if patient appears toxic; elevated WBC count

- Management/Treatment
  1. Antibiotics
     a. Amoxicillin 500 mg orally t.i.d. for 10 days; alternative is amoxicillin 875 mg b.i.d. for 10 days
        (1) Advantage—inexpensive
        (2) Disadvantage—ineffective against beta-lactamase-producing pathogens
        (3) Contraindicated in those with penicillin allergy
     b. For recurrent otitis media with resistant pathogens or characterized by fever > 102° F and/or otalgia
        (1) Amoxicillin clavulanate
        (2) Cephalosporins—cefixime, cefaclor
        (3) Macrolides—azithromycin or clarithromycin if beta lactam allergy
  2. If perforation is present, combined therapy of oral antibiotic and topical Cortisporin Otic Solution—4 drops in each ear t.i.d. or q.i.d. for 10 days
  3. Pain management
     a. Acetaminophen
     b. Topical local anesthetic otic solution—pain reliever
        (1) A/B Otic 2 gtts t.i.d. for 4 days
        (2) Auralgan 2 gtts t.i.d. for 4 days
  4. Refer/consult with MD or otolaryngologist
     a. No response to treatment after 48–72 hours
     b. Persistent hearing loss after adequate treatment
     c. Complications
        (1) Mastoiditis
        (2) Facial nerve palsy
        (3) Chronic perforation
        (4) Recurrent infections
     d. Surgical procedures—myringotomy, tympanostomy tubes for recurrent infection

◘ SEROUS OTITIS MEDIA (SOM)

- Definition—effusion in middle ear—also known as chronic otitis media with effusion (OME)

- Etiology/Incidence
  1. Patency of eustachian tube is impaired; prevents equalization of pressure
  2. Associated with
     a. Subacute infection
     b. Allergic manifestations
     c. Barotrauma
     d. Deviated septum
     e. Hypertrophic adenoids
     f. Benign or malignant neoplasms
  3. More common in children than adults

- Signs and Symptoms
  1. Hearing loss
  2. Popping sensation with yawning/swallowing
  3. Fullness in ear
  4. Occasional dizziness
  5. Often asymptomatic

- Differential Diagnosis
  1. Acute otitis media
  2. Conductive hearing loss
  3. Meniere's disease

- Physical Findings
  1. Tympanic membrane—retracted
  2. Air fluid level present, often with yellow/blue tinged fluid posterior to TM or bubbles of air may be seen through tympanic membrane
  3. Decreased membrane mobility with insufflation
  4. Conductive hearing loss
     a. Weber test—lateralize to affected side
     b. Rinne test—bone conduction may be greater than air conduction, BC > AC

- Diagnostic Tests/Findings
  1. Audiometry—decreased hearing
  2. Tympanometry—shows middle ear effusion

- Management/Treatment
  1. If mild symptoms, may spontaneously resolve in 2–3 weeks
  2. Topical decongestants—phenylephrine 1–2 sprays to each nostril every 8–12 hours for 3 days only
  3. Oral decongestants may be helpful
  4. Antihistamines usually are ineffective
  5. Patient education on Valsalva maneuver or chewing gum—to relieve eustachian tube blockage
  6. Follow up in 4–6 weeks
  7. Refer if persistent hearing loss

◘ OTITIS EXTERNA

- Definition—inflammation of external auditory canal; commonly known as "swimmer's ear"

- Etiology/Incidence
  1. Infectious agents include
     a. *Pseudomonas aeruginosa* (most common)
     b. *Staphylococcus aureus* or streptococcus
     c. *Proteus mirabilis*
     d. Fungi
  2. Inflammation develops from
     a. Frequent exposure to water (most common)
     b. Mechanical trauma from bobby pins, cotton applicators, ear plugs, hearing aids
     c. Eczema, skin disorders
  3. Common in summer months, especially in hot, humid climates
  4. More common in swimmers than nonswimmers

- Signs and Symptoms
  1. Otalgia—gradual or acute onset
  2. Pruritus
  3. Purulent discharge
  4. Occasional hearing loss, "plugged ear"

- Differential Diagnosis
  1. Furuncle
  2. Otitis media
  3. Mastoiditis
  4. Foreign body
  5. Eczema
  6. Cellulitis

- Physical Findings
  1. Erythema and edema of ear canal
  2. Pain on manipulation of auricle or pressure on tragus
  3. Purulent or white "cheesy" exudate may be present
  4. Preauricular adenopathy
  5. Edema may impair visualization of tympanic membrane; TM usually not affected

- Diagnostic Tests/Findings—culture of discharge if no response to treatment or recurrent infection

- Management/Treatment
  1. Pharmacologic
     a. Combined antibiotic, hydrocortisone, and propylene glycol will effectively treat infection and reduce inflammation—Cortisporin Otic Solution 4–5 gtts in ear(s) t.i.d. or q.i.d. for 7 days
     b. If unable to determine if TM is perforated or intact—ofloxacin 0.3% solution, instill 5–10 drops b.i.d. for 7–10 days
     c. Antifungal and antibacterial—acetic acid otic drops
     d. Saturated cotton wick with medication facilitates entry of medication in ear canal; moisten with antibiotic as directed

e. Severe cases often require systemic antibiotics

f. Analgesics

2. General measures

a. Protect ear from additional moisture

b. Eliminate trauma to ear canal

c. Prevent recurrences—instill 2% acetic acid 2–3 drops in ear canals b.i.d. after contact with water (commercial OTC products also available)

d. Improvement in 48 hours after initiating treatment

e. Instruction on proper technique to clean ears

☐ HEARING LOSS

- Definition—diminished ability to detect pure tones in decibels of 30 or greater

- Etiology/Incidence
  1. 10% of U.S. population has hearing problems
  2. Particularly common among the elderly
  3. Hearing loss may result from interference in sound conduction (conduction loss) or impaired transmission through nervous system (sensorineural) or both (mixed hearing loss)
  4. Conductive loss—decreased ability of external and middle ear to conduct sound waves to inner ear due to
     a. Cerumen impaction
     b. Foreign body
     c. Otitis media
     d. Otosclerosis—hereditary, bony ankylosis of stapes
     e. Scarring or perforation of TM
     f. Congenital problems
     g. Cholesteatoma
  5. Sensorineural loss—results from changes to cochlea and/or involvement of the acoustic nerve; causes include
     a. Acoustic neuroma
     b. Meniere's disease
     c. Presbycusis—hearing loss associated with aging
     d. Excessive noise exposure
     e. Viral syndrome—rubella, mumps
     f. Drugs—acetylsalicylic acid (ASA), gentamicin, furosemide, erythromycin
     g. Syphilis
     h. Multiple sclerosis

- Signs and Symptoms
  1. Conductive hearing loss—decreased ability to detect low tones and vowels; often history of ear disease, patient speaks softly
  2. Sensorineural—impaired high tone perception, poor speech discrimination, difficulty with background noise, and high-pitched female voice; patient speaks loudly
  3. Presbycusis—hearing loss is bilateral; gradual in onset; loss of high frequencies first, then lower frequency sounds; tinnitus is common

- Differential Diagnosis—see etiology/incidence

- Physical Findings
  1. Otoscopic examination of ear—usually normal
  2. Gross hearing/whisper test—diminished (acoustic nerve)
  3. Rinne test—compares air to bone conduction
     a. Normal—AC > BC
     b. Conductive loss—decreased AC:BC ratio, BC may be > AC in affected ear(s)
     c. Sensorineural loss—AC > BC (remains normal)
  4. Weber test
     a. Normal—sound midline
     b. Conductive loss—lateralize to affected ear
     c. Sensorineural loss—lateralize to normal ear
  5. Red flags for immediate referral
     a. Cholesteatoma in conductive loss
     b. Acoustic neuroma in sensorineural loss

- Diagnostic Tests/Findings
  1. Pure tone audiometry by audiologist
     a. Intensity is measured in decibels (dB), frequency is measured in hertz
     b. Threshold of normal hearing 0–20 dB
        (1) Mild loss—20–40 dB (soft-spoken voice)
        (2) Moderate loss—40–60 dB (normal-spoken voice)
        (3) Severe loss—60–80 dB (loud-spoken voice)
  2. Speech discrimination testing
     a. Detects clarity of hearing—impaired in sensorineural loss
     b. Results recorded as percentage correct
     c. 90–100% is normal
  3. CT scan or MRI—to detect tumors

- Management/Treatment—dependent on etiology
  1. Refer for formal audiogram
  2. Refer to otolaryngologist—particularly for sensorineural loss and conductive loss unresponsive to treatment
  3. Prevention
     a. Avoid loud music, machines (causes loss of high tones)
     b. Monitor ototoxic drugs carefully; if tinnitus or hearing loss, discontinue use
     c. U.S. Preventive Services Task Force recommends routine screening after 65 years of age
  4. Hearing aids—hearing amplification beneficial to patients with correctable hearing loss

◧ VERTIGO

- Definition—abnormal sensation of movement (may be peripheral or central); disturbances of peripheral/central vestibular system, which maintains spatial orientation/posture and is symptomatic of an underlying etiology

- Etiology/Incidence
  1. Peripheral vertigo (causes external to the brain stem and cerebellum)
     a. Meniere's disease
     b. Recurrent vestibulopathy
     c. Labyrinthitis
     d. Positional vertigo
     e. Traumatic vertigo
     f. Perilymphatic vertigo
     g. Medications—especially aspirin and alcohol
     h. Infections—middle/inner ear, viral illness
     i. Otoliths
  2. Central vertigo
     a. Neoplasm
     b. Vascular disease
     c. CNS disease—multiple sclerosis, syphilis
     d. Cranial nerve VIII abnormality
  3. Incidence
     a. 50% of vertigo is benign positional
     b. 25% of vertigo is vestibular neuronitis
     c. 10% of vertigo is Meniere's disease

- Signs and Symptoms
  1. "Room spinning" or "head spinning"/weaving sensation
  2. Nausea, vomiting, diaphoresis
  3. Imbalance
  4. Tinnitus
  5. Hearing loss
  6. Vague lightheadedness

- Differential Diagnosis
  1. Ataxia
  2. Syncope or near syncope

- Physical Findings
  1. Nystagmus with testing of extraocular movements
  2. Hearing loss
  3. Changes in blood pressure—associated with positional hypotension
  4. Carotid bruits—suggests impaired cerebral flow
  5. Cranial nerves—especially auditory changes, 5, 7, 8
  6. Romberg test—often abnormal
  7. Barany maneuver—stimulates vestibular system, reproduces vertigo

8. Additional findings consistent with specific cause
   a. Peripheral vertigo typically associated with
      (1) Hearing loss
      (2) Ear pain
      (3) Tinnitus
   b. Central vertigo typically associated with
      (1) Visual or sensory loss
      (2) Diplopia
      (3) Abnormalities in coordination

- Diagnostic Tests/Findings
  1. Audiogram if hearing impaired
  2. CT scan/MRI—to rule out tumor/neurological dysfunction
  3. VDRL and FTA—reactive in syphilis
  4. TSH, CBC with differential and glucose—to rule out infections and systemic disease
  5. Serum B_{12} to rule out pernicious anemia

- Management/Treatment
  1. Immediate referral, if abnormal neurological signs
  2. Bed rest for acute episodes, e.g., viral labyrinthitis
  3. Epley maneuvers for suspected otoliths
  4. Antivertigo medications most helpful in central disease
     a. Meclizine—12.5–25 mg orally t.i.d.; causes dry mouth and sedation
     b. Dramamine 50 mg orally t.i.d.
     c. Scopolamine transdermal patch
  5. Antiemetic for nausea/vomiting—promethazine 25 mg q.i.d.; or prochlorperazine 5–10 mg q.i.d.
  6. Do not perform tests for positional vertigo on geriatric patients
  7. Refer if vertigo persists

◧ EPISTAXIS

- Definition—bleeding from nostril, nasal cavity, or nasopharynx

- Etiology/Incidence
  1. Anterior nosebleed most common, occurring in the vascular plexus of septum (Kiesselbach plexus)
  2. Disruption of nasal mucosa due to
     a. Trauma
     b. Infection
     c. Allergies
     d. Dry environment
     e. Medications
     f. Cocaine use
     g. Neoplasm

    h. Occasionally systemic disease (hypertension, blood dyscrasia)
    i. Coagulopathy or anticoagulant therapy
  3. 10% of population will experience one significant nosebleed

- Signs and Symptoms
  1. Anterior epistaxis
    a. Unilateral bleeding from nostril
    b. Recurrent episodes last few minutes to ½ hour
    c. Venous source of blood
  2. Posterior epistaxis—occurs more in the elderly, often difficult to correct
    a. Intermittent brisk bleeding
    b. Arterial source
    c. Blood flows into pharynx, may cause nausea and coffee ground emesis

- Differential Diagnosis—epistaxis is a sign/symptom, not a disease; assess for significant pathology
  1. Coagulation disorders
  2. Nasal malignancy
  3. Hereditary telangiectasia
  4. Malignant hypertension

- Physical Findings
  1. Visual site—usually bleeding from one nostril; bilateral bleeding suggests trauma
  2. Skin, mucous membranes, and conjunctivae with evidence of the following suggests a pathological condition
    a. Rash
    b. Pallor
    c. Purpura
    d. Petechiae
    e. Telangiectasis

- Diagnostic Tests/Findings—dependent on suspected etiology
  1. Hemoglobin and hematocrit are decreased if severe blood loss
  2. Low platelet count and abnormal prothrombin time/partial thromboplastin time (PT/PTT) suggests a bleeding disorder

- Management/Treatment
  1. Position patient sitting up and leaning forward
  2. Apply continuous pinching pressure to anterior nasal septum for 10–15 minutes
  3. If inadequate blood clotting, place a small cotton pledget of 1:1000 epinephrine or vasoconstrictor nasal drops (phenylephrine) into vestibule of nose; apply pressure for 5–10 minutes; this will stop most anterior venous bleeds
  4. Application of ice may assist with clot formation

  5. Refer to emergency room or otolaryngologist if bleeding persistent/continuous or if posterior bleed is suspected
  6. General measures/prevention
    a. Warn against habitual nose picking, rubbing nose, forceful blowing
    b. Advise increased humidity, especially in winter months
    c. Use petrolatum-based ointment in nostril—promotes hydration
    d. Instruct patient on how to manage simple nosebleeds
  7. Recurrent episodes of epistaxis require additional investigation

◘ COMMON COLD

- Definition—minor, self-limiting viral nasopharyngitis

- Etiology/Incidence
  1. Caused by rhinoviruses or corona viruses
  2. Most common reason for "sick day"
  3. Incidence decreases with age
    a. Children average 6–8 colds per year
    b. Adults average 2–4 colds per year
  4. Transmission through hand-to-hand contact and airborne droplets

- Signs and Symptoms
  1. General malaise and fatigue
  2. Coryza
  3. Sore throat
  4. Low-grade fever
  5. Nasal congestion/stuffiness
  6. Watery eyes
  7. Headache
  8. Nonproductive cough
  9. Symptoms typically of short duration—3–7 days on average
  10. Symptom progression predictable—migrate from one region to the next, e.g., nose to throat to cough

- Differential Diagnosis
  1. Influenza
  2. Atypical pneumonia
  3. Otitis media
  4. Sinusitis
  5. Rhinitis
  6. Allergies

- Physical Findings
  1. Mildly elevated temperature
  2. Conjunctivae clear, possible erythema
  3. Injected nasal and pharyngeal mucosa
  4. Lungs clear
  5. Clear rhinorrhea may progress to cloudy/purulent

- Diagnostic Tests/Findings—none indicated; throat culture if streptococcal pharyngitis suspected

- Management/Treatment—palliative
  1. Rest, maintain fluid hydration
  2. Acetaminophen or ibuprofen for fever and headache
  3. Topical decongestants for nasal congestion; use 3–4 days only to avoid "rebound congestion"
  4. Oral decongestants for congestion
  5. First generation antihistamines/decongestant combination for cough
  6. OTC decongestants are used cautiously in diabetes, hypertension, and glaucoma patients
  7. Zinc, echinacea, Vitamin C—may reduce days of illness; begin within first day of symptoms for best results
  8. Zinc contraindicated in pregnancy
  9. Frequent hand washing to prevent viral spread
  10. Symptoms lasting longer than 2 weeks may indicate secondary bacterial infection

◘ INFLUENZA

- Definition—acute, contagious, febrile respiratory, viral infection

- Etiology/Incidence
  1. Influenza viral type A, B, C
  2. Type A influenza is most virulent, causing increased mortality
  3. Incubation 1–5 days
  4. Infections usually occur during epidemics in winter months
  5. Transmitted by airborne droplets

- Signs and Symptoms
  1. High fever, chills (sudden onset)
  2. Headache
  3. Myalgia (often severe)
  4. Malaise
  5. Sore throat
  6. Nonproductive cough
  7. Nausea and vomiting less common but may occur
  8. Coryza

- Differential Diagnosis
  1. Upper respiratory infection (URI)
  2. Bronchitis
  3. Pertussis
  4. Pneumonia
  5. Infectious mononucleosis
  6. Early HIV infection
  7. Illness associated with biological warfare such as inhalation anthrax, smallpox, tularemia, plague

- Physical Findings
  1. Elevated temperature, rapid pulse
  2. Skin flushed
  3. Watery eyes
  4. Clear nasal discharge
  5. Occasional tender cervical lymph nodes
  6. Pharyngeal erythema
  7. Lungs—clear (occasional wheezes or rales)

- Diagnostic Tests/Findings
  1. Usually none
  2. Complete blood count (CBC) or white blood count (WBC)—mild leukopenia
  3. Chest radiography—normal
  4. Culture of nasopharyngeal secretions

- Management/Treatment
  1. Supportive measures
     a. Increase fluid intake
     b. Humidified air
     c. Salt water gargles
     d. Analgesics and rest (for fever and myalgia)
  2. Antiviral medications
     a. Zanamivir 2 inhalations every 12 hours for 5 days
        (1) Effective against influenza type A and B
        (2) Administer within 48 hours of onset of symptoms
        (3) Contraindicated in patients with asthma, chronic obstructive pulmonary disease (COPD)
     b. Oseltamivir 75 mg orally b.i.d. for 5 days
        (1) Effective against uncomplicated cases of influenza type A and B
        (2) For patients 18 years of age and older
        (3) Administer within 48 hours of onset of symptoms
  3. Monitor for complications—especially in the elderly
     a. Bacterial pneumonia
     b. Otitis media
     c. Reye's syndrome
     d. Myocarditis (rare)
     e. Bronchitis
  4. Prevention
     a. Trivalent inactivated influenza vaccination (TIV) 0.5 cc IM deltoid
        (1) Administer every fall, prior to winter months
        (2) CDC recommends administration to everyone > 6 months old
        (3) Priority populations
           (a) Over age 65
           (b) Nursing home patients
           (c) Patients with chronic cardiac/respiratory disorders

(d) Immunocompromised patients (i.e., asplenic persons, HIV infection)

(e) Persons living in institutional settings

(f) Pregnant females in second and third trimesters

(g) Healthcare providers

(4) Contraindicated in persons with severe allergy to eggs

(5) Administer concomitantly with pneumococcal vaccine in high-risk patients

b. Live attenuated influenza vaccine (LAIV)

(1) Administer—½ dose in each nostril (intranasal route)

(2) Approved for healthy persons, age 5–49 years

(3) Contraindications—severe egg allergy, chronic medical and respiratory conditions (asthma, COPD), and immunosuppression

(4) Expensive compared to TIV

◻ PHARYNGITIS

- Definition—inflammation of pharynx, tonsils, or both (sore throat)

- Etiology/Incidence
  1. Viral pharyngitis (most common)
     a. Respiratory viruses—adenovirus
     b. Rhinovirus
     c. Herpangina—due to Coxsackie virus
     d. Epstein-Barr virus (EBV), cytomegalovirus (CMV)—causes infectious mononucleosis
  2. Bacterial pharyngitis
     a. Group A and B beta hemolytic streptococcus
     b. *Neisseria gonorrhoeae*
     c. *Corynebacterium diphtheriae*
     d. *Haemophilus influenzae*
     e. *Neisseria meningitidis*
  3. Other sources
     a. *Chlamydia trachomatis*
     b. *Mycoplasma pneumoniae*
     c. *Candida albicans*
     d. Trauma/irritating substance
     e. Mouth breathing/allergies
  4. Accounts for 10% of all office visits in primary care
  5. Occurs in all age groups

- Signs and Symptoms
  1. Sore throat
  2. Enlarged tonsils
  3. Dysphagia
  4. Fever
  5. Malaise

- Differential Diagnosis (see etiology/incidence section for pathogens)
  1. Peritonsillar abscess
  2. Pharyngeal abscess
  3. Epiglottitis
  4. Stomatitis
  5. Meningitis
  6. Thyroiditis

- Physical Findings
  1. Elevated temperature
  2. Viral presentation (respiratory)
     a. Tonsillar enlargement with or without exudate
     b. Injected "cobblestone" appearance post-pharynx
     c. Rhinorrhea
  3. Bacterial—group A beta hemolytic *streptococcus* (GAS)
     a. Erythema
     b. Often exudative tonsils
     c. Enlarged tender anterior cervical lymph nodes
     d. Occasionally petechiae
     e. Scarlatina rash
  4. *Corynebacterium diphtheriae* (infrequent in immunized patients)
     a. Gray adherent membrane on tonsils and pharynx
     b. Bleeding when membrane removed

- Diagnostic Tests/Findings
  1. Viral (respiratory) pharyngitis—by clinical diagnosis *only*
  2. Throat culture—if suspect
     a. Group A beta hemolytic *streptococcus*
     b. *Neisseria gonorrhoeae* (request separately)
  3. Rapid Strep Antigen Test—positive result, detects only GAS (5–10% false negatives)
  4. CBC with differential—WBC count elevated in bacterial infection
  5. Heterophil/monospot—negative

- Management/Treatment
  1. General measures
     a. Increase fluids
     b. Gargle with warm salt water
     c. Lozenges
     d. Acetaminophen or ibuprofen for pain relief
  2. Strep throat (GAS)
     a. Penicillin V 500 mg b.i.d. or t.i.d. for 10 days
     b. Benzathine penicillin 1.2 million units IM one time only
        (1) Advantage—full treatment completed
        (2) Disadvantage—five- to tenfold increase in anaphylactic reaction

    c. Alternative for penicillin allergy—erythromycin 250 mg orally q.i.d. for 10 days

    d. Post-treatment cultures—for recurrent strep infection or rheumatic fever

    e. Complications—if no or inadequate antibiotic treatment

       (1) Scarlet fever

       (2) Peritonsillar abscess (immediate referral)

       (3) Suppurative adenitis

       (4) Rheumatic fever

       (5) Acute glomerulonephritis

    f. Tonsillectomy—for recurrent severe infections

  3. Gonococcal pharyngitis

    a. Ceftriaxone 125 mg IM single dose *or* cefixime 400 mg orally single dose *or* ofloxacin 400 mg orally single dose

    b. Co-treat for chlamydia—doxycycline 100 mg orally b.i.d. for 7 days *or* erythromycin 500 mg orally q.i.d. for 7 days *or* azithromycin 1 g orally single dose

  4. Diphtheria (refer)

    a. Equine antitoxin—to prevent myocarditis

    b. Penicillin or erythromycin

◻ INFECTIOUS MONONUCLEOSIS

- Definition—acute viral syndrome associated with fever, pharyngitis, and adenopathy; often known as "kissing" disease

- Etiology/Incidence
  1. Epstein-Barr virus—herpes-type virus causes 90% of cases
  2. Cytomegalovirus—rare
  3. Transmission via saliva
  4. Usually occurs in adolescents and young adults (ages 10–35 years) in middle- and upper-socioeconomic populations
  5. Prolonged period of communicability—approximately 2–6 months after infection

- Signs and Symptoms—variable, but typically include
  1. Fever
  2. Fatigue/malaise
  3. Nausea/anorexia
  4. Swollen lymph nodes
  5. Sore throat

- Differential Diagnosis
  1. Streptococcal pharyngitis
  2. CMV
  3. Toxoplasmosis
  4. Hepatitis A or B
  5. Lymphoma/leukemia
  6. HIV infection

- Physical Findings
  1. Marked erythema and edema of pharynx
  2. Tonsillar enlargement with exudate, occasionally palatal petechiae
  3. Enlarged lymph nodes—especially posterior cervical nodes
  4. Splenic enlargement—50% of cases
  5. Hepatomegaly
  6. Occasionally periorbital edema
  7. Maculopapular rash

- Diagnostic Tests/Findings
  1. Complete blood count with differential
     a. WBC—leukocytosis (range of 10,000–20,000/mm^3)
     b. Increased lymphocytes (greater than 50% of leukocyte count)
     c. Atypical lymphocytes—common characteristic
     d. Thrombocytopenia (range 100,000–140,000/mm^3) 2–4 weeks after onset of illness
  2. Positive monospot or elevations in heterophil titer—1:224 or greater is diagnostic
  3. Liver function tests—elevations in aspartate aminotransferase (AST), alanine aminotransferase (ALT), bilirubin, and lactic dehydrogenase (LDH)
  4. Throat culture—frequently secondary infection with streptococcus (GAS)
  5. CT scan imaging—may reveal splenomegaly and/or hepatomegaly
  6. EBV—antibody titers
     a. IgG—past infections
     b. IgM—recent infections

- Management/Treatment
  1. Supportive/palliative measures
  2. Rest during acute phase of illness
  3. Avoidance of contact sports for at least 1 month with splenomegaly; CT scan to determine resolution of splenomegaly
  4. Avoid alcohol (ETOH) with elevated liver enzymes/hepatomegaly
  5. Corticosteroids often prescribed for significant pharyngeal edema and obstructive tonsillar enlargement
  6. Analgesics for pain relief
  7. Antiviral medications not effective
  8. Ampicillin/amoxicillin should be avoided, as patients frequently develop a maculopapular rash
  9. Existence of chronic EBV infection (chronic fatigue syndrome) is very controversial

◘ ALLERGIC RHINITIS

- Definition—a noninfectious symptom complex that includes perennial or seasonal manifestations

- Etiology/Incidence
  1. Seasonal allergies—symptoms at same time each year, related to pollens
     a. Trees (April to July)
     b. Grasses (May to July)
     c. Ragweed (August to October)
  2. Perennial allergies—year-round symptoms related to molds, animal dander, feathers, dust mites, cockroaches
  3. Most common allergens—pollens, molds, dust mites, animal dander
  4. 8–12% of U.S. population affected; onset usually before age 30

- Signs and Symptoms
  1. Nasal congestion
  2. Sneezing
  3. Clear, watery nasal discharge
  4. Itchy nose, throat, eyes
  5. Cough from postnasal drip
  6. Mouth breather/snoring
  7. Loss/alteration of smell

- Differential Diagnosis
  1. Vasomotor rhinitis
  2. Foreign body
  3. Nasal polyps/tumor
  4. Sinusitis
  5. Medications—especially overuse of topical decongestants ("rebound"); oral contraceptives
  6. Deviated septum
  7. Hypothyroidism and pregnancy cause nasal congestion

- Physical Findings
  1. Pale, boggy nasal mucosa
  2. Enlarged turbinates
  3. Injected conjunctiva, tearing
  4. "Allergic shiner" under eyes
  5. No sinus tenderness

- Diagnostic Tests/Findings
  1. Nasal smear for eosinophils—elevated
  2. Serum IgE—elevated in 30–40% of patients
  3. Allergy testing—identify specific allergens
  4. CBC if infection suspected

- Management/Treatment
  1. Preventive measures
     a. Allergen avoidance
     b. Air conditioning/air filters
     c. Environmental control—vacuum, dust, remove carpeting, feather pillows, stuffed animals
     d. Minimize contact with animals
  2. Pharmacological
     a. Antihistamines—mainstay of treatment for acute symptom relief
        (1) Both sedating and nonsedating available OTC
        (2) Nonsedating antihistamines in prescriptive doses
            (a) Fexofenadine 60 mg orally b.i.d.
            (b) Desloratadine 5 mg orally q.d.
            (c) Cetirizine 5–10 mg orally q.d.
            (d) Also available in ophthalmic and otic forms
     b. Decongestants (oral or topical)—vasoconstriction; decrease mucosal edema
     c. Topical corticosteroids—mainstay of chronic control
        (1) Beclomethasone dipropionate—2 sprays each nostril b.i.d.
        (2) Flunisolide—2 sprays each nostril b.i.d.
        (3) Steroid sprays (slow onset) up to 2 weeks before significant results appear
     d. Cromolyn sodium—1 spray each nostril up to 6 times per day
     e. Leukotriene modifiers
     f. Omalizumab for serious refractory cases; required documented treatment failure to typical therapies, eosinophilia, and elevated IgE—prescribed by allergist
     g. Immunotherapy desensitization for management failures; patients receiving desensitization must know signs/symptoms of anaphylaxis

◘ SINUSITIS

- Definition—inflammation of one or more paranasal sinuses

- Etiology/Incidence
  1. Bacterial infections
     a. *Streptococcus pneumoniae*
     b. *Haemophilus influenzae*
     c. *Moraxella catarrhalis*
  2. Preceding sinus inflammation often a factor
     a. Viruses—majority of cases are either viral in origin or postviral URI inflammation
     b. Allergies
  3. Anatomical predisposition to bacterial collection—deviated septum
  4. Classified as acute or chronic based upon duration of infection

5. Maxillary sinuses most common site of infection, followed by ethmoid, sphenoid, and lastly frontal involvement

- Signs and Symptoms
  1. Nasal congestion and pressure
  2. Mucopurulent nasal discharge/postnasal drip
  3. Cough more prevalent in the A.M. due to increased posterior sinus drainage when supine
  4. Malaise and fever
  5. Headache
  6. Pain—dull to throbbing
     a. Over cheeks, worse with bending (maxillary sinus)
     b. Above and behind eye—ethmoid sinus
     c. Above eyebrows—frontal sinus
  7. Periorbital edema

- Differential Diagnosis
  1. Rhinitis—viral or allergic
  2. Dental abscess
  3. Nasal polyp/tumor
  4. URI
  5. Migraine/cluster headache

- Physical Findings
  1. Mild to moderate elevated temperature
  2. May have purulent discharge in nasal cavity
  3. Percussion/palpation over frontal and maxillary sinuses—may exacerbate pain/tenderness
  4. Transillumination of sinuses—may show impaired light transmission
  5. Percussion of maxillary teeth—may reveal dental root infection

- Diagnostic Tests/Findings
  1. None for typical presentation
  2. Maxilofacial CT scan when diagnosis is in question or patient unresponsive to treatment—will demonstrate opacity, air fluid levels, thick mucosa
  3. Nasal culture—sinus fluid to determine actual organisms
  4. CBC with differential, if patient appears toxic—elevated WBC

- Management/Treatment
  1. Antibiotics
     a. Amoxicillin—500 mg orally t.i.d. for 10–14 days
     b. Amoxicillin/clavulanate 500–875 mg b.i.d. for 10 days
     c. Several cephalosporin options for 14 days
     d. Alternative for PCN allergy
        (1) Macrolides—clarithromycin
        (2) Trimethoprim/sulfamethoxazole—1 double strength tablet b.i.d. for 14 days (PCN alternative)

        e. Respiratory fluoroquinolones for moderate/severe cases or those unresponsive to above therapies
  2. General measures
     a. Increase fluids
     b. Steam inhalation
     c. Avoid smoking
     d. Analgesics for pain relief
     e. Nasal decongestant—improves sinus drainage
  3. Topical steroids—reduce mucosal inflammation
  4. Refer to ENT if no improvement after 72 hours of appropriate treatment and maxilofacial CT scan supports diagnosis
  5. Instruct patient to report symptoms of complications
     a. Stiff neck (meningitis)
     b. Periorbital edema (orbital cellulitis)
     c. Severe dental pain (abscess)

◘ QUESTIONS

Select the best answer.

1. The common cold is caused by:

   a. *Haemophilus influenzae*
   b. Rhinoviruses
   c. *Streptococcus*
   d. Herpes virus

2. Nasal congestion is a characteristic of upper respiratory infection (URI). It is best treated with:

   a. Antihistamines
   b. Nasal corticosteroids
   c. Topical decongestants
   d. Antibiotics

3. Prevention of influenza epidemics is best achieved by administration of annual "flu" vaccine. Contraindications to administering the vaccine include:

   a. Immunosuppressed patients
   b. Severe allergy to eggs
   c. Chronic respiratory disease
   d. Allergy to aspirin products

4. Zanamivir and osteltamivir are used in the treatment of influenza. Which of the following statements is true about these drugs?

   a. They are preferred to influenza vaccination in persons with penicillin allergy
   b. Both agents are effective against types A and B influenza
   c. Both agents are contraindicated in COPD
   d. They are contraindicated under the age of 5 and over the age of 49

5. Group A beta hemolytic strep (GAS) is a common pathogen in bacterial pharyngitis. It is also an infectious agent in which of the following medical conditions?

   a. Acute pyelonephritis
   b. Rheumatic fever
   c. Viral meningitis
   d. Acute mononucleosis

6. What is the most common physical finding associated with strep pharyngitis?

   a. Unilateral tonsillar edema
   b. Exudative tonsils
   c. Ulcerations on buccal mucosa
   d. Injected uvula

7. Infectious mononucleosis is caused by:

   a. Coxsackie virus
   b. Herpes simplex
   c. Viral hepatitis A
   d. Epstein-Barr virus

8. Earl Thomas, an 18-year-old college student, presents with fever of 101°F, sore throat, dysphagia, and fatigue. Physical exam reveals periorbital edema, exudative tonsils, enlarged tender posterior cervical nodes, and no hepatosplenomegaly. Your preliminary diagnosis is infectious mononucleosis. What diagnostic tests would you order to confirm your diagnosis?

   a. Throat culture
   b. Hetrophil antibody
   c. Electrolytes
   d. CMV titer

9. A 40-year-old male accountant presents with a 3-day history of left eye irritation. On physical examination, there is moderate conjunctival injection, watery discharge, palpable preauricular lymph nodes, and visual acuity, 20/20 both eyes. What is the most likely diagnosis?

   a. Acute glaucoma
   b. Bacterial conjunctivitis
   c. Blepharitis
   d. Viral conjunctivitis

10. In the history of a patient presenting with red eye, it is important to ask about:

    a. Photophobia
    b. Itchiness
    c. Cold symptoms
    d. Myopia

11. What are the two most important tests in assessment of a corneal abrasion?

    a. Pupillary reaction and extraocular movements
    b. Funduscopic exam and peripheral vision
    c. Visual acuity and fluorescein stain
    d. Cover/uncover test and accommodation

12. Miss Shell presents with sinus pain, pressure, and yellow nasal discharge. Your examination of this patient would include palpation and transillumination of the:

    a. Ethmoid and frontal sinuses
    b. Maxillary and sphenoid sinuses
    c. Frontal and maxillary sinuses
    d. Sphenoid and ethmoid sinuses

13. Which of the following conditions may predispose a patient to sinusitis?

    a. Tumor, gingivitis, deviated septum
    b. Nasal polyps, allergies, upper respiratory infection
    c. Temporomandibular joint syndrome, rhinitis, otitis
    d. Common cold, pharyngitis, meningitis

14. Ototoxic drugs are a potential cause of sensorineural hearing loss. Which of the following drugs may cause hearing loss?

    a. Gentamicin
    b. Penicillin
    c. Cephalexin
    d. Minocycline

15. A 60-year-old male suddenly develops headache, blurred vision, and severe eye pain upon entering a dark movie theater. What is the most likely diagnosis?

    a. Angle closure glaucoma
    b. Uveitis
    c. Giant cell arteritis
    d. Open angle glaucoma

16. Absent red reflex may indicate which of the following ophthalmologic conditions:

    a. Foreign body
    b. Cataracts
    c. Glaucoma
    d. Uveitis

17. Presbycusis—hearing impairment associated with aging is characterized by:

    a. Acoustic nerve damage
    b. Cerumen impaction
    c. High-frequency loss
    d. Conductive loss

18. Macular degeneration is manifested by:

    a. Loss of peripheral vision
    b. Irregular pupils
    c. Loss of central vision
    d. Excessive tearing

19. Which condition is most likely associated with conductive hearing loss?

    a. Syphilis
    b. Meniere's disease
    c. Acute otitis media
    d. Hypothyroidism

20. A physical characteristic that differentiates otitis externa from otitis media is:

    a. Hearing loss
    b. Pain with movement of pinna
    c. Excessive cerumen
    d. Enlarged submaxillary node

21. What is the most common pathogen of acute otitis media in adults?

    a. *Pseudomonas aeruginosa*
    b. *Streptococcus pneumoniae*
    c. *Mycoplasma pneumoniae*
    d. *Escherichia coli*

22. A 30-year-old housewife presents with long-standing nasal stuffiness, clear watery nasal discharge, and annoying sneezing. What is the most likely diagnosis?

    a. Chronic sinusitis
    b. Nasal polyps
    c. Common cold
    d. Allergic rhinitis

23. Microscopic examination of nasal secretions of a patient with allergic rhinitis may reveal:

    a. Lymphocytes
    b. Neutrophils
    c. Eosinophils
    d. Basophils

24. What is the primary treatment for allergic rhinitis?

    a. Allergy avoidance and antihistamines
    b. Systemic steroids and decongestants
    c. Topical nasal sprays and antibiotics
    d. Humidified air and cough suppressants

25. What is the most common cause of vertigo?

    a. Malignant neoplasm
    b. Otoliths
    c. Vascular disease of the cerebellum
    d. Benign positional vertigo

26. Topical steroids are contraindicated in patients with corneal abrasions because:

    a. They inhibit tearing
    b. They increase risk of bacterial infection
    c. They increase intraocular pressure
    d. They may lead to iritis

27. Which of the following in not a cause of epistaxis?

    a. Hypertension
    b. Diabetes mellitus
    c. Neoplasms
    d. Trauma

28. A special diagnostic test/procedure for vertigo is:

    a. Tonometry
    b. Barany maneuver
    c. Pneumatic otoscopy
    d. EEG

29. Mr. Jones, a 32-year-old salesman, presents with a complaint of frequent nosebleeds for the last 2 months. He states they occur spontaneously 3 times a week and usually stop within 10 minutes. He denies any other acute or chronic medical problems. Which of the following diagnostic tests is indicated at this time?

    a. CBC
    b. Hemoglobin electrophoresis
    c. Prothrombin time
    d. Clotting time

30. Upon further evaluation of Mr. Jones, you find he has nasal congestion, postnasal drip, and scratchy throat. He uses an antihistamine at night for nasal symptoms and sleep. Your initial treatment plan for Mr. Jones should be:

    a. Add a decongestant to alleviate nasal congestion
    b. Increase humidity to moisten nasal mucosa
    c. Have patient elevate head of bed to promote sleep
    d. Discontinue antihistamine due to drying effect on nasal mucosa

31. Kyle Smith, a 21-year-old law student, presents with fatigue for 3–4 months, low-grade fever, and intermittent sore throat. You order a complete blood count. The result of the CBC is as follows: Hgb and Hct normal, elevated WBC, and atypical lymphocytes. What is the most likely diagnosis?

    a. Hepatitis A
    b. Infectious mononucleosis
    c. Herpangina
    d. Toxoplasmosis

32. Which of the following is not a common cause of vertigo?

    a. Otoliths
    b. Viral labyrinthitis
    c. Meniere's disease
    d. Transient ischemic attack

33. What is the antibiotic of choice in the treatment of gonococcal pharyngitis?

    a. Erythromycin
    b. Ampicillin
    c. Ceftriaxone
    d. Amantadine

34. Hearing loss caused by cerumen impaction is a:

    a. Conductive loss
    b. Sensorineural loss
    c. "Mixed" loss
    d. Congenital loss

35. Zeke Gilbert, a 72-year-old retired factory worker, has hearing loss in his right ear due to excessive noise exposure. When performing a Weber test, you would expect to find:

    a. Sound lateralizes equally to both ears
    b. Sound lateralizes to the left ear
    c. Sound lateralizes to the right ear
    d. Sound lateralizes to neither ear

36. What is the most sensitive test for diagnosing sinusitis?

    a. CBC
    b. Nasal culture
    c. CT scan
    d. Sinus radiography

37. What is the most common cause of otitis externa?

    a. Fungus
    b. *Staphylococcal epidermidis*
    c. Alpha streptococcus
    d. *Pseudomonas aeruginosa*

38. A physical finding that differentiates conjunctivitis from glaucoma is:

    a. Injected conjunctiva
    b. Excessive tearing
    c. Clear cornea
    d. Nystagmus

39. When prescribing topical corticosteroids for patients with allergic rhinitis, it is important to discuss that:

    a. Topical steroid use may predispose to infections
    b. It may take up to 2 weeks before they experience significant reduction in symptoms

    c. Steroids must be taken with antihistamines to be effective
    d. After 48 hours of use, patient will experience reduction in symptoms

40. It is important to highlight the short-term use of topical nasal decongestant because of this adverse effect:

    a. Rhinorrhea
    b. Confusion
    c. Somnolence
    d. Rebound congestion

ANSWERS

1. **b**		21. **b**	
2. **c**		22. **d**	
3. **b**		23. **c**	
4. **b**		24. **a**	
5. **b**		25. **d**	
6. **b**		26. **b**	
7. **d**		27. **b**	
8. **b**		28. **b**	
9. **d**		29. **a**	
10. **a**		30. **d**	
11. **c**		31. **b**	
12. **c**		32. **d**	
13. **b**		33. **c**	
14. **a**		34. **a**	
15. **a**		35. **b**	
16. **b**		36. **c**	
17. **c**		37. **d**	
18. **c**		38. **c**	
19. **c**		39. **b**	
20. **b**		40. **d**	

◘ BIBLIOGRAPHY

Andreoli, T. E., Carpenter, C. J., Griggs, R.C., & Ivor, B. (Eds.). (2007). *Cecil essentials of medicine* (7th ed.). Philadelphia: W. B. Saunders.

Barker, L. R., Fiebach, N.H., Kern, D. E., Thomas, P. A. & Ziegelstein, R. C. (Eds.). (2006). *Principles of ambulatory medicine* (7th ed.). Baltimore: Lippincott Williams & Wilkins.

Bickley, L. S., & Szilagyi, P. G. (Eds.). (2007). *Bates guide to physical examination and history taking* (9th ed.). Philadelphia: J. B. Lippincott.

Centers for Disease Control and Prevention National Immunization Program. (2008). *The pink book: Epidemiology and prevention of vaccine-preventable diseases* (10th ed.). Washington, DC: Author.

Distelhorst, J. S., & Highes G. M. (2003). Open-angle glaucoma. *American Family Physician, 67*(9), 1937–1944.

Johnson, T. D. (2008). *Control of communicable diseases manual* (19th ed.). Washington, DC: American Public Health Association.

Lustig, L. R., & Schindler, J. (2012). Ear, nose, and throat disorders. In S. J. McPhee, M. A. Papadakis, & M. W. Rabow. (Eds.), *Current medical diagnosis and treatment* (51st ed., pp. 196–237). New York: McGraw-Hill.

Riordan-Eva, P. (2009). Disorders of the eye and lids. In S. J. McPhee, M. A. Papadakis, & M. W. Rabow. (Eds.). *Current medical diagnosis and treatment* (51st ed., pp. 164–193). New York: McGraw-Hill.

Sinus and Allergy Health Partnership (2004). Antimicrobial treatment guidelines for acute bacterial rhinosinusitis. *Otolaryngology, Head & Neck Surgery, 130*, 1–45.

Uphold, C. R., & Graham, M. V. (2003). *Clinical guidelines in family practice* (4th ed.). Gainesville, FL: Barmarrae Books.

Weber, P. C. (2010). Evaluation of hearing loss in adults. *UpToDate*. Retrieved from http://www.uptodate.com/contents/evaluation-of-hearing-loss-in-adults

5

Respiratory Disorders

Margaret Hadro Venzke

◘ PULMONARY FUNCTION TESTS

Proper assessment of most patients with pulmonary disease requires the use of pulmonary function testing. Pulmonary function tests objectively measure the respiratory system's ability to perform gas exchange via assessment of ventilation, diffusion, and mechanical properties. Understanding these tests is important for correct interpretation of results and accurate patient diagnosis.

- Indications for Use of Pulmonary Function Tests (PFT)
  1. Evaluation of dyspnea, cough, pulmonary dysfunction
  2. Early detection of lung dysfunction
  3. Disability assessment, including evaluation of risk factors in work settings
  4. Evaluation of response to therapy
  5. Reevaluation of progress of restrictive or obstructive disease
  6. Preoperative evaluation
  7. Contribute to diagnostic criteria for asthma and chronic obstructive pulmonary disease (COPD)

- Types of Pulmonary Function Tests
  1. Spirometry—measures airflow rates and forced vital capacity (FVC)
     a. Forced vital capacity (FVC)—volume of air forcefully expelled from lungs after maximal inhalation
     b. Forced expiratory volume (FEV_1)—the volume of air expelled in the first second of FVC
     c. Forced expiratory flow 25–75 (FEF_{25-75})—maximal midexpiratory airflow rate
     d. Peak expiratory flow rate (PEFR)—the maximum airflow rate on forceful expulsion after maximum inspiration
     e. Maximum voluntary ventilation (MVV)—maximum volume of gas that can be breathed in 1 minute
  2. Lung volumes
     a. Total lung capacity (TLC)—volume of air in the lungs after maximum inspiration
     b. Functional residual capacity (FRC)—air left in lungs after a normal unforced expiration
     c. Residual volume (RV)—air remaining in lungs after maximum expiration
     d. Slow vital capacity (SVC)—volume of gas slowly exhaled after maximal inspiration
     e. Expiratory reserve volume (ERV)—the gas volume difference between the FRC and RV

- General Relationship of PFT to Pulmonary Disease
  1. Obstructive pulmonary disease is characterized by reduced airflow rates; causes include
     a. Asthma
     b. Emphysema
     c. Chronic bronchitis
     d. Cystic fibrosis
  2. Restrictive pulmonary disease is associated with reduced lung volumes; examples include
     a. Pulmonary infiltrate
     b. Lung resection
     c. Chest wall disorders
     d. Neuromuscular disease

◘ ACUTE BRONCHITIS

- Definition—acute inflammation of trachea, bronchi, and bronchioles

- Etiology/Incidence
  1. Common causes
     a. Rhinovirus, coronavirus—usually short course of afebrile illness
     b. Adenovirus, influenza, *Mycoplasma pneumoniae*—more severe febrile bronchitis
     c. *Bordetella pertussis*
     d. *Chlamydia pneumoniae*
  2. Associated with secondary bacterial infections
     a. Atypical pathogens, e.g., *M. pneumoniae* and *C. pneumoniae*
     b. *Haemophilus influenzae*—more common in smokers
  3. Mucous membranes become hyperemic, edematous with increased bronchial secretions
  4. Frequency and severity increase with cigarette smoking

- Signs and Symptoms
  1. Cough—persistent, deep, and pervasive (hallmark symptom)
     a. Initially dry
     b. Later productive with mucopurulent sputum
  2. Fever (may be absent)
  3. Fatigue, malaise
  4. Chest burning or substernal pain
  5. Headache
  6. Occasional dyspnea
  7. Wheezing
  8. Generally self-limiting illness but may last several weeks or even months—longer in smokers

- Differential Diagnosis
  1. Pneumonia
  2. Asthma
  3. Influenza
  4. Pertussis
  5. Upper respiratory infection (URI)
  6. Allergies
  7. Cystic fibrosis
  8. Tuberculosis
  9. Gastroesophageal reflux disease (GERD)
  10. Postinfectious cough

- Physical Findings
  1. Temperature less than 101° F
  2. Chest and lungs—lung consolidation rules out diagnosis
     a. Clear to auscultation
     b. Resonant to percussion
     c. Wheezes
     d. Diffuse bronchi (often clear with coughing)
     e. Occasional crackles

- Diagnostic Tests/Findings
  1. Diagnosis based on clinical presentation
  2. If diagnosis uncertain or symptoms severe
     a. Chest radiograph—normal in acute bronchitis
     b. Sputum cultures—not helpful in the diagnosis
     c. CBC/WBC—normal or slightly elevated
  3. Purified protein derivative (PPD)—clinical suspicion exists for tuberculosis exposure.

- Management/Treatment
  1. No treatment with antibiotics in otherwise healthy persons
  2. Palliative measures
     a. Rest
     b. Increase fluid intake to thin secretions
     c. Humidity/steam
     d. Expectorants—not recommended, no demonstrable benefit
     e. First generation antihistamine/decongestant combination for cough
     f. Cough suppressants—dextromethorphan or codeine for patients who cannot tolerate cough without hypoxia or interference with activities of daily living
     g. Decrease environmental irritants
     h. Analgesics for pain/fever
  3. Smoking cessation
  4. Bronchodilator for wheezing/cough
  5. Recovery usually in 7–14 days; postinfectious cough may persist for weeks
  6. Follow-up visit if no improvement or worsening symptoms after 72 hours
  7. Secondary bacterial infections associated with high fever, productive cough with purulent sputum; treat with antimicrobial therapy to cover atypical pathogens, more likely in patients who smoke cigarettes or have underlying chronic airway disease
     a. Azithromycin 500 mg orally once on first day followed by 250 mg daily for 4 days
     b. Doxycycline 100 mg b.i.d. for 10 days for coverage of *C. pneumoniae*, *M. pneumoniae* organisms
  8. Refer/consult with physician if no improvement after 4–6 weeks

◘ PNEUMONIA

- Definition
  1. Acute inflammation of lung parenchyma including alveoli and interstitial tissues; usually secondary to infection
  2. Categorized as either community acquired or hospital acquired (nosocomial) regardless of causative organism

a. Hospital acquired occurs > 72 hours after admission

b. Community acquired encompasses all others occurring as an outpatient or within first 72 hours of hospitalization

- Etiology/Incidence
  1. Community acquired—activation of colonized infection (*Streptococcus pneumonia)* and inhalation of pathogens (atypical pathogens) most common
  2. Hospital acquired—aspiration of secretions, inhalation of pathogens and/or hematogenous dissemination
  3. Common pathogens in outpatient setting
     a. Bacteria
        (1) *S. pneumoniae* (pneumococcus)—most common
        (2) Atypical pathogens *M. pneumoniae* and *C. pneumoniae* second-most-common cause of bacterial pneumonia in the outpatient setting
        (3) *Haemophilus influenzae*—ranked second to streptococcal pneumonia in hospitalized patients; not as prevalent in outpatient setting
     b. Viruses (4–39% of adult pneumonias, more prevalent in children)
        (1) Influenza
        (2) Parainfluenza
        (3) Adenovirus
        (4) Varicella
  4. Common pathogens in inpatient setting in addition to *S. pneumoniae* and *H. influenzae*
     a. *Staphylococcus aureus*
     b. *Klebsiella pneumoniae*
     c. *Legionella pneumophila*—1–4% of community-acquired pneumonia
     d. *Moraxella catarrhalis*
     e. *Chlamydia pneumoniae*
     f. *M. pneumoniae* (most common in adolescents/young adults)
     g. *Pseudomonas aeruginosa*
     h. *Escherichia coli*
  5. Hospital-acquired pneumonia (nosocomial)—occurs more than 72 hours after hospital admission, more common in patients requiring intensive care and mechanical ventilation
  6. Increasingly common in the elderly and patients with coexisting illness or disease
  7. Ranked first for cause of death from infectious disease
  8. Sixth leading cause of death in the United States
  9. Biological warfare pathogens such as anthrax, tularemia, plague
  10. Severe acute respiratory syndrome (SARS)—SARS coronavirus (first identified 2002 in China)

- Signs and Symptoms
  1. Fatigue, malaise
  2. Pleuritic chest pain—worsens with inspiration
  3. Fever
  4. Chills
  5. Dyspnea
  6. Cough
  7. Purulent mucus production—more common in hospital acquired

- Differential Diagnosis
  1. Types of pneumonia (see Etiology/Incidence)
  2. Atelectasis
  3. Pneumothorax
  4. Lung abscess
  5. Congestive heart failure
  6. Neoplasms
  7. Chronic obstructive pulmonary disease (COPD)
  8. Tuberculosis

- Physical Findings
  1. Elevated temperature and pulse
  2. Observe respiratory status, may have
     a. Cyanosis
     b. Nasal flaring/grunting
     c. Tachypnea
     d. Intercostal retractions
  3. Diminished localized breath sounds
  4. Evidence of consolidation
     a. Dullness to percussion
     b. Increased fremitus
     c. Egophony "e to a" changes
     d. Whispered pectoriloquy
     e. Rales
  5. Fine crepitant rales—do not clear with cough

- Diagnostic Tests/Findings
  1. Chest radiograph may show any variety of lower airway consolidation—findings lack specificity
  2. CBC with differential—WBC often elevated
     a. WBC differential with left shift—bacterial origin
     b. Differential useful in evaluating severity and prognosis
  3. Gram stain and sputum culture—consider that atypical pathogens will not gram stain; typically not useful unless induced via bronchoscopy
     a. Gram positive—*S. pneumoniae, S. aureus*
     b. Gram negative—*H. influenzae, K. pneumoniae*
  4. Serum electrolytes, hepatic enzymes—important in severe cases (when considering hospitalization); hyponatremia
  5. Blood cultures—severely ill, toxic patients
  6. Refer for thoracentesis if pleural effusion
  7. PPD to rule out tuberculosis
  8. Serum cold agglutinins—for mycoplasma
  9. Pulse oximetry

- Management/Treatment
  1. General measures
     a. Increase fluid intake
     b. Analgesics for fever and headache
     c. Avoid cough suppressants and cigarettes
     d. Humidification
  2. Empiric antimicrobial treatment of community-acquired pneumonia (CAP)
     a. Patients without comorbidity
        (1) A macrolide antibiotic (erythromycin, azithromycin, or clarithromycin) *or*
        (2) Doxycycline
     b. Patients with comorbidity
        (1) Beta lactam with macrolide or doxycycline *or*
        (2) Respiratory fluoroquinolone or beta lactam antibiotic + either an advanced-generation macrolide or doxycycline
        (3) Consider the need to cover drug-resistant streptococcus
        (4) Consider the need for hospitalization with CURB-65 criteria
     c. CURB-65 criteria—hospitalize for treatment if patient has at least three of the five criteria:
        (1) **C**onfusion
        (2) **U**remia (BUN > 19)
        (3) **R**espiratory rate > 30
        (4) **B**lood pressure < 90 mm Hg SBP or 60 mm Hg DB
        (5) **65** years old
  3. Prevention
     a. Pneumococcal 23 valent vaccine (Pneumovax) 0.5 cc IM—indicated for patients over age 65 and those with immunosuppression or chronic disease
     b. Influenza vaccine annually—may administer with pneumovax at the same time, at different sites
  4. Refer/consult with physician regarding
     a. Seriously ill, toxic patients
     b. Suspected biological warfare pathogens or SARS (infectious disease consult)

▣ ASTHMA

- Definition—complex disorder characterized by variable and recurring symptoms, airflow obstruction, bronchial hyperresponsiveness, and an underlying inflammation; airflow obstruction is widespread but variable, and is often reversible either spontaneously or with treatment

- Etiology/Incidence
  1. Caused by a single or multiple triggers such as
     a. Allergies
        (1) Airborne pollens
        (2) Molds
        (3) House dust
        (4) Animal dander
        (5) Food additives/preservatives
        (6) Feather pillows
     b. Nonallergic factors
        (1) Smoke and other pollutants
        (2) Infections
        (3) Medications—ASA, NSAID, beta-blockers
        (4) Exercise
        (5) Gastroesophageal reflux
        (6) Emotional factors
        (7) Hormones
        (8) Menses, pregnancy
        (9) Thyroid disease
  2. Affects men and women equally, approximately 5% of the U.S. population
  3. Chronic disease with acute exacerbations

- Signs and Symptoms
  1. Cough—often the only symptom
  2. Diffuse, bilateral wheezing is common—may be absent in severe exacerbation when air movement is essentially absent
  3. Dyspnea
  4. Chest tightness
  5. Exercise intolerance
  6. URI symptoms
  7. Conditions associated with asthma
     a. Rhinitis
     b. Sinusitis
     c. Nasal polyps
     d. Eczema/atopic dermatitis

- Differential Diagnosis
  1. Heart disease—congestive heart failure
  2. Foreign body aspiration (FOB)
  3. Chronic obstructive pulmonary disease (COPD)
  4. Acute infection—bronchitis/pneumonia
  5. Pulmonary embolism
  6. Cough secondary to beta-blockers or angiotensin converting enzyme (ACE) inhibitors
  7. Anaphylaxis due to allergen

- Physical Findings
  1. General appearance—note distress or decreased responsiveness
  2. Nasal flaring
  3. Use of accessory respiratory muscles, retraction
  4. Lungs
     a. Tachypnea
     b. Prolonged expiration
     c. Expiratory wheezing—unilateral wheezing suggests mechanical obstruction
     d. Generalized decreased or distant breath sounds
  5. Red flags—indicate potentially life-threatening severe exacerbation requiring immediate emergency treatment

a. Pulsus paradoxus—an exaggerated fall in systolic blood pressure during inspiration
b. Diaphoresis
c. Inaudible breath sounds
d. Inability to lie flat
e. Cyanosis

- Diagnostic Tests/Findings
1. Diagnosis is made based upon a symptom assessment, frequency of bronchodilator use, and pulmonary function testing
2. Pulmonary function tests/spirometry—forced expiratory volume 1 (FEV_1) at least < 80% of predicted norm for age, gender, height; degree of decrease correlates with staging of asthma
3. CBC
   a. Slight increase in WBC during acute attack
   b. Eosinophil increase related to allergic response
4. Chest radiograph—normal, rarely hyperinflation
5. Arterial blood gases (ABG)
   a. Hypoxia in severe cases
   b. Hypocapnia
   c. Normal pCO_2 indicates very ill patient
   d. Hypercapnia is a medical emergency
6. Sputum examination—positive for eosinophilia
7. Nasal secretion—positive for eosinophilia
8. Allergy testing
9. Broncho-provocation with methacholine, histamine, or exercise challenge induces symptoms

- Management/Treatment
1. The treatment-naïve patient is classified based upon the subjective and objective assessment as either intermittent or mild, moderate, or severe persistent asthma
2. A six-step treatment algorithm is utilized to determine initial management strategies based upon classification
   a. Step 1—short-acting beta-adrenergic agonists p.r.n.
   b. Step 2—low-dose daily inhaled corticosteroids (ICS) as preferred treatment; alternatives include mast-cell stabilizers and leukotriene receptor antagonists
   c. Step 3—medium-dose ICS preferred, may add long-acting beta-adrenergic agonists (LABA) to a low-dose ICS
   d. Step 4—medium-dose ICS with LABA; alternatives available
   e. Step 5—high-dose ICS with LABA
   f. Step 6—high-dose ICS with LABA and oral corticosteroid; consider omalizumab
3. Patients are reassessed after treatment begins and classified as either well controlled, not well controlled, or very poorly controlled, based

upon a symptom analysis, spirometry, and use of a validated asthma control questionnaire
4. Nonpharmacologic interventions
   a. Avoidance of triggers
   b. Environmental management
      (1) Do not open windows before 10:00 A.M.
      (2) Remove carpets from sleeping rooms
      (3) Wash bed linens frequently in very hot water
      (4) Annual influenza vaccination
5. Goals of treatment
   a. Activity without symptoms; sleep through the night
   b. Prevention of chronic troublesome symptoms
   c. Sports and exercise participation
   d. Optimal pharmacotherapy with minimal/no adverse effects
   e. Maintain nearly normal pulmonary function
   f. Meet patient/family's expectations of, and satisfaction with, asthma care

◩ CHRONIC OBSTRUCTIVE PULMONARY DISEASE (COPD)

- Definition—a disease state characterized by airflow obstruction due to emphysema, chronic bronchitis, or both; may be partially reversible
1. Emphysema—permanent abnormal distention of the terminal air spaces due to loss of elastic recoil; characterized by destruction of alveolar walls and resultant air trapping
2. Chronic bronchitis—excessive sputum production with chronic or recurring cough on most days for 3 months or more during 2 consecutive years

- Etiology/Incidence
1. Occupational exposure to irritants
2. Heredity—alpha$_1$ protease inhibitor deficiency may cause emphysema; suspect in patients under age 35 who have COPD
3. 10–15% of smokers develop COPD
4. Affects 5% of the adult population in the United States
5. Third leading cause of death in the United States
6. Predominantly seen over age 40
7. 70-pack year smoking history is the best predictor of airflow obstruction
8. Affects men more than women, but prevalence in women is rising

- Signs and Symptoms
1. Emphysema (pink puffer)
   a. Early stage
      (1) Mild dyspnea
      (2) Cough uncommon
      (3) Fatigue

b. Later stage
   (1) Severe dyspnea
   (2) Dyspnea on exertion
   (3) Pursed-lip breathing
   (4) Muscle wasting
   (5) Weight loss
   (6) Flushed appearance
   (7) Mild cough with clear mucoid sputum
2. Chronic bronchitis (blue bloater)
   a. Mild
      (1) Productive cough of mucopurulent sputum, especially in the mornings
      (2) Intermittent dyspnea
      (3) Copious mucus production, causing nocturnal awakening
      (4) Frequent infections
   b. Severe
      (1) Cyanosis
      (2) Edema
      (3) Recurrent respiratory failure

- Differential Diagnosis
  1. Asthma
  2. Congestive heart failure (CHF)
  3. Tuberculosis (TB)
  4. Acute bronchitis
  5. Chronic sinusitis
  6. Lung cancer

- Physical Findings
  1. Emphysema
     a. Thin
     b. Hypertrophied accessory muscles
     c. Increased anteroposterior chest diameter (barrel chest)
     d. Lungs
        (1) Hyperresonance to percussion
        (2) Diminished breath sounds
     e. Absence of cyanosis, clubbing
  2. Chronic bronchitis
     a. Central cyanosis
     b. Normal chest diameter
     c. Lungs
        (1) Normal resonance to percussion
        (2) Wheezes, bronchi
     d. Enlarged heart

- Diagnostic Tests/Findings
  1. A combination of history, physical exam, and spirometric testing produces most sensitive diagnosis; the combination of the following three items assures diagnosis, where the absence of all three virtually rules it out
     a. 55-pack year smoking history
     b. Wheezing on auscultation
     c. Self-report of wheezing

2. FEV_1 to FVC ratio < 70% postbronchodilator therapy classically considered diagnostic criteria for all stages
3. COPD stage based upon assessment of isolated FEV_1
   a. Stage I—FEV_1 > 80% predicted
   b. Stage II—FEV_1 > 50% but < 80% predicted
   c. Stage III—FEV_1 > 30% but < 50% predicted
   d. Stage IV—FEV_1 < 30% predicted or < 50% predicted in the setting of chronic respiratory failure
4. Arterial blood gases
   a. Hypercapnia
   b. Hypoxemia earlier in chronic bronchitis; present in later stages of both chronic bronchitis and emphysema
5. Increased hematocrit indicative of polycythemia in advanced chronic bronchitis
6. Chest radiograph
   a. Hyperinflation, occasional bullae/blebs in emphysema
   b. Increased markings and cardiac enlargement in chronic bronchitis
   c. Increased retrosternal airspace
   d. Flattened diaphragm
7. ECG may show right ventricular hypertrophy

- Management/Treatment
  1. Refer patients with signs and symptoms of respiratory failure to physician
  2. Avoid irritants, discontinue smoking—consider pharmacologic interventions if necessary
  3. Avoid airway irritants and temperature extremes
  4. Maintain hydration and indoor humidity
  5. Pharmacologic therapy in accordance with the joint guidelines of the American College of Physicians (ACP), American College of Chest Physicians (ACCP), American Thoracic Society (ATS), and the European Respiratory Society (ERS)
     a. Spirometry should be obtained in all patients with respiratory symptoms
     b. All stages of COPD should have annual influenza immunization and a pneumococcal vaccination
     c. Stable patients with symptoms and FEV_1 between 60% and 80% predicted may be prescribed p.r.n. bronchodilators
     d. Stable patients with FEV_1 < 60% predicted should be treated with inhaled bronchodilator
     e. Bronchodilator therapy should be monotherapy with either long-acting anticholinergic or long-acting beta-adrenergic agonist
     f. Combination therapy among inhaled long-acting anticholinergics, long-acting

beta-adrenergic agonists, or inhaled corticosteroids may be used (evidence not as strong as for monotherapy with either long-acting bronchodilator

    g. Pulmonary rehabilitation should be prescribed for symptomatic patients with $FEV_1 < 50\%$ predicted; may consider for exercise-limited patients with higher FEV_1

    h. Continuous oxygen therapy for patients with resting hypoxemia ($paO_2 < 55$ mm Hg or $saO_2 < 88\%$)

◘ TUBERCULOSIS (TB)

- Definition—chronic bacterial infectious disease most commonly infecting the lungs; may occur in lymph nodes, bones, kidneys, and meninges, and can disseminate throughout body

- Etiology/Incidence
  1. Mycobacteria of "tuberculosis complex," primarily *Mycobacterium tuberculosis*, a gram positive, acid-fast bacillus
  2. Usually spread by airborne droplet nuclei
  3. 10–15 million infected in the United States
  4. Incidence of TB is greatest in Asians, Pacific Islanders, American Indians, Alaska natives, and Hispanics
  5. 90–95% of primary TB infections remain in a latent or dormant stage
  6. High-risk populations include
     a. HIV-infected individuals
     b. Close contacts of infected persons
     c. Low-income populations
     d. Alcoholics and IV drug abusers
     e. Elderly
     f. Immigrants from Asia and Central/South America
     g. Persons in correctional institutions and in long-term care facilities
     h. Individuals with chronic disease

- Signs and Symptoms (90% asymptomatic at the time of primary infection)
  1. Fatigue
  2. Anorexia, weight loss
  3. Fever
  4. Night sweats
  5. Productive cough with purulent sputum
  6. Hemoptysis
  7. Pleuritic chest pain

- Differential Diagnosis
  1. Pneumonia
  2. Malignancy
  3. Pleurisy
  4. Histoplasmosis
  5. Silicosis
  6. COPD

- Physical Findings
  1. Typically none early in disease
  2. Later may appear chronically ill, weak, and cachectic
  3. Lungs
     a. Auscultation—apical rales, often a positive whispered pectoriloquy
     b. Palpation—increased tactile fremitus over consolidated areas
     c. Percussion—dull

- Diagnostic Tests/Findings
  1. PPD
     a. Positive with active disease or prior exposure
     b. History of Bacillus Calmette-Guérin (BCG) vaccine does not impact interpretation of PPD
     c. Patients with AIDS and other mechanisms of immunosuppression may have diminished reactivity
  2. PPD interpretation (record induration, not erythema)
     a. A reaction of 5 mm is considered positive in patients with
        (1) Recent close contact with infected person
        (2) Evidence of inactive disease
        (3) HIV infection
     b. A reaction of 10 mm is considered positive in patients with
        (1) Diabetes mellitus, cancer, or end-stage renal disease
        (2) Immigrants from Asia, Africa, Latin America
        (3) Medically underserved, low-income populations
        (4) High-risk minorities
        (5) Residents of nursing homes and prisons
        (6) Healthcare workers
     c. A reaction of 15 mm is considered positive for all populations
     d. False-negative result
        (1) PPD administered after live virus vaccine (e.g., postponed for 4–6 weeks following measles vaccination)
        (2) Immunosuppressed
        (3) Elderly
     e. False-positive result—nontuberculosis mycobacterium
  3. QuantiFERON-TB Gold
     a. May be used in all circumstances in which PPD screening currently indicated

b. Requires venipuncture and processing within 12 hours

c. Results not subject to reader bias

d. Not impacted by BCG vaccine

4. Sputum for acid-fast bacilli (AFB) provides presumptive diagnosis and is an indication to begin treatment; is not definitive diagnosis

5. Sputum culture
   a. Essential to confirm diagnosis of TB—three specimens advised
   b. Takes 3–6 weeks for results to be obtained

6. Gastric aspirate culture
   a. Alternative to bronchoscopy
   b. Use for culture only—not stained smear

- Management/Treatment
  1. Prevention
     a. Bacillus Calmette-Guérin (BCG) vaccine intended for prophylaxis of noninfected persons; not routinely used in the United States
     b. Positive PPD converter or QuantiFERON—prescribe isoniazid 300 mg orally and vitamin B_6 50 mg orally every day for 9 months
  2. Pharmacotherapy—consult/refer to physician or health department for management
     a. Medication options include (for sensitive organisms)
        (1) Isoniazid daily 5 mg/kg up to 300 mg per day for 2 months, together with
        (2) Rifampin daily 10 mg/kg up to 600 mg per day for 2 months
        (3) Pyrazinamide 15–30 mg/kg up to 2 grams per day for 2 months
     b. Order baseline liver function tests prior to initiating antituberculosis medications
     c. Perform baseline color vision (red-green) test prior to ethambutol therapy and an audiology examination prior to streptomycin treatment
  3. Follow up on contacts of persons with active disease
  4. Reportable disease—report to state and local health departments
  5. After therapy completion, follow up in 1 year; monitor for recurrence
  6. Stress importance of compliance; Directly Observed Therapy (DOT)—one method of ensuring adherence
  7. Review symptoms of drug side effects and toxicity
     a. Isoniazid
        (1) Peripheral neuropathy (prevent with daily pyridoxine)
        (2) Hepatitis
        (3) Hypersensitivity
     b. Rifampin
        (1) Orange discoloration of secretions and urine
        (2) Permanent orange stain to contact lenses
        (3) Nausea
        (4) Vomiting
     c. Pyrazinamide
        (1) Hepatotoxicity
        (2) Hyperuricemia
     d. Ethambutol
        (1) Fever
        (2) Rash
        (3) Optic neuritis
     e. Streptomycin—ototoxicity
  8. Stress importance of nutritious diet and education regarding selection of food

◻ LUNG CANCER

- Definition—primary malignant neoplasm of the lung; cell types involved include squamous cell, adenocarcinoma, large cell carcinoma, and small cell carcinoma

- Etiology/Incidence
  1. Cigarette smoking accounts for 95% of lung cancer in men and 85% of lung cancer in women
  2. Cigarette smoke in combination with other environmental pollutants (e.g., asbestos) associated with increased incidence
  3. Most common in 50–70 year olds
  4. Occurs in males more frequently than females
  5. Leading cause of cancer death in men and women in the United States

- Signs and Symptoms—depend on the area of tumor location and involvement of nodes or other organs; only 10–25% of patients are asymptomatic at time of diagnosis; symptoms occur with advanced disease
  1. "Smoker's cough"—most common early symptom
  2. Anorexia/weight loss
  3. Dyspnea—related to obstruction of major bronchus
  4. Hemoptysis—20% of all patients with hemoptysis have lung cancer
  5. Wheezing
  6. Fever
  7. Chest pain—related to extension beyond parenchyma
  8. Fatigue
  9. Hoarseness
  10. Bone pain
  11. Neurological deficits

- Differential Diagnosis
  1. Pneumonia
  2. Lung abscess
  3. Bronchitis
  4. Tuberculosis

- Physical Findings
  1. Examination may not reveal significant changes
  2. Tumor obstructing bronchus—may cause atelectasis
  3. Visible or palpable supraclavicular lymph nodes
  4. Hepatomegaly

- Diagnostic Tests/Findings
  1. Chest radiograph
     a. Negative in 15% of patients with lung cancer
     b. Not diagnostic in itself, but indicates need for additional workup
     c. Manifestations—hilar or enlarging mass, infiltrate, atelectasis, cavitation, or pleural effusion
  2. Laboratory
     a. CBC
     b. Liver function tests
     c. Serum electrolytes and calcium
  3. Definitive diagnosis requires cytologic or histologic evidence
  4. Sputum for cytology—positive in 40–60% of patients
  5. Bronchoscopy with biopsy
  6. MRI/CT scan

- Management/Treatment
  1. Surgery—25% of patients with lung cancer are candidates for surgery
  2. Chemotherapy
  3. Radiation therapy—generally palliative
  4. Refer to physician when lung cancer suspected
  5. Encourage patient to stop smoking
  6. Decrease exposure to pollutants
  7. Realistic assessment for patient and family of prognosis, pros and cons of therapy—essential to patient's decision for treatment
  8. Discuss side effects of chemotherapy/radiation
  9. Encourage nutritious diet
  10. Effective pain control
  11. Hospice care

❑ QUESTIONS

Select the best answer.

1. Which of the following drugs is contraindicated in patients with severe asthma?

   a. Propranolol
   b. Theophylline
   c. Amoxicillin
   d. Albuterol

2. What is the most common organism causing community-acquired pneumonia?

   a. *Eschericia coli*
   b. *Staphylococcus aureus*
   c. *Streptococcus pneumoniae*
   d. *Klebsiella pneumoniae*

3. Which of the following is not a differential diagnosis of chronic cough?

   a. Tuberculosis
   b. Asthma
   c. Allergies
   d. Pneumonia

4. What is the most common side effect of isoniazid?

   a. Idiopathic splenomegaly
   b. Seizures
   c. Gynecomastia
   d. Peripheral neuropathy

5. Alpha$_1$ antitrypsin deficiency is associated with which of the following conditions?

   a. Chronic bronchitis
   b. Asthma
   c. Emphysema
   d. Cystic fibrosis

6. A 25-year-old nurse presents to employee health for her annual physical examination. Her previous PPD, 1 year ago, was negative. A PPD is repeated and results 3 days later shows 14 mm of induration. The nurse is asymptomatic and her chest radiograph is normal. The most appropriate management at this time would be:

   a. Repeat chest radiograph yearly
   b. Prescribe isoniazid for 9 months
   c. Prescribe ethambutol for 6–12 months
   d. Repeat PPD in 2 months

7. Which of the following statements is true in the treatment of moderate persistent asthma?

   a. Inhaled corticosteroids are the cornerstone of therapy
   b. Beta-blockers should be used vigorously
   c. Cromolyn is used during acute attacks
   d. Long-acting beta-adrenergic agonists are contraindicated

8. Which of the following signs/symptoms are not associated with chronic bronchitis?

   a. Productive cough
   b. Obesity
   c. Dyspnea
   d. Pursed-lip breathing

9. What is the most important measurement of pulmonary function in asthma?

   a. The total lung capacity
   b. The forced vital capacity
   c. The residual volume
   d. The forced expiratory volume (FEV$_1$)

10. What is the most common cause of pneumonia in adolescents and young adults?

    a. Pneumococcus
    b. Mycoplasma
    c. Varicella
    d. Chlamydia

11. Which of the following represents the best choice of antibiotic for outpatient treatment of pneumonia in a 50-year-old healthy male?

    a. Amoxicillin
    b. Trimethoprim/sulfamethoxazole
    c. Azithromycin
    d. Cephalexin

12. Physical findings in bacterial pneumonia would include:

    a. Hyperresonance to percussion
    b. Rales that clear with cough
    c. Decreased fremitus
    d. Positive egophony

13. Max Murphy is a 55-year-old postal worker who was recently diagnosed with stage I COPD. Initial therapy must include:

    a. A daily inhaled corticosteroid
    b. A long-acting anticholinergic inhaler
    c. Annual influenza vaccination
    d. Pulmonary rehabilitation

14. Pneumococcal vaccine is considered a preventive measure to bacterial pneumonia. For which population(s) is it indicated?

    a. Patients with acute bronchitis
    b. Patients with COPD
    c. Adolescents and young adults
    d. Persons over age 45

15. Indicators of a severe asthma attack requiring emergency treatment include:

    a. Prolonged expiration
    b. Bilateral rales
    c. Chest tightness
    d. Inaudible breath sounds

16. When ordering a CBC in a person with acute exacerbations of asthma, you would expect to see:

    a. Moderate elevation in WBCs and atypical lymphocyte
    b. Decrease in WBCs and lymphocytosis
    c. Increased hematocrit and increased platelets
    d. Mild elevation in WBCs and eosinophilia

17. Albuterol is an example of:

    a. Antihistamine
    b. β$_2$ adrenergic agonist
    c. Corticosteroid
    d. Antitussive

18. Which of the following is not a risk factor for lung cancer?

    a. Radon exposure
    b. Passive cigarette smoking
    c. Allergen irritant
    d. Asbestos exposure

19. What is the leading cause of cancer deaths in the United States?

    a. Gastric cancer
    b. Malignant melanoma
    c. Breast cancer
    d. Lung cancer

20. What is the drug of choice in treatment of chronic bronchitis?

    a. Theophylline
    b. Erythromycin
    c. Cromolyn sodium
    d. Ipratropium bromide

21. Pulsus paradoxus is:

    a. Increase in diastolic blood pressure on expiration
    b. Decrease in systolic blood pressure on inspiration
    c. Increase in systolic blood pressure on expiration
    d. Decrease in diastolic blood pressure on inspiration

22. Mary is a 24-year-old female with mild persistent asthma since she was 7. She has been maintained on low-dose inhaled corticosteroids for several years, but an assessment of asthma control reveals that her condition is not well controlled. Which of the following is the next step in her pharmacologic management?

    a. A leukotriene receptor antagonist
    b. A medium-dose, inhaled corticosteroid
    c. A long-acting beta-adrenergic agonist
    d. Oral corticosteroids

23. Which of the following groups is *not* at high risk for tuberculosis?

    a. HIV-infected individuals
    b. Asian immigrants
    c. Homeless individuals
    d. College students

24. The serum cold agglutinins test is used to diagnose:
    a. *Haemophilus influenzae* pneumonia
    b. Legionella pneumonia
    c. Rickettsia infection
    d. Mycoplasma pneumonia

25. The problem with diagnosing early stage lung cancer is that:
    a. The CBC lab result is normal
    b. It mimics the symptoms of asthma
    c. Patients are often asymptomatic until late in the disease
    d. Pulmonary function tests are normal

26. Signs and symptoms of COPD correlate with which one of the following:
    a. Emphysema with decreased total lung capacity (TLC)
    b. Asthma and right-sided heart failure
    c. Chronic bronchitis and airway obstruction
    d. Hemoptysis and hypoxemia

27. Assessment findings in a patient with COPD would include:
    a. Increased egophony and increased rhonchi
    b. Decreased tactile fremitus and hyperresonance to percussion
    c. Bilateral wheezes and pleuritic chest pain
    d. Fever during exacerbations

28. Diagnostic criteria for COPD must include:
    a. A history of smoking or other irritant exposure
    b. The presence of dyspnea, chronic cough, and sputum
    c. A FEV_1/FVC ratio of 70%
    d. An FVC of < 80% predicted

29. Young Chow, an 18-year-old Chinese exchange student, presents to student health for an immunization update. He states he had BCG vaccine as a young child and therefore will never get tuberculosis. You administer a PPD and the result is positive. Your next best action would be to:
    a. Assume the positive result is due to BCG vaccine; no further evaluation needed
    b. Assume the positive result is related to TB exposure or infection; order a chest radiograph
    c. Begin isoniazid therapy immediately
    d. Repeat PPD test in 1 month to verify results

30. The most common side effect of the antituberculin drug rifampin is:
    a. Hepatotoxicity
    b. Optic neuritis
    c. Fever
    d. Orange discoloration of secretions

Answers

1.	**a**	16.	**d**
2.	**c**	17.	**b**
3.	**d**	18.	**c**
4.	**d**	19.	**d**
5.	**c**	20.	**d**
6.	**b**	21.	**b**
7.	**a**	22.	**b**
8.	**d**	23.	**d**
9.	**d**	24.	**d**
10.	**b**	25.	**c**
11.	**c**	26.	**c**
12.	**d**	27.	**b**
13.	**c**	28.	**c**
14.	**b**	29.	**b**
15.	**d**	30.	**d**

❑ BIBLIOGRAPHY

American Thoracic Society, CDC, & Infectious Disease Society of America. (2003). Treatment of tuberculosis. *Morbidity and Mortality Weekly Report, 52*(RR11), 1–77.

Braman, S. (2006). Postinfectious cough: ACCP evidence-based clinical practice guidelines. *Chest, 129*(1 supp), 138S–146S.

Chestnutt, M. S., & Prendergast, T. J. (2012). Pulmonary disorders. In S. J. McPhee, & M. A. Papadakis (Eds.), *Current medical diagnosis and treatment* (48th ed.). New York: McGraw-Hill.

Gross, N. (2008). Chronic obstructive pulmonary disease: An evidence-based approach to treatment with a focus on anticholinergic bronchodilation. *Mayo Clinic Proceedings, 83*(11), 1241–1250.

Hart, A. M. (2007). An evidence-based approach to the diagnosis and management of acute respiratory infections. *The Journal for Nurse Practitioners, 3*(9), 607–611.

Mandell, L. A., Wunderink, R. G., Anzueto, A., Bartlett, J. G., Campbell, G. D., Dean, N. C., . . . Whitney, C. G. (2007). Infectious Diseases Society of America/American Thoracic Society consensus guidelines on the management of community-acquired pneumonia in adults. *Clinical Infectious Diseases 44*, S27–S72.

National Asthma Education and Prevention Programs. (2007). *Expert Panel Report 3: Guidelines for the Diagnosis and Management of Asthma.* U.S. Dept. of Health and Human Services publication #NIH08-5846. Bethesda, MD: National Institutes of Health, National Heart, Lung, and Blood Institute.

Qassim, A., Wilt, T. J., Weinberger, S. E., Hanania, N. A., Criner, G., van der Molen, T., . . . Shekelle, P. (2011). Diagnosis and management of stable chronic obstructive pulmonary disease: A clinical practice guideline update from the American College of Physicians, American College of Chest Physicians, American Thoracic Society, and European Respiratory Society. *Annals of Internal Medicine, 155,* 179–191.

U.S. Preventive Services Task Force. (2006). *The Guide to Clinical Preventive Services: Recommendations of the United States Preventive Services Task Force.* Retrieved from http://www.ahrq.gov/clinic/pocketgd .pdf

Cardiovascular Disorders

Sally K. Miller

6

◻ HYPERTENSION (HTN)

- Definition—(1) persons with persistent elevation of systolic blood pressure (SBP) > 140 mm Hg or diastolic blood pressure (DBP) > 90 mm Hg based upon an average of two or more properly measured, seated blood pressure readings on each of two or more office visits, or (2) persons taking antihypertensive medication; important to perform blood pressure measurements under nonstressful circumstances, e.g., well rested, empty bladder, no immediate psychosocial stressors; hypertension should not be diagnosed based upon one blood pressure measurement unless that measurement is greater than 180/110 mm Hg or is accompanied by end organ damage (National Heart, Lung, and Blood Institute, 2003)
  1. Blood Pressure Classification Guidelines

Classification	SBP		DBP
Normal	< 120	and	< 80
Prehypertension	120–139	or	80–89
Hypertension			
Stage 1	140–159	or	90–99
Stage 2	> 160	or	> 100

- Etiology/Incidence—95% of cases due to unknown etiology—unknown etiology is defined as primary, essential, or idiopathic hypertension; remaining 5% of cases are attributable to secondary causes

1. | Theories of Etiology of HTN | Etiology of Secondary HTN |
|---|---|
| Volume-related | Chronic kidney disease |
| Renin-mediated | Renal vascular disease |
| Neurogenic | Hyperaldosteronism |
| | Cushing's syndrome |
| | Pheochromocytoma |
| | Coarctation of the aorta |
| | Pregnancy |
| | Sleep apnea |
| | Thyroid or parathyroid disease |

2. Incidence
   a. 10–15% of Caucasian adults
   b. 20–30% of African-American adults
   c. Heredity
   d. Cigarette smoking
   e. Increased salt intake
   f. Obesity
   g. Affects over 70 million Americans

- Signs and Symptoms
  1. Often no symptoms—known as "silent killer"
  2. Symptoms of underlying cause may present in secondary hypertension
     a. Flushing
     b. Palpitations
     c. Pallor
     d. Tremor
     e. Profuse perspiration

3. Suboccipital pulsating headache occurring early in morning and improving throughout the day in severe hypertension
4. Chronic hypertension may result in ventricular hypertrophy and associated symptoms of heart failure
5. Oliguria, nocturia, or hematuria may be present
6. Epistaxis in severe hypertension
7. Severe hypertension may present with signs and symptoms of hypertensive encephalopathy
    a. Nausea and vomiting
    b. Somnolence and confusion
    c. Visual disturbances

- Differential Diagnosis—secondary causes of hypertension must be ruled out
  1. Renal disorders
      a. Medical renal disease
      b. Diabetic nephropathy
      c. Acute tubular necrosis
  2. Endocrine disorders
      a. Cushing's syndrome
      b. Hyperaldosteronism
      c. Pheochromocytoma
      d. Diabetes mellitus (DM)
      e. Acromegaly
      f. Hyperthyroidism
  3. Structural/anatomic disorders
      a. Coarctation of the aorta
      b. Carotid artery stenosis
      c. Renal artery stenosis
      d. Sleep apnea
  4. Pregnancy

- Physical Findings
  1. Most significant is elevated blood pressure noted in definition
  2. S_4 gallop due to decreased left ventricular compliance is common
  3. Displaced point of maximal impulse (PMI) when left ventricular hypertrophy present
  4. Diffuse anterior chest wall heave when right ventricular hypertrophy present
  5. Peripheral pulses may be abnormal in some secondary cases
      a. Coarctation of the aorta
      b. Stenosis of major arteries
  6. Systolic murmur of aortic stenosis may be heard
  7. Dependent edema in chronic, uncontrolled disease
  8. Renal artery bruit in cases of renal artery stenosis
  9. Neurologic evidence of previous cerebral infarcts may be present

10. Flame hemorrhages and/or fluffy exudate on ophthalmoscopic examination

- Diagnostic Tests/Findings
  1. Laboratory findings usually normal in uncomplicated essential hypertension
  2. Microalbuminuria is earliest indication of target organ damage
  3. Hematuria and/or proteinuria in secondary renal disease
  4. Rapid sequence intravenous pyelogram (IVP) to rule out renal vascular disease
  5. Chest radiograph
      a. Rule out coarctation of the aorta via chest radiograph
      b. Cardiac hypertrophy in chronic, uncontrolled disease
  6. Plasma lipids may be elevated
  7. Hormone levels to evaluate underlying endocrine cause
      a. Elevated serum aldosterone levels—primary hyperaldosteronism
      b. Elevated adrenocorticotropic hormone or serum cortisol—Cushing's syndrome
      c. Low thyroid stimulating hormone and elevated T_3—hyperthyroidism
      d. Elevated serum and urine catecholamines—pheochromocytoma
  8. Sleep studies as indicated by history

- Management/Treatment
  1. Assessment of baseline status
      a. All hypertensive and prehypertensive patients should have a thorough review of systems and a physical examination documented to assess for target organ damage
      b. Those requiring pharmacologic therapy should have baseline diagnostic testing to assess for target organ damage
      c. Electrocardiogram/chest radiograph frequently performed; utility questionable
      d. Serum multichemical analysis with renal function tests
      e. Urinalysis and microalbuminuria
      f. Hemoglobin
      g. Fasting blood sugar
      h. Serum lipid profile
      i. Serum uric acid
  2. Assessment of medical history
      a. Screening for presence of compelling indications for specific pharmacologic agents
          (1) Heart failure—thiazide diuretics (thiazide), beta-adrenergic antagonists/blocker (BB), angiotensin-converting enzyme inhibitors (ACEI), angiotensin receptor antagonist blocker (ARB), aldosterone antagonists (aldo antag)

(2) Post myocardial infarction (MI)—beta blockade (BB), ACEI, aldosterone antagonist
(3) High cardiovascular disease (CVD) risk—thiazide, BB, ACEI, calcium channel antagonist (blockers) (CCB)
(4) Diabetes—ACEI, angiotensin receptor blocker (ARB)
(5) Chronic kidney disease—ACEI, ARB
(6) Recurrent stroke prevention—thiazide, ACEI

b. Screening for presence of contraindications to specific pharmacologic therapy
(1) Thiazides—gout
(2) Beta adrenergic blockade reactive airway disease (RAD), second- or third-degree atrioventricular (AV) block
(3) Calcium channel blockade—congestive heart failure (CHF)
(4) ACEI second-, third-trimester (TM) pregnancy, angioedema

- Goals of Therapy
1. Reduction of cardiovascular and renal morbidity and mortality
2. Reduction of blood pressure to < 140/90 mm Hg
3. Reduction of blood pressure to < 130/80 mm Hg in patients with diabetes mellitus or chronic kidney disease

- Lifestyle Modifications
1. Weight reduction—10 kg weight loss can reduce systolic blood pressure by 20 mm Hg
2. Dietary Approaches to Stop Hypertension (DASH) diet—increase fruits, vegetables; decrease fats
3. Dietary sodium restriction to < 2.4 g/day
4. Physical activity—30 minutes of moderately vigorous activity (brisk walking) 5 days weekly or vigorous activity (jogging) 20 minutes 2 days weekly
5. Moderate alcohol consumption; no more than 2 drinks/day men, 1 drink/day women

- Pharmacologic Management
1. Indicated for all patients not at goal blood pressure
2. Thiazide diuretics reduce overall morbidity and mortality—initial drug choice for stage 1 and stage 2 hypertension unless contraindication (gout) or compelling indication to use another drug
3. Alternate drug therapy for stage 1 and additional drug therapy for stage 2 based upon the presence or compelling indication

4. Joint National Committee (JNC) VII algorithm

Not at Goal BP?
(140/90 or 130/80 for DM and Chronic Kidney Disease (CKD)

Without Compelling Indications		With Compelling Indications
		Drugs for Compelling Indications
Stage 1	Stage 2	
Thiazides for most; may use ACEI, ARB, BB, CCB, or combo	Two drug therapy; Thiazide + 1 ACEI, ARB, BB, CCB	Antihypertensives as needed (see "compelling indications" for each individual drug class; other antihypertensives as needed)

*If not at goal, consider specialty referral

5. Counseling regarding medication side effects, compliance, follow-up, and lifestyle modifications
6. Consult physician when instituting pharmacologic therapy and when patient does not respond to first-line pharmacotherapy

◘ CORONARY ARTERY DISEASE (CAD)

- Definition—clinical syndrome also known as angina pectoris that occurs from atherosclerotic changes to the coronary vasculature; the result is decreased blood flow through vessels either due to partial obstruction (sclerosis) or vasospasm (may happen in a nonsclerotic vessel); when tissue ischemia and pain occur as a result of decreased blood flow, angina occurs

- Etiology/Incidence
1. Hypertension
2. Tobacco use
3. Serum lipid abnormalities
4. Diabetes mellitus
5. Insulin resistance and metabolic syndrome
6. Family history with a first-degree relative (particularly when age of onset < 50 years)
7. Sedentary lifestyle
8. Use of oral contraceptives
9. Gender prevalence depends upon age
   a. Overall more prevalent in men by a 4:1 ratio
   b. Under age 40, ratio is 8:1
   c. Over age 70, ratio is 1:1
10. Obesity
11. Personality type is less-certain risk factor

- Types of Angina
1. Exertional—occurs with activity, generally subsides with rest

2. Variant threshold occurs at various times, including rest
3. Prinzmetal's angina occurs only at rest
    a. Chest pain occurs without the usual precipitating factors
    b. Often affects women under age 50
    c. Characteristically occurs in early morning, awakening patient from sleep
    d. Tends to involve right coronary artery

- Signs and Symptoms
    1. Characteristic chest discomfort
        a. Sensation of tightness, squeezing, burning, pressure
        b. 80–90% of cases discomfort is felt behind or slightly to the left of the mid-sternum
        c. Radiates most often to left shoulder and upper arm, traveling down inner aspect of arm to elbow, forearm, wrist, and fourth or fifth finger
        d. May be felt in lower jaw, back of neck, or upper left side of back
        e. Typically lasts 15–20 minutes, may resolve more quickly but usually lasts at least several minutes; pain lasting > 30 minutes is unstable angina
    2. Anxiety
    3. Dyspnea

- Differential Diagnosis
    1. Gastroesophageal reflux (heartburn)
    2. Anxiety
    3. Depression
    4. Costrochondral pain
    5. Pneumothorax
    6. Congestive heart failure
    7. Pneumonia
    8. Pericarditis
    9. Asthma
    10. Aortic dissection
    11. Myocardial infarction

- Physical Findings
    1. Systolic and diastolic blood pressures usually elevated during attack
    2. May hear apical systolic murmur due to transient mitral regurgitation
    3. Transient S_3 and/or S_4 may be present
    4. May detect signs of disease that contribute to or accompany CAD
        a. Diabetes mellitus
        b. Hypertension
        c. Aortic stenosis
        d. Hypertrophic cardiomyopathy
        e. Mitral valve prolapse
    5. Pulse and respirations may be elevated

6. May see tobacco stained teeth or fingers
7. May see signs of peripheral artery disease
    a. Diminished distal pulses
    b. Pale skin
    c. Poor hair growth
8. Levine's sign (clenched fist over sternum) highly suggestive of angina
9. May not have any remarkable physical findings

- Diagnostic Tests/Findings
    1. Serum lipid levels
        a. LDL cholesterol must be lowered to at least 100 mg/dL; < 70 mg/dL preferable
        b. HDL cholesterol should be increased to > 40 mg/dL
    2. Electrocardiogram (ECG)
        a. Normal in 25% patients with angina
        b. Characteristic finding is downward sloping of S-T segment or T wave peak or inversion during attack; reverses after attack
        c. May show signs of old myocardial infarction or hypertrophy
    3. Exercise electrocardiography (stress testing)
        a. Ischemic changes or angina during exercise test—clinically diagnostic
        b. Markedly positive test is any one of the following
            (1) S-T segment depression after start of exercise
            (2) > 2 mm of new S-T segment depression in multiple leads
            (3) New S-T segment elevation
            (4) Decreased systolic blood pressure with exercise
            (5) Development of heart failure with exercise
            (6) Inability to exercise for > 2 minutes
            (7) Prolonged interval after exercise for return to normal ECG
    4. Nuclear medicine studies to evaluate presence, location, and extent of coronary disease
        a. Exercise thallium imaging
            (1) Especially useful in patients with preexisting ECG abnormalities and patients taking digoxin
            (2) Areas of diminished uptake indicate hypoperfusion
            (3) Should be conducted at experienced center
        b. Radionuclide ventriculography
            (1) Images left ventricle and measures ejection fraction
            (2) Resting abnormalities represent infarction
            (3) Abnormalities with exercise indicate stress-induced ischemia

c. Coronary angiography
  (1) Definitive test for diagnosis of CAD
  (2) Indicated in high-risk patients
    (a) With refractory unstable angina
    (b) With spontaneous or exercise-induced ischemia after myocardial infarction

- Management/Treatment (see **Table 6-1**)
  1. Treatment of acute attack
    a. Sublingual or buccal spray nitroglycerin
    b. Dose may be repeated 3 times at 5-minute intervals
    c. Pain unrelieved after 3 doses is unstable and should be evaluated in emergency room

2. Prevention of further attacks
  a. Reduction of risk factors when possible
    (1) Weight reduction
    (2) Smoking cessation
    (3) Exercise program
    (4) Daily ASA
  b. Lowering LDL cholesterol to < 100 mg/dL is of paramount importance
    (1) If LDL cholesterol is between 100 and 130 mg/dL, diet modification program may be implemented
    (2) If LDL cholesterol is > 130 mg/dL, pharmacologic therapy should be instituted
      (a) Hydroxymethylglutaryl coenzyme A (HMG CoA) reductase inhibitors

■ **Table 6-1** Treatment Algorithm for Stable Angina

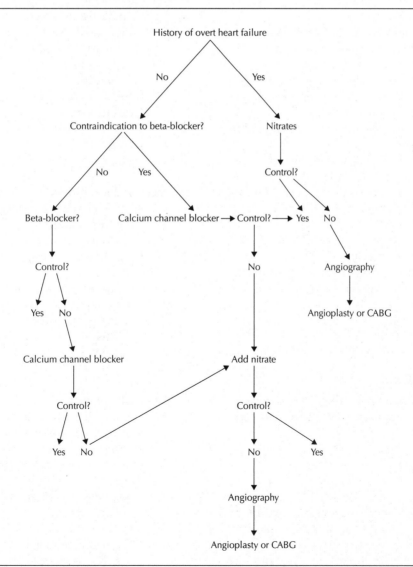

are the drug of choice for LDL reduction unless contraindicated

- (b) Niacin
- (c) Bile acid binding resins
- (d) Cholesterol absorption inhibitors
- (e) All patients whose risk for CAD warrants pharmacologic therapy should also take aspirin daily

c. Beta-blockers prevent angina by reducing myocardial oxygen requirements
  - (1) Metoprolol 50–200 mg daily in 2 divided doses
  - (2) Atenolol 25–200 mg once daily
  - (3) Major contraindications are bronchospastic disease, bradydysrhythmias, and heart failure

d. Calcium channel blockers prevent angina by reducing myocardial oxygen demand and inducing coronary vasodilation
  - (1) Nifedipine 30–120 mg daily
  - (2) Verapamil 180–480 mg in 1 or 2 doses daily
  - (3) Diltiazem 360 mg in 2 daily doses

e. Long-acting nitrates prevent angina by inducing coronary vasodilation
  - (1) Isosorbide dinitrate 10–40 mg 3 daily
  - (2) Sustained release nitroglycerin 6.25–25 mg daily in 2–4 divided doses

f. Coronary revascularization is indicated in the following
  - (1) Unacceptable symptoms despite medical therapy to its tolerable limits
  - (2) Left main coronary artery stenosis greater than 50% with or without symptoms
  - (3) Three-vessel disease with left ventricular dysfunction
  - (4) Unstable angina with ischemia on exercise stress test after symptom control
  - (5) Post–myocardial infarction with continued angina or ischemia on noninvasive testing

g. Counseling regarding medication side effects

3. Physician consultation
   a. When pharmacologic therapy initiated
   b. Failure to respond to pharmacologic therapy

◘ DYSLIPIDEMIA

- Definition
  1. A general term used to describe any one or combination of lipid abnormalities that serve as a marker for coronary artery disease risk; while elevated total cholesterol (TC) and low

levels of high-density lipoproteins (HDL) are linked to increased incidence of coronary artery disease, and conversely high HDL appears to be cardioprotective, elevated low-density lipoproteins (LDL) remain the primary target of lipid-lowering strategies in all levels of prevention

2. With respect to cardiovascular risk, dyslipidemia is quantified as follows
   a. Optimal LDL—< 100 mg/dL
   b. Near optimal LDL—> 100 < 129 mg/dL
   c. Borderline high LDL—> 130 < 159 mg/dL
   d. High LDL—> 160 < 189 mg/dL
   e. Very high LDL—> 190 mg/dL
   f. Optimal TC—< 200 mg/dL
   g. Borderline high TC—> 200 < 239 mg/dL
   h. High TC—> 240 mg/dL
   i. Low HDL—< 40 mg/dL
   j. High HDL—> 60 mg/dL

- Etiology/Incidence
  1. Familial hypercholesterolemia
  2. Endocrine disease
     a. Thyroid disorders
     b. Hypercortisolism
     c. Diabetes
  3. Nephrotic syndrome
  4. Hepatic disease
  5. Sedentary lifestyle
  6. Obesity
  7. Malignancy

- Signs and Symptoms
  1. Asymptomatic in most cases
  2. Diagnosis occurs as a function of screening or the laboratory evaluation of patients with heart disease

- Differential Diagnosis (of underlying causes)
  1. Familial syndrome
  2. Endocrine disease
  3. Liver disease
  4. Malignancy
  5. Obesity

- Physical Findings
  1. No specific findings in most cases
  2. May show findings consistent with vascular disease
  3. May show findings of underlying endocrine disease
  4. In extreme dyslipidemias
     a. Corneal arcus
     b. Xanthomas
     c. Lipemia retinalis
     d. Earlobe crease

- Diagnostic Tests/Findings
  1. Elevated LDL (see Definition)
  2. HDL < 40 mg/dL is a cardiac risk factor
  3. HDL > 60 mg/dL is cardioprotective and negates another risk factor
  4. Serum triglycerides > 150 mg/dL—no link to heart disease, but may cause pancreatic disease
  5. As indicated to rule out underlying secondary causes

- Management/Treatment
  1. Cholesterol-lowering diet
     a. Total fat < 25–30% of intake
     b. Saturated fat < 7% of intake
     c. Dietary cholesterol < 200 mg/day
  2. Pharmacologic therapy
     a. HMG CoA reductase inhibitors
        (1) Drug of choice in patients with existing CAD
        (2) Primary utility is LDL reduction—may reduce up to 60%
        (3) Contraindicated in severe liver disease
        (4) Caution rhabdomyolysis
     b. Cholesterol absorption inhibitors
        (1) Ezetimibe is currently only available drug in this class
        (2) Used as adjunct therapy when additional LDL reduction needed
        (3) Relatively benign adverse effect profile
        (4) No utility as monotherapy
     c. Bile acid sequestrants
        (1) Prevent GI reabsorption of 90% of bile salts
        (2) No significant systemic effects
        (3) May reduce LDL up to 30%
        (4) Monotherapy in those unable to take other agents; adjunct for LDL reduction with HMG CoA reductase therapy
        (5) Safe in pregnancy
     d. Niacin
        (1) Utility in polylipid abnormalities
        (2) Reduces LDL up to 30%, improves HDL to 25%, triglyceride reduction to 50%
        (3) May be used as monotherapy in the absence of CAD
        (4) Vasomotor and GI effects may impact adherence; pretreatment with ASA and slow titration to therapeutic doses may be helpful
     e. Fibric acid derivatives
        (1) May be useful in those whose primary problem is low HDL
        (2) May be linked to increased cancer deaths

        (3) Potentially hepatotoxic, particularly in combination with other lipid-lowering agents
  3. Implementation of therapy depends upon the presence of other CAD risk factors
     a. Those with existing CAD—begin pharmacologic therapy if LDL > 130 mg/dL; if LDL 100–130 mg/dL, may trial therapeutic lifestyle changes for up to 6 months before beginning drug therapy to a target of < 100 mg/dL
     b. Those with two or more CAD risk factors but no existing CAD, goal of therapy is LDL of 130 mg/dL—may trial therapeutic lifestyle changes for up to 6 months before beginning pharmacologic therapy
     c. Those with zero or one risk factor, goal of therapy is 160 mg/dL—may trial therapeutic lifestyle changes for up to 6 months before beginning pharmacologic therapy

◘ MYOCARDIAL INFARCTION (MI)

- Definition—myocardial necrosis due to inadequate blood flow, usually a result of atherosclerotic stenosis but may be the result of prolonged vasospasm

- Etiology/Incidence
  1. Risk factors and epidemiology same as for CAD
  2. Leading cause of death in adults in the United Sates; 1.5 million deaths annually

- Signs and Symptoms
  1. One-third of patients give history of alteration in typical pattern of angina
  2. Pain similar to angina but more severe
  3. Diaphoresis, dyspnea, cough, and wheeze
  4. Anxiety
  5. Nausea and vomiting
  6. Weakness or light-headedness
  7. Often prefer not to lie quietly—continuously seek comfortable position
  8. Women may present with atypical symptoms, i.e., burning sensation in chest, indigestion, weakness

- Differential Diagnosis
  1. Angina
  2. Gastroesophageal reflux
  3. Pulmonary embolus
  4. Costochondral pain
  5. Pericarditis
  6. Dissecting aortic aneurysm
  7. Anxiety

- Physical Findings
  1. Heart rate may range from bradycardia to tachycardia
  2. Dysrhythmias common
  3. Low-grade fever may appear after 12 hours and persist for several days
  4. S_4 and murmur of mitral regurgitation common
  5. S_3 less common—when present indicates severe left ventricular dysfunction
  6. Blood pressure may be elevated or abnormally low
  7. May see findings consistent with heart failure; jugular vein distention, rales
  8. Cyanosis and cold temperature indicate low cardiac output

- Diagnostic Tests/Findings
  1. ECG is essential—most patients have ECG changes in a regional distribution
     a. Convex S-T segment elevation with peaked upright or inverted T waves indicative of transmural (S-T elevation) MI (STEMI)
     b. S-T segment depression may indicate subendocardial MI (NSTEMI); develops inverted T waves in chronic phase
     c. Development of clinically significant Q waves (at least 1-mm deep and 1-mm wide) generally considered diagnostic of MI; develops in chronic phase of STEMI
     d. Regional distribution
        (1) Inferior wall—leads II, II, aVF
        (2) Lateral wall—leads I, aVL
        (3) Anterior wall—leads V_1 through V_6
  2. Leukocytosis 10,000–20,000/μL on second day
  3. Cardiac isoenzymes progressively increase as necrosis evolves
     a. Creatine kinase muscle-brain (CK-MB) increases within 4–6 hours of pain onset, peaks in 10–20 hours, returns to baseline in 36–48 hours
     b. Troponin T and troponin I demonstrate high specificity and sensitivity and remain elevated for 5–7 days post-MI
     c. Lactic dehydrogenase (LDH) elevations detectable 12 hours after pain onset, peak in 24–48 hours, and remain elevated for 10–14 days—LDH_1:LDH_2 ratio > 1.0 consistent with MI
  4. Echocardiography for assessment of cardiac wall motion and valvular/structural defects post-MI
  5. Technetium 99m pyrophosphate scintigraphy used in diagnosis of MI for patients hospitalized late in the course
  6. Radionuclide ventriculography allows assessment of regional wall motion and ejection fraction

  7. Coronary angiography is definitive test to visualize the coronary vasculature

- Management/Treatment—immediate hospitalization
  1. Immediate goals are to provide oxygen, relieve pain, and treat dysrhythmia
     a. Oxygen by nasal cannula, face mask, or endotracheal tube
     b. Morphine sulfate 2–4 mg at 5–10 minute intervals p.r.n.
     c. Nitroglycerin sublingual or intravenously
     d. Heparin 5,000-unit bolus followed by intravenous infusion
     e. Chewable aspirin 160 mg
     f. Treat dysrhythmia as indicated
  2. Thrombolytics for coronary artery reperfusion within 4–6 hours of pain onset in STEMI
  3. Percutaneous transluminal coronary artery angioplasty (PTCA)
  4. Other medications have varying levels of effectiveness in the acute setting
     a. Beta-blockers
     b. Calcium channel blockers
     c. ACEI
  5. Patient education regarding cardiac rehabilitation and risk factor reduction
  6. Physician consultation when acute MI suspected

◘ CONGESTIVE HEART FAILURE (CHF)

- Definition—clinical syndrome that results when cardiac output is insufficient to meet metabolic demands of body; any condition that affects heart rate or contractile function can precipitate CHF

- Etiology/Incidence
  1. Acute myocardial infarction; dysrhythmia
  2. Chronic hypertension
  3. Valvular stenosis or regurgitation
  4. Cardiomyopathy
  5. Medication toxicity
  6. 5,000,000 estimated cases in the United States —500,000 new cases diagnosed annually

- Types of CHF
  1. Acute
     a. Abrupt onset usually follows acute MI or valve rupture
     b. Also known as "left-sided failure"
     c. Symptoms are produced by acute diffusion of water into the pulmonary air spaces
  2. Chronic
     a. Develops as a result of inadequate compensatory mechanisms that have been employed over time to improve cardiac output

    b.   Also known as "right-sided failure"

    c.   Symptoms are produced by increased hydrostatic pressure in the venous system and subsequent diffusion of water into the interstitium

  3. Systolic—contractile dysfunction results in decreased cardiac output

  4. Diastolic—inability to relax and fill with blood results in decreased cardiac output; accounts for half of all cases of CHF

- Signs and Symptoms
  1. Acute CHF
     a. Dyspnea at rest
     b. Frothy cough worse in the recumbent position
     c. Feeling of anxiety and/or impending doom
  2. Chronic CHF
     a. Dyspnea on exertion; easily fatigued
     b. Chronic nonproductive cough
     c. Abdominal fullness
     d. Weight gain
     e. Paroxysmal nocturnal dyspnea
     f. Oliguria, nocturia
     g. Peripheral cyanosis

- Differential Diagnosis
  1. Acute MI
  2. Pulmonary embolus
  3. Pneumonia
  4. Asthma
  5. Chronic venous insufficiency

- Physical Findings
  1. Acute
     a. Coarse rales over all lung fields
     b. Wheezing over all lung fields
     c. S_3 gallop very common
     d. Appears generally healthy except for the acute event
     e. Systolic murmur of mitral regurgitation
     f. Usually no edema or systemic signs of fluid overload
  2. Chronic
     a. Lungs may be clear or may exhibit rales at the bases
     b. Dependent edema
     c. Appears chronically ill
     d. Jugular venous distention
     e. Hepatosplenomegaly
     f. Point of maximal impulse displaced to the left
     g. Diffuse anterior chest wall heave
     h. S_3 and/or S_4
     i. Any variety of stenotic or regurgitant murmurs

- Diagnostic Tests/Findings
  1. Acute
     a. B-type natriuretic peptide (BNP) levels above 80 pg/mL—may be as high as > 1000 pg/mL
     b. Hypoxemia and hypocapnia on arterial blood gas
     c. Serum basic metabolic panel (BMP) 7 (sodium, potassium, chloride, carbon dioxide, blood urea nitrogen, creatinine, and glucose) usually normal
     d. Urinalysis usually normal
     e. Chest radiograph shows pulmonary edema, Kerley's lines, effusions
     f. Echocardiogram will show contractile, relaxation, and valve function
  2. Chronic
     a. Basic metabolic panel (BMP) may show electrolyte abnormalities
     b. Mild hypoxemia on arterial blood gas— pCO_2 usually normal
     c. Chest radiograph shows redistribution of flow, enlarged heart
     d. Echocardiogram will show contractile, relaxation, and valve function

- Management/Treatment
  1. Of primary importance is identification and treatment of underlying cause
  2. Nonpharmacologic interventions
     a. Sodium/fluid restriction
     b. Rest/activity balance
     c. Weight reduction in the obese
  3. Pharmacologic interventions
     a. Diuretics for all symptomatic patients and those who are not adequately managed with an ACEI/beta-adrenergic antagonist combination
        (1) Furosemide 20–160 mg in 1 or 2 daily doses, treatment of choice
        (2) Hydrochlorothiazide more questionable utility; may augment loops in doses > 25 mg daily
     b. ACEI are mainstays of chronic management
        (1) Captopril 6.25–50 mg 3–4 times daily
        (2) Enalapril 2.5–40 mg daily in 2 divided doses
        (3) Lisinopril 2.5–10 mg daily
     c. Beta-adrenergic antagonists are mainstays of chronic management
        (1) Carvedilol to 25 mg b.i.d.
        (2) Toprol XL to 190 mg q.d.
        (3) Improve function by blocking excessive adrenergic stimulation
     d. Inotropic
        (1) Beneficial in moderate to severe systolic failure
        (2) Digoxin 0.125–0.25 mg daily

    e. Neurohormonal antagonists
      (1) Spironolactone 25 mg daily
      (2) Mediate major effects of renin-an-giotensin-aldosterone activation, e.g., remodeling
    f. Vasodilators—useful as adjunct therapy in heart failure refractory to initial therapies

  4. Application of interventions according to stage
    a. Stage A
      (1) Patients at risk due to disease, cardio-toxins, or family history but no structural disease
      (2) Manage underlying disease
      (3) Control other risk factors
      (4) ACEI as indicated
    b. Stage B
      (1) Patients with structural disease but no symptoms
      (2) All interventions under stage A
      (3) ACEI and beta-adrenergic antagonists as indicated
    c. Stage C
      (1) Patients with structural heart disease and symptoms of failure
      (2) All measures under stage B
      (3) Inotropic agents as indicated
      (4) Dietary sodium restriction 2–2.5 g/day
    d. Stage D
      (1) Refractory heart failure
      (2) All measures under stage C
      (3) Assist devices, heart transplant, hospice as indicated
  5. Patient counseling
    a. Lifestyle modification
    b. Medication toxicities and side effects
  6. Physician consultation
    a. When pharmacologic therapy initiated
    b. When patient unresponsive to initial medications

◘ PERIPHERAL ARTERIAL DISEASE (PAD)

- Definition—narrowing and eventual obstruction of the arterial lumen usually caused by atherosclerosis; occlusion tends to be segmental; result is decreased blood supply to limbs

- Etiology/Incidence—same as those for coronary artery disease

- Signs and Symptoms
  1. Intermittent claudication usually presenting symptom
  2. Distance patient can walk is indicative of degree of circulatory impairment
  3. Cold and/or numbness of the extremity
  4. Pain or ache at night/rest suggestive of severe disease

- Differential Diagnosis
  1. Sciatica
  2. Myopathies
  3. Acute arterial emboli

- Physical Findings
  1. Reduced or absent pulses distal to obstruction
  2. Dependent rubor
  3. Skin pallor or cyanosis
  4. Poor hair/nail growth
  5. Dry ulceration/gangrene in severe disease

- Diagnostic Tests/Findings
  1. Radiography of affected extremity may show calcification
  2. Doppler ultrasound will demonstrate reduced pressures distal to occlusion
  3. Arteriography will show location and extent of block

- Management/Treatment
  1. Control risk factors as much as possible
  2. Tobacco cessation
  3. Walk daily to develop collateral circulation—walking to point of pain followed by a 3-minute rest should be done 8 times daily
  4. Aspirin 80–325 mg has theoretical value and should be given to all patients with severe disease
  5. Cilostazol 100 mg orally b.i.d.—contraindicated in heart failure
  6. Pentoxifylline 400 mg orally t.i.d.
  7. Surgical revascularization

◘ THROMBOPHLEBITIS

- Definition—partial or complete occlusion of a vein by a thrombus with secondary inflammation of venous wall—may be superficial or deep

- Etiology/Incidence
  1. Virchow's triad
    a. Vessel injury
    b. Venous stasis
    c. Hypercoagulation states
  2. Prolonged bed rest
  3. Use of oral contraceptives (particularly in smokers)
  4. Postoperative period
  5. More prevalent in females
  6. Occurs in 800,000 new patients annually

- Signs and Symptoms
  1. Sudden onset of pain (superficial)
  2. Pain, tenderness, ache, or tightness especially with activity (deep)

- Differential Diagnosis
  1. Muscle strain or contusion
  2. Cellulitis
  3. Arterial disease
  4. Lymphatic obstruction

- Physical Findings
  1. Localized heat and erythema (superficial)
  2. Edema distal to occlusion (deep)
  3. Distention of superficial venous collateral vessels
  4. Low-grade temperature
  5. Cool skin
  6. Palpable cords

- Diagnostic Tests/Findings
  1. Doppler ultrasound and impedance plethysmography to evaluate venous flow
  2. Contrast venography is definitive study to identify location and extent

- Management/Treatment
  1. Prevention
     a. Elevation of lower extremities 15–20 degrees
     b. Leg exercises when immobility required
     c. Compression stockings
     d. Anticoagulation
        (1) Low-dose unfractionated heparin
        (2) Low molecular weight heparin
  2. Elevation of extremity and warm compress (superficial)
  3. Bed rest with extremity elevated (deep)
  4. Anticoagulation therapy for deep thrombosis
     a. Heparin infusion for 7–10 days
     b. Coumadin therapy for 12 weeks

CHRONIC VENOUS INSUFFICIENCY

- Definition—impaired venous return with resultant chronic lower-extremity edema

- Etiology/Incidence
  1. Destruction of valves in deep venous channels of lower legs secondary to deep thrombophlebitis
  2. Neoplastic obstruction of pelvic veins
  3. Leg trauma
  4. Sustained elevation of venous pressure
  5. More common in women than men

- Signs and Symptoms
  1. Aching of lower extremities relieved by elevation
  2. Edema at end of day or after prolonged standing
  3. Night cramps

- Differential Diagnosis
  1. Lymphedema
  2. Congestive heart failure
  3. Renal disease
  4. Liver disease

- Physical Findings
  1. Edema of lower extremities
  2. Trophic changes with brownish discoloration
  3. Cool to touch
  4. Thin, shiny, atrophic skin
  5. Wet ulcerations on the medial or anterior aspect of the leg

- Diagnostic Tests/Findings
  1. BUN/creatinine to rule out renal disease
  2. Liver function tests to rule out liver disease
  3. Chest radiograph to rule out congestive heart failure
  4. Doppler ultrasound to rule out thrombosis

- Management/Treatment
  1. Bed rest with legs elevated to diminish chronic edema
  2. Use of elastic stockings
  3. Weight reduction in the obese
  4. Hydrocortisone cream for stasis dermatitis

QUESTIONS

Select the best answer.

1. When is it appropriate to diagnose and treat hypertension based upon one blood pressure reading?

   a. When there is a strong family history
   b. When the diastolic pressure is > 100 mm Hg
   c. When there is target organ damage
   d. When there is suboccipital headache

2. Which of the following is not a cause of secondary hypertension?

   a. Exercise
   b. Thyroid disease
   c. Sleep apnea
   d. Coarctation of the aorta

3. What is the percentage of Caucasian adults afflicted with hypertension?

   a. < 10%
   b. 10–15%
   c. 20–30%
   d. > 50%

4. The patient with chronic hypertension presents with lower-extremity edema, abdominal pain, and fatigue. Physical exam findings reveal a diffuse chest wall heave and displaced point of maximal impulse. This makes you suspicious that the patient has:

   a. Biventricular hypertrophy
   b. Renal vascular stenosis
   c. Hypertensive encephalopathy
   d. Malignant hypertension

5. Which of the following endocrine disorders is not a cause of secondary hypertension?

   a. Cushing's syndrome
   b. Diabetes mellitus
   c. Hyperthyroidism
   d. Addison's disease

6. Pharmacologic therapy should be started in any patient who is diagnosed with hypertension and has end organ damage. Pharmacologic therapy should begin with:

   a. Beta-blockers
   b. Calcium channel blockers
   c. Diuretics
   d. Angiotensin-converting enzyme inhibitors

7. Which of the following medications is the drug of choice for the patient with hypertension and comorbid diabetes mellitus?

   a. Lisinopril 5 mg p.o. q.d.
   b. Furosemide 20 mg p.o. q.d.
   c. Metoprolol 50 mg p.o. b.i.d.
   d. Diltiazem 90 mg p.o. b.i.d.

8. Which of the following is not a risk factor for coronary artery disease?

   a. Stage 2 hypertension
   b. Serum cholesterol of 300 mg/dL
   c. A parent with history of myocardial infarction
   d. African-American ancestry

9. Prinzmetal's angina typically occurs:

   a. During periods of emotional stress
   b. Early in the morning
   c. In men under age 50
   d. In extremes of temperature

10. Your patient complains of chest pain just to the left of the mid-sternal area that occurred while mowing the lawn. As you pursue the history of present illness in an effort to rule out angina, which of the following characteristics of the pain experience makes angina less likely?

    a. The pain was also felt in the back of the neck
    b. The pain felt like a burning sensation
    c. The pain lasted 15 minutes
    d. The pain was a stabbing, knife-like sensation

11. Aortic stenosis can be a contributing cause of coronary artery disease. Which of the following heart sounds is suggestive of aortic stenosis?

    a. A systolic murmur loudest at the second intercostal space, right sternal border
    b. A diastolic murmur loudest at the second intercostal space, left sternal border
    c. An extra heart sound heard early in diastole
    d. An extra heart sound heard early in systole

12. Exercise electrocardiography (ECG) is clinically diagnostic for coronary artery disease. Which of the following is not a positive finding on exercise ECG?

    a. > 2 mm of new S-T segment depression in multiple leads
    b. Decreased systolic blood pressure with exercise
    c. S-T segment depression after start of exercise
    d. Inability to exercise for > 5 minutes

13. You diagnosed coronary artery disease in Mrs. J. 6 months ago. At that time her LDL cholesterol was 130 mg/dL and so your teaching interventions included ways to lower fat in her diet. Today her LDL cholesterol is 125 mg/dL. The most appropriate intervention is to:

    a. Begin lovastatin 10 mg q.d. and reevaluate in 1 month
    b. Continue diet modification and reevaluate in 3 months
    c. Begin enteric coated aspirin 325 mg q.d. and reevaluate in 1 month
    d. Begin cholestyramine 12 gm b.i.d. and reevaluate in 3 months

14. Which of the following pharmacological agents prevents angina by reducing myocardial oxygen demand and inducing coronary vasodilation?

    a. Diltiazem
    b. Isosorbide dinitrate
    c. Atenolol
    d. Aspirin

15. Mr. L. is a 64-year-old patient with difficult-to-control angina. His initial therapy was atenolol 25 mg q.d., and his dose was increased until it was 200 mg daily. When angina persisted, diltiazem 180 mg b.i.d. was added to the regimen, but even the combination of medications is not controlling symptoms. At this point the next appropriate step would be to:

    a. Recommend cardiac angiography
    b. Begin nifedipine 30 mg q.d.
    c. Begin isosorbide dinitrate 10 mg t.i.d.
    d. Recommend radionuclide ventriculography

16. Patients having a myocardial infarction (MI) may report that the chest pain they are experiencing is different from their usual anginal pain. Which of the following is also suspicious for MI rather than angina?

    a. Pain lasting > 15 minutes
    b. Nausea and vomiting
    c. Elevated systolic blood pressure
    d. Presence of S_3 or S_4 heart sounds

17. Which of the following diagnostic findings is most suggestive of myocardial infarction?

    a. 15,000/μL leukocytes
    b. Development of Q waves
    c. S-T segment elevation
    d. Hypoxia on ABG

18. Acute congestive heart failure produces symptoms as a function of the diffusion of water into the pulmonary air spaces. Acute failure is most commonly caused by:

    a. Chronic hypertension
    b. Valvular stenosis
    c. Medication toxicity
    d. Myocardial infarction

19. When increased hydrostatic pressure in the venous system causes water to diffuse into the interstitium, resultant physical findings would most likely include:

    a. Weight gain
    b. S_3 gallop
    c. Coarse rales in all lung fields
    d. Dyspnea at rest

20. Kerley's lines on chest radiography are suggestive of:

    a. Inadequate compensatory mechanisms when cardiac output fails
    b. Hydrostatic pressure increase in the peripheral vascular system
    c. Diffusion of water into pulmonary air spaces
    d. Prinzmetal's angina

21. Congestive heart failure is a syndrome that results when the cardiac output is insufficient to meet the metabolic demands of the body. This can be either an acute or chronic state. Causes of chronic failure include:

    a. Hypertension
    b. Mitral valve rupture
    c. Myocardial infarction
    d. Cardiac ischemia

22. Typical laboratory findings in acute CHF include:

    a. Red blood cells in urinalysis
    b. Blood urea nitrogen (BUN) 70 mg/dL; serum creatinine 2.0 mg/dL
    c. PaO_2 64 mm Hg by arterial blood gas
    d. Redistribution of flow by chest radiography

23. Cardiac glycosides may be useful therapy in congestive heart failure when:

    a. Failure is unresponsive to angiotensin-converting enzyme inhibitors
    b. Failure is severe and refractory to first-line therapies
    c. Failure is due to cardiomyopathy
    d. Failure is severe and refractory to vasodilators

24. Dependent rubor is a physical finding associated with:

    a. Chronic venous insufficiency
    b. Arteriosclerotic occlusive disease
    c. Deep vein thrombosis
    d. Superficial thrombophlebitis

25. Which of the following physical findings is not associated with thrombophlebitis?

    a. Low-grade temperature
    b. Cool skin
    c. Heat and erythema
    d. Reduced or absent peripheral pulses

26. Edema of the lower extremities is a physical finding associated with a variety of medical conditions. A diagnosis of chronic venous insufficiency is made when other causes are ruled out. When chronic venous insufficiency is diagnosed, the appropriate treatment includes:

    a. Heparin infusion for 7–10 days
    b. Use of elastic stockings
    c. Aspirin 325 mg daily
    d. Surgical revascularization

27. Mr. H. is a 32-year-old male who presents for a job-related physical. Cholesterol screening reveals serum LDL of 190 mg/dL. The appropriate action would be:

    a. Implement diet and lifestyle changes and reevaluate in 3 months
    b. Begin drug therapy with an HMG coenzyme A reductase inhibitor
    c. Repeat the lipid panel in 1 week before beginning interventions
    d. Begin drug therapy with niacin

Answers

1.	**c**	15.	**c**
2.	**a**	16.	**b**
3.	**b**	17.	**b**
4.	**a**	18.	**d**
5.	**d**	19.	**a**
6.	**c**	20.	**c**
7.	**a**	21.	**a**
8.	**d**	22.	**c**
9.	**b**	23.	**a**
10.	**d**	24.	**b**
11.	**a**	25.	**d**
12.	**d**	26.	**b**
13.	**a**	27.	**a**
14.	**a**		

◻ BIBLIOGRAPHY

Adams, K. F., Lindenfeld, J., Arnold, J. M. O., Baker, D. W., Barnard, D. H., Baughman, K. L., Boehmer, J. P. . . . Wagoner, L. E. (2006). Executive summary: HFSA 2006 comprehensive heart failure practice guideline. *Journal of Cardiac Failure 12*(1), 10–38.

American College of Cardiology/American Heart Association. (2005). ACC/AHA 2005 guideline update for the diagnosis and management of chronic heart failure in the adult: A report of the American College of Cardiology/American Heart Association task force on practice guidelines (writing committee to update the 2001 guidelines for the evaluation and management of heart failure). Retrieved from http://www.acc.org /clinical/guidelines/failure/update/index.pdf

Bashore, T. M., Granger, C. B., Hranitzky, P., & Patel, M. R. (2012). Heart disease. In S. J. McPhee, & M. A. Papadakis (Eds.), *Current medical diagnosis and treatment* (51st ed.). New York: McGraw-Hill.

Chobanian, A. V. (2007). Isolated systolic hypertension in the elderly. *New England Journal of Medicine, 357,* 780–796.

Crawford, M. H. (2009). *Current diagnosis and treatment in cardiology* (3rd ed.). New York: McGraw-Hill.

Gey, D. C., Lesho, E. P., & Manngold, J. (2004). Management of peripheral arterial disease. *American Family Physician, 69,* 525–532, 533.

Harmel, A. P., & Berra, K. (2003). Impact of new national cholesterol education program (NCEP) guidelines on patient management. *Journal of the American Academy of Nurse Practitioners, 15*(8), 350–360.

Levy, P. J. (2002). Epidemiology and pathophysiology of peripheral arterial disease. *Clinical Cornerstone, 4,* 1–15.

Mann, S. J. (2004). Interview—An overlooked cause of refractory hypertension. *The Clinical Advisor, 7*(2), 28–36.

National Cholesterol Education Program. (2004). Third report of the Expert Panel on Detection, Evaluation, and Treatment of High Blood Cholesterol in Adults (Adult Treatment Panel III) 2004 update. Retrieved from http://www.nhlbi.nih.gov/guidelines/cholesterol /index.htm

National Heart, Lung, and Blood Institute. (2003). Seventh report of the Joint National Committee on Prevention, Detection, Evaluation, and Treatment of High Blood Pressure (JNC 7) Express. NIH Publication No. 5233. Bethesda, MD: National Institutes of Health.

Sutters, M. (2012). Systemic hypertension. In S. J. McPhee, & M. A. Papadakis (Eds.), *Current medical diagnosis and treatment* (51st ed.). New York: McGraw-Hill.

Zepf, B. (2001). Diagnosis and treatment of venous stasis ulcers. *American Family Physician, 64,* 1452.

7

Hematological and Oncological Disorders

Sister Maria Salerno

◘ COMMON ANEMIAS

- Anemia describes a symptom of abnormally low red blood cell (RBC) count, quality of hemoglobin, and/or volume of packed cells. The World Health Organization defines it in terms of peripheral blood hemoglobin < 13 grams (g) [hematocrit < 45%] for men and < 12 grams [hematocrit < 37%] for women. Anemias are classified based upon red cell morphology (microcytic, normocytic, or macrocytic) and are further described based upon the amount of pigment red blood cells contain (hypochromic, normochromic) and/or underlying etiology.

◘ MICROCYTIC ANEMIAS (MCV < 80μ³)

- Because the majority of the mature RBC volume is hemoglobin, abnormalities of hemoglobin cause a low mean cell volume (MCV); consequently, microcytic anemias are anemias characterized by hemoglobin abnormalities.

◘ IRON DEFICIENCY ANEMIA

- Definition—a microcytic, hypochromic anemia with an MCV < 80μ³ caused by insufficient iron for hemoglobin synthesis

- Etiology/Incidence
  1. Slow, persistent blood loss is the most common cause of iron deficiency anemia in adults; specific causes include menorrhagia, gastritis, aspirin ingestion, polyps, GI neoplasms, peptic ulcer disease, and esophageal varices
  2. Inadequate iron intake (< 1–2 mg/day), e.g., infants on milk-only diets, persons on vegetarian diets, alcoholics, pregnant women, or adolescents whose demand is increased
  3. Impaired absorption of iron, e.g., after gastrectomy, in Celiac disease
  4. Slow, persistent blood loss, e.g., menorrhagia, gastritis, aspirin ingestion, polyps, GI neoplasms, peptic ulcer disease, esophageal varices, hemorrhoids; in adult males and postmenopausal females, acute or chronic hemorrhage is most common cause
  5. One of the most common anemias throughout the world; particularly prevalent in women of childbearing age; estimated 20% of adult women, 50% of pregnant women, and 3% of adult males in the United States have iron deficiency

- Signs and Symptoms
  1. Depend on
     a. Rate at which anemia develops
     b. Age of the individual
     c. Individual's compensatory mechanisms
     d. Activity level
     e. Underlying disease state
     f. Severity of the anemia
  2. General signs and symptoms
     a. Easily fatigued
     b. Dyspnea on exertion

   c.   Dizziness
   d.   Listlessness
   e.   Pallor (conjunctiva, nail beds, mucous membranes)
   f.   Faintness
   g.   Weakness
   h.   Headaches
   i.   Tachycardia
   j.   Wide pulse pressure
   k.   Heart murmurs
   l.   Myocardial hypertrophy
   m.   Angina
   n.   Anorexia
   3.   Findings specific to iron deficiency anemia
   a.   Pica
   b.   Brittle, dry hair
   c.   Flat or concave nail beds

- Differential Diagnosis
   1.   Thalassemia
   2.   Sideroblastic anemia
   3.   Anemia of chronic disease
   4.   Lead poisoning

- Physical Findings
   1.   May be normal without overt findings in mild anemia
   2.   General appearance—pale, lethargic
   3.   Vital signs—pulse and respirations may be increased in moderate to severe anemia; in severe cases postural hypotension may be evident
   4.   Integumentary—pallor and dryness of skin and mucous membranes; brittle, flattened, ridged, concave, or spoon-shaped nails (koilonychia); brittle, fine hair
   5.   Cardiovascular—tachycardia, mild cardiac enlargement; functional systolic murmurs in severe anemias
   6.   Abdominal—may be some hepatic enlargement
   7.   Neurological—usually within normal limits

- Diagnostic Tests/Findings
   1.   See **Tables 7-1** and **7-2** for laboratory tests used in diagnosis of common anemias
   2.   Routine CBC (with peripheral smear)
   a.   Hemoglobin—< 13 g/dL in males; < 12 g/dL in females
   b.   Hematocrit (Hct)—< 45% in males; < 37% in females
   c.   Low MCV (microcytic) and mean corpuscular hemoglobin concentration (MCHC) (hypochromic)
   d.   Increased red cell distribution width (RDW) (>15%)
   3.   Iron status determinants—serum ferritin is considered the most sensitive and most specific for iron deficiency; bone marrow studies

are done if the diagnosis is unclear and/or there is a lack of response to a 3-week therapeutic trial
   a.   High total iron binding capacity (TIBC)— usually normal or low in anemia of chronic disease (ACD)
   b.   Low serum ferritin < 12 μg/L—infection, chronic disease, and liver disease may raise ferritin levels and mask coexisting iron deficiency; in these cases a serum ferritin level < 30 μg/L is consistent with iron deficiency
   c.   Serum iron—low < 50 μg/dL; may be normal in early stages (oral contraceptives may cause false elevation)
   d.   Low serum transferrin saturation—< 20%
   e.   Bone marrow studies
      (1)   Show depletion of iron (on staining), normocytic hyperplasia
      (2)   Usually not part of initial workup

- Management/Treatment
   1.   Diagnostic
   a.   Once diagnosis is established underlying cause must be identified and, if possible, corrected; bleeding must be suspected in the absence of clearly identifiable nutritional intake deficiency or increased body need
   b.   Search for infection, trauma, neoplasm, GI disorders
   c.   Stool guaiac, bilirubin, and additional studies may be needed to establish etiology
   d.   Obtain physician consult on any patient with
      (1)   Hct < 25%
      (2)   Positive stool guaiac or history of bleeding
      (3)   Family history of anemia
      (4)   Suspected underlying inflammatory, infectious, or malignant disease
      (5)   Failure to respond to iron supplementation
   2.   Therapeutic
   a.   Oral iron replacement
      (1)   Oral is safer and much less expensive than IM or IV
      (2)   Begin 6-month trial of ferrous sulfate tablets, 300–325 mg (depending on brand) 3 times a day after meals
      (3)   Determine effectiveness of iron replacement therapy during the first 2 weeks of therapy (increased reticulocyte count)
      (4)   Refer those on oral iron replacement therapy to a physician if 2 g/100 mL increase in Hgb is not seen in 3–4 weeks;

■ **Table 7-1** Common Laboratory Tests Used in Diagnosing Anemia

Hematocrit (Hct)	Relative amount of plasma to total red blood cell mass; measure of RBC concentration. Normal 40–54% males; 38–47% females (Hct typically 3 × Hgb, e.g., Hgb 12 g/dL = Hct 36%)
Hemoglobin (Hgb)	Basic screening test for anemia; main component of erythrocytes; vehicle for transport of O_2 and CO_2; normal 13.5–18 g/100 mL males; 12–15 g/100 mL females
Red blood cell count (RBC)	Measure of number of Hgb-carrying red blood cells (RBC, erythrocytes); needed to calculate other RBC indices
Mean corpuscular volume (MCV)	Mathematical measure of average RBC size; expressed in micro cubic millimeters; value classifies cells as microcytic, normocytic, macrocytic; normal 80–100μ^3
Mean corpuscular Hgb (MCH)	Mathematical measure of hemoglobin concentration of average RBC; expressed in picograms; calculated by dividing Hgb in grams by number of RBC; allows for classification of RBC as hypochromic, normochromic; normal 27–31 pg/cell
Mean corpuscular Hgb concentration (MCHC)	Mathematical measure of concentration of Hgb in grams per 100 mL of RBC; normal 32–36 g/dL or 32–36%; little help in identifying hypochromia or microcytosis
Red cell distribution width (RDW)	Mathematical coefficient of width variation in red cell size—RDW increase indicates greater variation in cell size; normal RDW 11–15%
Serum iron (SI)	Concentration of iron bound to transferrin; inverse correlation with TIBC; normal 50–150 μg/dL in adults; insensitive to early iron deficiency
Total iron binding capacity (TIBC)	Measures amount of iron that transferrin can still bind; inverse correlation with serum iron; normal 250–450 μg/dL in adults
Bilirubin (indirect)	Fractionation of total bilirubin; reflects breakdown of hemoglobin; elevated levels indicate hemolysis
% Transferrin saturation w(% SAT)	100 × SI/TIBC; low sensitivity for iron deficiency; normal 20–50%
Serum ferritin	Correlates roughly with total iron stores; no diurnal variation; not affected by exogenous ingestion or injection, or specimen contamination; most sensitive and specific for iron deficiency; normal males 12–300 μg/L; females 12–150 μg/L (McPherson & Pinkus, 2007)
Coombs indirect	Detects free antibodies in patient's serum and certain RBC antigens
Peripheral blood smear	Smear of whole blood stained with Wright's stain; variations in cell morphology and staining characteristics important to diagnosis of hematologic conditions
Bone marrow	Marrow aspirated for microscopic examination; indicated when anemia not obviously due to iron deficiency; iliac crest preferred to sternum site

NOTE: Laboratory reference ranges differ among laboratories. Check normal values in each laboratory where tests are conducted.

■ **Table 7-2** Select Morphological and Etiologic Categories of Anemia and Related Laboratory Findings

	Macrocytic (MCV > 100)		Microcytic (MCV < 80)		Normocytic (MCV 80–100)
	B_{12} Deficiency	*Folate Deficiency*	*Iron Deficiency*	*Thalassemia*	*Anemia of Chronic Disease*
MCH	normal	normal	low	low	normal
Fe	high	high	normal/low	normal/sl, high	low-high
TIBC	normal	normal	high	normal	normal/low
Ferritin	high	high	low	normal	normal/high
B_{12}	low	normal	normal	normal	normal
Folate	normal	low	normal	normal/low	normal/low

in uncomplicated iron deficiency, a 1 g per week increase is expected
  (5) Levels return to normal within 2 months, 3–6 months more needed to replace stores
  (6) Response failure usually due to non-compliance
 b. Parenteral iron is indicated if patient can not tolerate or absorb oral iron or if iron loss exceeds oral replacement; IM or IV iron dextran is used (very rarely needed or used)
  (1) More expensive
  (2) Associated with significant side effects
   (a) Anaphylaxis
   (b) Phlebitis
   (c) Regional lymphadenopathy
   (d) Serum-sickness-type reaction
   (e) Staining of IM injection sites
  (3) Dose based on the patient's weight
3. Education
 a. Cause of iron deficiency and treatment plan
 b. Purpose, dosage, side effects, toxic effects of iron replacement
  (1) Side effects of nausea, GI irritation, constipation, diarrhea, and black stools
  (2) Food and fluid taken concurrently may interfere with absorption but may be warranted to alleviate gastric distress
  (3) Taking with orange juice or other source of vitamin C (ascorbic acid) will enhance absorption
  (4) Milk and antacids will interfere with absorption
  (5) Monitor and discuss with patients concurrent use of over-the-counter medications—some products such as urine and stool deodorizers often used by elderly with incontinence problems can lead to iron overdose and heart failure
  (6) Therapy should continue for 6 or more months to replenish tissue stores
 c. Medication should be kept out of reach of children as iron overdose can be fatal to them
 d. Nutrition—foods high in iron include organ and lean meats, egg yolk, shellfish, apricots, peaches, prunes, grapes, raisins, green leafy vegetables, iron-fortified breads and cereals
 e. Activity—frequent rest periods as needed

◘ THALASSEMIA

- Definition—thalassemia is a group of genetic inherited syndromes of abnormal hemoglobin synthesis
- Etiology/Incidence
 1. Inherited, autosomal recessive disorder that results in impaired synthesis of either one or more of the alpha or beta chain of adult hemoglobin; four genes control alpha chain production, two control beta chain production
 2. Second most common cause of microcytic anemia
  a. Alpha thalassemia more common in African-Americans, Chinese, Vietnamese, Cambodians, and Laotians
  b. Beta thalassemia more common in those of Mediterranean descent (Italians, Greeks, some Arabs, and Sephardic Jews)
 3. In United States more common than iron deficiency in African-Americans, Asian Americans, and Italian Americans

- Signs and Symptoms—the severity of the anemia can range from mild to severe depending on the number of hemoglobin-controlling genes involved; forms seen in adults include
 1. Alpha trait (carrier state) (one of four alpha chain-forming genes affected)—usually asymptomatic
 2. Alpha-thalassemia minor (two of four alpha chain-forming genes affected) and Beta-thalassemia minor (heterozygous form)—both are usually asymptomatic and have mild presentations with mild to moderate microcytic, hypochromic anemia, enlarged liver and spleen, bronze coloring of the skin, and bone marrow hyperplasia
 3. Beta-thalassemia major (homozygous form affecting both beta chain-forming genes) also called Cooley's anemia—severe anemia with significant cardiovascular burden; high output congestive failure is common; fractures related to bone marrow expansion; retarded growth and maturation; in addition to general signs and symptoms presented in section on Iron Deficiency Anemia
 4. Hemoglobin H disease (three of four alpha hemoglobin chain-forming genes affected)—occurs predominantly in Chinese; moderate to severe microcytic anemia with splenomegaly

- Differential Diagnosis
 1. Iron deficiency anemia
 2. Sideroblastic anemia
 3. Anemia of chronic disease
 4. Lead poisoning—not common in adults unless occupation related

- Physical Findings—will generally be within normal limits unless the more severe forms of thalassemia are encountered
 1. General appearance—pallor or bronze appearance; mild listlessness
 2. Abdominal—enlarged liver, enlarged spleen

3. Cardiovascular—tachycardia, widened pulse pressure, systolic murmur if anemia is moderate or severe
4. Respiratory—may have increased respiratory rate
5. Musculoskeletal—some bone deformity of the face (chipmunk deformity) related to expansion of bones caused by hyperplastic marrow
6. Neurologic—within normal limits

- Diagnostic Tests/Findings
  1. Hgb—decreased
  2. MCV—lower than in iron deficiency
  3. Serum iron—normal or increased
  4. TIBC—normal
  5. Ferritin—normal or increased
  6. RDW—normal
  7. Hemoglobin electrophoresis—demonstrates decreased alpha or beta hemoglobin chains
  8. Peripheral smear will show microcytosis, variable hypochromia, target cells (thin, fragile RBC), basophilic stippling
  9. Skull and skeletal radiographs—widened marrow spaces in skull and long bones; osteoporosis

- Management/Treatment
  1. No specific treatment for mild to moderate forms
  2. Iron supplementation generally contraindicated in all thalassemias since iron overload can result—patients with alpha trait and co-existing iron deficiency should be referred to physician for iron supplementation
  3. Chronic folate supplementation is used in certain circumstances; should be initiated by hematology
  4. Severe forms should be referred to a hematologist for treatment, which often includes transfusions and chelation therapy to avoid fatal iron overload (hemochromatosis)
  5. Refer for genetic counseling
  6. Stress overall good nutrition without additional iron supplementation
  7. Discuss signs and symptoms of iron overload
     a. Weakness/lassitude
     b. Loss of body hair
     c. Weight loss
     d. Palmar erythema
     e. Gynecomastia
     f. Loss of libido
     g. Abdominal pain
     h. Thinning, darkening skin
     i. Pain and or stiffness in joints
     j. Blurred vision or other symptoms related to onset of diabetes
     k. Shortness of breath
     l. Swelling in ankles

8. Document findings to avoid
   a. Unnecessary repeated workups
   b. Inappropriate iron supplementation

▢ MACROCYTIC ANEMIAS (MCV > 100μ³)

- Unlike microcytic anemias, macrocytic anemias are not characterized by hemoglobin abnormalities—hemoglobin synthesis is unimpaired; the etiology centers around inadequate red blood cell synthesis, and consequently macrocytic anemias are typically characterized by a low red blood cell count—each existing red blood cell is packed to excess with hemoglobin, resulting in macrocytosis.

▢ PERNICIOUS ANEMIA

- Definition—a megaloblastic, macrocytic, normochromic anemia caused by a deficiency of intrinsic factor produced by the stomach that results in malabsorption of vitamin B_{12} necessary for DNA synthesis and maturation of RBC

- Etiology/Incidence
  1. Typically occurs secondary to other factors, which lead to decreased production of intrinsic factor or decreased absorption of B_{12}
     a. Loss of parietal cells post-gastrectomy
     b. Overgrowth of intestinal organisms
     c. Ileal resection or abnormalities
     d. Fish tapeworm
     e. Congenital enzyme deficiencies
  2. Less commonly due to an autoimmune reaction involving the gastric parietal cell that results in nonproduction of intrinsic factor and atrophy of gastric mucosa
  3. Vegans with no oral B_{12} supplementation also at risk
  4. Common in Caucasians of Northern European descent
  5. Both sexes equally affected
  6. Usually presents around age 60
  7. Increased incidence in those with other autoimmune disease, e.g., hypothyroidism

- Signs and Symptoms
  1. Weakness
  2. Sore tongue or glossitis
  3. Peripheral paresthesia—numbness, burning, tingling
  4. Palpitations
  5. Dizziness
  6. Swelling of legs
  7. Anorexia
  8. Diarrhea
  9. Mucositis
  10. Dementia and spinal cord degeneration in advanced stages

- Differential Diagnosis
  1. Folate deficiency
  2. Anemia of liver disease
  3. Myelodysplastic syndromes

- Physical Findings
  1. Vital signs—temperature may be slightly elevated, wide pulse pressure, pulse and respirations may be elevated if anemia is severe
  2. General appearance—premature aging; premature graying of hair
  3. HEENT—smooth beefy red tongue; sclera and skin may be slightly icteric
  4. Cardiovascular—systolic flow murmur, tachycardia, and cardiomegaly if anemia is severe
  5. Abdomen—hepatomegaly and splenomegaly may be evident
  6. Neurological—deep tendon reflexes increased or decreased; diminished position sense; poor or absent vibratory sense in lower extremities; ataxia; poor finger-nose coordination; positive Romberg and Babinski; mental status changes ranging from mild forgetfulness and irritability to psychotic behavior (only form of anemia to produce neurologic findings early in disease; neurologic changes may precede anemia)

- Diagnostic Tests/Findings
  1. Hgb and Hct—decreased
  2. RBC—decreased
  3. Reticulocytes—normal or low with anisocytosis and poikilocytosis
  4. MCV—increased > 100 μ^3 (usually markedly increased)
  5. MCHC—normal
  6. Serum B_{12}— may be decreased < 100 pg/mL; however, normal serum B_{12} does not preclude diagnosis
  7. Increased LDH
  8. Serum folate and/or RBC level—normal or decreased
  9. Elevated methylmalonate (MMA) levels
  10. Parietal cell antibodies may be present
  11. Urinalysis—increased urobilinogen
  12. WBC and platelet count decreased in severe cases

- Management/Treatment
  1. Diagnostic—consult with physician regarding those
     a. With other autoimmune diseases
     b. With a history of B_{12} replacement
     c. Suspected of having pernicious anemia for further testing, e.g., those with neurological symptoms but without macrocytosis or overt anemia; might include

     (1) GI radiographic studies
     (2) Gastric analysis—absence of free hydrochloric acid after histamine or pentagastrin injection
     (3) Bone marrow aspiration—hyperplastic, megaloblastic marrow
  2. Therapeutic
     a. B_{12} (cyanocobalamin) 100 μg IM daily for 1 week; decrease frequency and administer a total of 2,000 μg during the first 6 weeks of therapy; maintenance treatment requires lifelong administration of 100 μg IM monthly
     b. In select cases, oral cobalamin in high doses (1,000 μg per day) can replace parenteral for maintenance, but must be taken daily and consistently
     c. If anemia is severe may need K^+ supplementation to avoid hypokalemia
     d. Follow up elderly and those with cardiovascular symptoms 48 hours after initiating therapy; rapid increase in RBC production can lead to hypervolemia in these persons
     e. Consider concomitant iron supplementation during first month of therapy; rapid blood cell regeneration increases iron requirement and may lead to iron deficiency
  3. Education
     a. Teach client about etiology and nature of the disease
     b. Discuss need for lifelong B_{12} replacement by injection
     c. Provide client with information on side effects of B_{12} injections
        (1) Pain and burning at injection site
        (2) Peripheral vascular thrombosis
        (3) Transient diarrhea
     d. CNS symptoms/signs are reversible if present < 6 months prior to treatment
     e. Teach client or family member to administer injections or refer to home care agency to provide injections
     f. Teach comfort and safety measures to clients with neurological involvement (can be arrested but not reversed with treatment)
  4. Follow-up—check initial hematologic response in 4–6 weeks; then every 6 months for Hct and stool for occult blood; endoscopy every 5 years; incidence of gastric cancer increased in persons with pernicious anemia

◘ FOLIC ACID DEFICIENCY ANEMIA

- Definition—macrocytic, normochromic, megaloblastic anemia caused by a deficiency of folic acid needed for DNA synthesis, RBC maturation, and maintenance of gastric mucosa

- Etiology/Incidence
  1. Inadequate intake may be relative to malabsorption syndrome or increased demand as in pregnancy and infancy; body stores depleted more rapidly than B_{12}
  2. Drugs that may cause decreased folic acid levels include oral contraceptives, phenytoin, antimalarials, estrogen, chloramphenicol, phenobarbital, trimethoprim/sulfamethoxazole, and sulfasalazine
  3. Found in all races and in all age groups
  4. More common than pernicious anemia, especially in alcoholics and other chronically malnourished persons, e.g., anorexics, many elderly, and those who do not eat fresh fruits and vegetables (especially green leafy) or overcook them

- Signs and Symptoms
  1. Similar to those of B_{12} deficiency but more severe; neurological signs are absent
  2. General signs and symptoms
     a. Easily fatigued
     b. Dyspnea on exertion
     c. Dizziness
     d. Listlessness
     e. Pallor (conjunctiva, nail beds, mucous membranes)
     f. Faintness
     g. Weakness
     h. Headaches
     i. Tachycardia
     j. Wide pulse pressure
     k. Heart murmurs
     l. Myocardial hypertrophy
     m. Angina
     n. Anorexia
     o. Pica

- Differential Diagnosis
  1. Pernicious anemia
  2. Anemia of liver disease
  3. Myelodysplastic syndromes

- Physical Findings—similar to those found in most anemias
  1. General appearance—pale, lethargic, or no overt signs if anemia is mild
  2. Vital signs—pulse and respirations may be increased in moderate to severe anemia; in severe cases postural hypotension may be evident
  3. Integumentary—pallor and dryness of skin and mucous membranes; brittle nails; brittle, fine hair
  4. HEENT—glossitis, angular stomatitis or cheilitis; pale conjunctiva and gums
  5. Cardiovascular—tachycardia; mild cardiac enlargement; functional systolic murmurs in severe anemias
  6. Abdominal—may be some hepatic enlargement
  7. Neurological—usually within normal limits

- Diagnostic Tests/Findings
  1. Hct—decreased
  2. MCV—elevated
  3. MCHC—normal
  4. RBC folate level—< 150 ng/mL and/or RBC level decreased
  5. Serum folate—< 3 ng/mL; less reliable than RBC folate
  6. MMA—normal
  7. Serum B_{12}—normal
  8. Parietal cell antibodies absent

- Management/Treatment
  1. Diagnostic—consult with physician regarding clients with suspected folate deficiency for differential diagnosis of concurrent B_{12} deficiency and treatment
  2. Therapeutic—folate 1 mg orally or parenterally per day
     a. Duration of treatment dependent on etiology and its elimination
     b. If related to malabsorption (e.g., sprue) up to 5 mg/day—very high doses of folate may be toxic and should only be ordered by hematology
     c. Large doses of folic acid will correct hematologic abnormalities of B_{12} deficiency but not arrest neurological abnormalities
  3. Education—especially important for women of childbearing age as deficiency during first trimester is associated with neural tube defects in the fetus
     a. Nature and cause of anemia
     b. Need for and purpose of therapeutic replacement
     c. Teach dietary sources of folic acid, which include asparagus, bananas, fish, green leafy vegetables, peanut butter, oatmeal, red beans, beef liver, wheat bran
        (1) Encourage daily intake from these foods
        (2) Instructions in preparation as overcooking can destroy folic acid
        (3) Provide client with list of foods high in folic acid
     d. Need for frequent rest periods until anemia is corrected
     e. Importance of good oral hygiene
  4. Follow-up
     a. Check initial hematologic response with Hct and in 4–6 weeks

(1) Hct begins to rise after the second week

(2) Total correction expected within 2 months

b.   Individuals with a good response can be followed every 6–12 months if they must continue therapy

◻ NORMOCYTIC ANEMIAS (MCV 80–100 μ³)

- Normocytic anemias are characterized neither by hemoglobin or red blood cell abnormalities; therefore cell volume is normal.

◻ ANEMIA OF CHRONIC DISEASE (ACD)

- Definition—a chronic, normochromic, normocytic, hypoproliferative anemia associated with chronic inflammatory disease, e.g., systemic lupus, rheumatoid arthritis; infection, e.g., bacterial endocarditis, tuberculosis, AIDS, Crohn's disease, and some malignancies; *often progresses to a hypochromic anemia*

- Etiology/Incidence
  1.   Etiology not fully understood but involves decreased erythrocyte life span, ineffective erythropoiesis, and disturbances of the iron cycle
  2.   Most common cause of hypoproliferative, normocytic anemia
  3.   Exact incidence unknown, however, association with so many other disorders probably ranks it second to iron deficiency in incidence

- Sign and Symptoms
  1.   General symptoms common to all anemias such as fatigue, weakness, exertional dyspnea, lightheadedness, and anorexia
  2.   Usually fewer and milder than most other anemias; Hgb rarely drops below 9 g/dL
  3.   Other signs and symptoms are usually related to the specific underlying disease and may be more overt than those of anemia

- Differential Diagnosis
  1.   Aplastic anemia
  2.   Pure red blood cell aplasia
  3.   Infiltration marrow diseases
  4.   Exclude reversible causes

- Physical Findings
  1.   General appearance—may appear thin, pale, toxic
  2.   Signs of underlying chronic disorder may dominate
  3.   Vital signs—increased pulse and respirations
  4.   Skin—may be pale, jaundiced, moist

  5.   HEENT—sclera may be icteric, tongue may be coated
  6.   Cardiovascular—cardiomegaly, tachycardia, systolic murmurs
  7.   Abdomen—splenomegaly, hepatomegaly

- Diagnostic Tests/Findings
  1.   Hct—low
  2.   Hgb—low (if < 9 g/dL consider other causes)
  3.   MCV—normal or slightly reduced
  4.   Serum iron—low
  5.   TIBC—normal or low
  6.   Serum ferritin—normal or increased
  7.   Percentage of iron saturation (Fe/TIBC)—30% or more rules out iron deficiency

- Management/Treatment
  1.   Treatment of associated disease
  2.   Adequate nutritional intake; use of B_{12}, folic acid, and liver extract have not been effective in treatment of this type of anemia
  3.   Adequate rest
  4.   Consult with physician regarding clients with suspected anemia of chronic disease for further testing (bone marrow biopsy), and treatment of underlying disorder
  5.   Education—patient education will most likely be centered on etiology and treatment of the underlying chronic disease and its relationship to anemia
  6.   Follow-up—will depend on identified etiology
  7.   Erythropoietin alfa intravenous or subcutaneous is reserved for those who are transfusion dependent or those for whom the quality of life would be greatly improved by the hematologic response

◻ SICKLE CELL ANEMIA

- Definition—a chronic hemolytic anemia characterized by sickle-shaped RBC

- Etiology/Incidence
  1.   Autosomal recessive genetic disorder; individual is homozygous for hemoglobin (Hb SS)
  2.   Abnormal hemoglobin (Hb S) develops in place of hemoglobin A (Hb A)
  3.   Some individuals may have sickle cell trait (heterozygous with about one-fourth of their hemoglobin in abnormal S form and remainder as normal A)
  4.   Mutation that causes Hb S to develop involves one amino acid; one valine amino acid is substituted for a glutamic acid
  5.   Prevalent in black persons of African or African-American ancestry; also found at a lower frequency in persons of Mediterranean ancestry

- Signs and Symptoms
  1. Sickle cell trait
     a. Essentially asymptomatic except in extreme conditions
     b. Symptoms from vaso-occlusion occur only in cases of severe hypoxia
  2. Sickle cell anemia
     a. Manifestations due to anemia, vaso-occlusive events, and to secondary end organ damage
        (1) Osteomyelitis
        (2) Retinopathy
        (3) Renal disease—hematuria
        (4) Cardiomegaly
        (5) Nonpalpable spleen in adults
     b. Increased susceptibility to infection
     c. Vaso-occlusive crises
        (1) Due to an increased rate of sickling
        (2) Precipitating factors include conditions that cause hypoxia or deoxygenation of the RBC, e.g., viral or bacterial infections, high altitudes, emotional or physical stress, surgery, blood loss, dehydration; occasionally crisis occurs spontaneously
        (3) Episodes characterized by sudden onset of excruciating pain in back, chest, or extremities
        (4) Occasionally low-grade fever may occur 1–2 days following attack
        (5) Pain may last from hours to days
        (6) Severe abdominal pain with vomiting may be present

- Differential Diagnosis
  1. Acute pulmonary infarction without sickle beta thalassemia
  2. Anemia from other causes
     a. Sickle thalassemia
     b. Hemoglobin C disorders
        (1) Milder onset and course than sickle cell anemia
        (2) No Hb S on electrophoresis
  3. Acute hepatitis
  4. Choledocholithiasis
  5. Cholecystitis

- Physical Findings
  1. During vaso-occlusive crises, there may be no external findings such as heat, swelling, or tenderness over the affected bones; if bone infarction occurs close to a joint, an effusion can develop
  2. Chronic findings
     a. Skin ulcers/jaundice
     b. Mild scleral icterus; retinal hemorrhage or detachment, neovascularization
     c. Cardiomegaly, systolic murmur
     d. Hepatomegaly
     e. Degenerative arthritis

- Diagnostic Tests/Findings
  1. Peripheral smear
     a. Sickle cell trait—normal
     b. Sickle cell anemia—partially or completely sickled cells
  2. Sickle cell preparation/sickledex
     a. Sickle cell trait—sickle cells
     b. Sickle cell anemia—sickle cells
     c. Used for initial screening
     d. Cannot differentiate between anemia/trait
  3. Hemoglobin electrophoresis
     a. Sickle cell trait—Hb S and Hb A
     b. Sickle cell anemia—Hb S
     c. Used for confirmation and discrimination between anemia/trait
  4. MCV normal (low if beta thalassemia is also present)

- Management/Treatment
  1. Physician referral for suspected cases and consultation for management
  2. Therapeutic—primarily supportive
     a. Chronic folic acid supplementation
     b. Use of cytotoxic agents to reduce frequency of painful episodes
     c. Antibiotic prophylaxis
  3. In acute painful episodes
     a. Analgesia
     b. Large volume IV fluids
     c. Oxygen to treat hypoxia
     d. Antibiotics to treat associated bacterial infections
     e. Blood transfusions reserved for aplastic or hemolytic crises and during third trimester of pregnancy
  4. Patient education
     a. Basis of disease and reasons for supportive care
     b. Methods to avoid crises
     c. Pain control
     d. Availability of support groups
  5. Referral for genetic counseling of identified heterozygotes (sickle cell trait) and prenatal diagnostic services for pregnancies at risk for sickle cell anemia

◘ LEUKEMIA

- Definition—acquired, neoplastic, myeloproliferative disorder of hematopoietic stem cells

- Etiology/Incidence
  1. In most cases no known cause can be found

2. Possible causes include
   a. Exposure to ionizing radiation and certain chemicals, e.g., benzene, prior exposure to alkylating agents
   b. Genetic and congenital factors
3. Incidence of all leukemias is approximately 13 per 100,000 per year
4. More frequent in males than females

- General features of the four common forms of leukemia are shown in **Table 7-3**

- Differential Diagnosis
  1. Viral-induced cytopenia, lymphadenopathy
  2. Immune or drug-induced cytopenia
  3. Aplastic anemia

- Diagnostic Tests/Findings (see Table 7-3)
  1. CBC/differential—subnormal RBC, neutrophils, and occasionally subnormal platelets
  2. Sedimentation rate—elevated
  3. Reticulocyte count—< 0.5%
  4. Bone marrow studies—confirmatory for final diagnosis
  5. Chest radiograph—identification of mediastinal mass
  6. Ultrasound or CT—organomegaly

- Management/Treatment
  1. Physician referral for suspected cases
     a. Goal of treatment is remission
     b. Chemotherapy
     c. Bone marrow transplantation

■ **Table 7-3** Comparison of Most Common Types of Leukemia

Type	Age of Onset	Signs and Symptoms Physical Findings	Diagnostic Tests/Findings	Prognosis
Acute lymphocytic (ALL)	Childhood; more gradual rise in frequency in later life; 20% of acute adult	Fever; pallor, bleeding; anorexia; fatigue; generalized lymphadenopathy and infection, joint pain, etc.	Cytopenia, pancytopenia WBC—H, L, or N RBC, Hgb, Hct-L Platelets-L Bone marrow-lymphoblasts	Good response to treatment; 80% of adults have complete remission
Acute myelogenous (AML) or nonlymphocytic (ANLL)	Increase with age; 50% under age of 50	Fatigue; weakness; headache; mouth sores; bleeding; fever; sternal tenderness; occasional lymphadenopathy	RBC, Hgb, Hct-L Platelet ct—very low WBC—H to L Myeloblasts—many	Remission rates range from 50–85%; patients > 50 years are less likely to achieve complete remission
Chronic lymphocytic (CLL)	Middle and old age	May be asymptomatic; may have fatigue, anorexia, weight loss, dyspnea on exertion; splenomegaly; lymphadenopathy; hepatomegaly	Hallmark is sustained absolute lymphocytosis 40,000–150,000/μL; bone marrow—increased lymphocytes	Median survival—approximately 10 yrs
Chronic myelogenous (CML) or chronic granulocytic (CGL)	Occurs most often at median age of 42	May be asymptomatic; or insidious onset of nonspecific symptoms, e.g., fatigue, weakness, anorexia, weight loss, fever, night sweats, splenomegaly; blurred vision; resp. distress; priapism, sternal tenderness	RBC, Hgb, Hct-L Platelet count—H early, L later; WBC-H; leukocytosis with immature granulocytes WBC—about 150,000–200,000/μL in symptomatic pt; bone marrow—Ph[1] chromosome presence is significant	No advantage to early therapy if asymptomatic; 60% of young adults with allogeneic bone marrow transplants complete cure; median survival in nontransplanted patients is 3–4 years

L = low; N = normal; H = high

2. Assistance in meeting psychosocial needs
3. Assistance for patient and families in adjusting to chronic effects of illness, e.g., dependence, withdrawal, changes in role responsibilities, alterations in body image
4. Patient education
   a. Importance of compliance with chemotherapy regimens; side effects and management
   b. Disease process and rationale for treatment
   c. Adaptation to any physical limitations

◘ NON-HODGKIN'S LYMPHOMA

- Definition—heterogenous group of lymphocytic malignancies with absence of giant Reed-Sternberg cells characteristic of Hodgkin's disease; characterized as indolent or aggressive

- Etiology/Incidence
  1. Etiology unclear; animal studies have suggested a viral etiology
  2. Other factors associated with increased incidence include
     a. Ionizing radiation
     b. Hereditary predisposition
     c. Congenital or acquired immunodeficiency
     d. Exposure to pesticides
  3. Approximately 55,000 new cases occur each year in the United States and appear to be increasing
  4. Most common neoplasm between ages of 20 and 40; with increased incidence of AIDS, number of cases has sharply increased

- Signs and Symptoms
  1. More than two-thirds of patients present with persistent painless peripheral lymphadenopathy
  2. Some patients may present with persistent cough and chest discomfort (mediastinal involvement)
  3. If abdominal contents involved, chronic pain, abdominal fullness, early satiety, or viscus obstruction may be presenting symptoms
  4. Diffuse disease may present with skin lesions, testicular masses
  5. Fever, night sweats, weight loss

- Differential Diagnosis
  1. Infectious mononucleosis
  2. Cytomegalovirus infection
  3. Human immunodeficiency virus involvement
  4. Toxoplasmosis
  5. Other malignant tumors
  6. Cat scratch disease
  7. Tuberculosis
  8. Syphilis
  9. Sarcoidosis

- Physical Findings
  1. Painless peripheral lymphadenopathy may be initial finding
  2. May present with abdominal mass, massive splenomegaly
  3. Early systemic findings usually absent

- Diagnostic Tests/Findings
  1. Requires skilled interpretation of adequate tumor tissue to determine tumor architecture and cell type
  2. B cell and T cell typing—complements pathologic interpretation
  3. Bone marrow biopsy—pathologic confirmation of disease process
  4. Staging procedures conducted once diagnosis established—no perfect classification system exists; various types include the Rappaport classification, Luke-Collins classification, the International Working Formulation National Cancer Institute (NCI), Ann Arbor staging system is most popular
  5. Chest radiograph may show mediastinal mass

- Management/Treatment—based on grade and extent of disease
  1. Radiotherapy
  2. Chemotherapy
  3. Bone marrow transplantation
  4. Newer modalities include monoclonal antibodies (MAbs) alone and combined with radionuclides or toxins to produce cytotoxic effects; cytokines, e.g., interferons, tumor necrosis factor, and interleukin 2 are currently under study
  5. General considerations
     a. Prognosis not usually as good as with Hodgkin's disease
     b. Both family and patient require supportive therapy during diagnosis and treatment stages
     c. Education and necessity of drug compliance important factor
     d. Increased susceptibility to infection

◘ HODGKIN'S DISEASE

- Definition—malignant disorder with lymphoreticular proliferation

- Etiology/Incidence
  1. Cause is unknown
  2. People with a history of infectious mononucleosis due to Epstein-Barr virus are at greater risk; virus may activate a cellular pathway that leads to proliferation
  3. Approximately 8,000 new cases are diagnosed each year in the United States

4. Most common malignancy in the 10–30 age group; average age is 28 years; peaks at 15–24 years and again after age 55
5. More common in males
6. Siblings have a three times higher risk than the general population
7. Mortality in the United States has fallen more rapidly for adult Hodgkin's lymphoma than for any other malignancy; largely related to improved treatment

- Signs and Symptoms
  1. Most patients present with a painless, enlarging mass, most often in the neck or occasionally in axilla or inguinal region; often the only manifestation at time of diagnosis
  2. Older patients may present with
     a. Fatigue
     b. Weight loss
     c. Persistent fever and/or night sweats
  3. Pruritus—may be mild and localized, but may also be progressive; rarely occurs in the absence of fever
  4. An unexplained symptom is immediate pain in diseased areas after consuming alcoholic beverages

- Differential Diagnosis
  1. Infectious mononucleosis
  2. Toxoplasmosis
  3. Cytomegalic inclusion disease
  4. Non-Hodgkin's lymphoma
  5. Leukemia
  6. Bronchogenic carcinoma
  7. Sarcoidosis
  8. Cat scratch disease

- Physical Findings
  1. Initial findings are usually enlargement of cervical, axillary, or inguinal lymph nodes (movable, nontender)
  2. Other findings may include hepatomegaly and splenomegaly; usually not present unless the disease is advanced

- Diagnostic Tests/Findings
  1. Presence of characteristic Reed-Sternberg giant cell on biopsy of lymph node tissue or other sites (needle aspiration not sufficient)
  2. WBC—polymorphonuclear leukocytosis may be present
  3. CBC—hypochromic, microcytic anemia in advanced disease

4. Low serum iron, low iron binding capacity
5. Chest radiologic examinations—to determine mediastinal involvement

- Management/Treatment
  1. Physician referral for suspected cases
     a. Radiotherapy
     b. Chemotherapy
     c. Autologous bone marrow transplant for chemotherapy failures
  2. For treatment to be precise, Hodgkin's disease needs to be staged, which involves determining the extent and involvement of the disease
  3. Psychosocial considerations for patient and family
  4. More than 75% of all newly diagnosed patients with adult Hodgkin's lymphoma can be cured with combination chemotherapy and/or radiation therapy
  5. Once patient is in remission, ongoing maintenance treatment is usually not needed; patients need to be instructed in the importance of returning for follow-up visits
  6. Patient education
     a. Gonadal side effects of treatment
     b. Consideration of sperm banking for males
     c. Risk of secondary malignancy

◘ QUESTIONS

Select the best answer.

Questions 1, 2, and 3 refer to the following scenario.

A 50-year-old male of Italian descent presents for a routine work-related health assessment. He has no complaints. His history and physical examination are unremarkable. A routine CBC reveals the following: Hgb 11.2 g/dL, MCV 72µ^3, WBC 5.7 × 10^3, Hct 35%, and MCH 25.

1. Based on this information how would his anemia be classified?

   a. Normocytic, normochromic
   b. Microcytic, hypochromic
   c. Macrocytic, hypochromic
   d. Microcytic, normochromic

2. Which aspect of this patient's history would provide the least useful information for diagnostic decision making?

a. Diet (including alcohol use)
b. Social history
c. Family history
d. Medical history

3. The patient in the preceding questions has a diet with regular daily intake of lean red meats, vegetables, and fruits and alcohol use once or twice a year. He admits to taking Maalox almost daily for indigestion. He says that weak blood runs in his family, although he has never had this problem. He has no surgical history and has never been treated for any medical problems except high cholesterol, which was treated with diet and exercise. This information helps rule out which of the following as cause for his anemia?

a. Folate deficiency
b. Inadequate dietary intake
c. GI bleeding
d. Malabsorption of vitamins and minerals

4. This patient's lack of abnormal physical signs and symptoms:

a. Probably indicates a lab error in the blood work
b. Is not unusual given the degree of his anemia
c. Is not unusual in a patient of this age
d. May be masked by use of Maalox

5. Your next step would be to:

a. Order B_{12} and folate serum levels
b. Order serum iron and TIBC
c. Obtain a urine culture
d. Order MMA test

6. What other test would be essential at this point?

a. Stool guaiac
b. GI series
c. Bilirubin
d. Liver function tests

7. Which is the most likely etiology of the type of anemia exhibited in this patient?

a. B_{12} or folate deficiency
b. Chronic disease
c. Dehydration
d. GI bleeding

8. If you obtain a negative stool guaiac in a male patient with a microcytic, hypochromic anemia who has a low serum iron and a high TIBC, you would:

a. Begin ferrous sulfate 300 mg orally t.i.d.
b. Order a Schilling test
c. Repeat the stool guaiac
d. Refer to a hematologist

Questions 9, 10, and 11 refer to the following scenario.

Mrs. M. is a 30-year-old graduate student from Morocco with a family and personal history of "weak blood" who presents with a complaint of abdominal pain, increasing fatigue, and weight loss. She has never needed treatment for her blood problem but has been supplementing her usually well-balanced diet with high-potency vitamin and mineral supplements because of the increased stress of graduate studies in a foreign country. A routine CBC indicates a mild microcytic, hypochromic anemia.

9. It is likely that this patient's "weak blood" is:

a. Thalassemia minor
b. Thalassemia major
c. Related to an unidentified chronic disease
d. Related to an iron deficiency from gastrointestinal bleeding

10. Which of the following do you need to consider as a strong etiology for her current symptoms?

a. Iron deficiency
b. Folate deficiency
c. Peptic ulcer
d. Iron overload

11. If further blood studies indicate a decreased TIBC and increased serum iron your next step should be which of the following?

a. Tell Mrs. M. to discontinue her vitamin/mineral supplements; obtain hematologic consult
b. Refer her for genetic counseling
c. Refer for hemoglobin electrophoresis
d. Begin chelation therapy and refer for a GI consult

Questions 12, 13, and 14 refer to the following scenario.

Ms. Z. is a 26-year-old, African-American female who comes in complaining of fatigue, shortness of breath, and lightheadedness. Her history reveals no significant medical problems but several years of fad dieting without vitamin supplementation. Physical findings are unremarkable except for pallor of the mucous membranes, tachycardia, and a systolic flow murmur.

12. Your next step would be to:

    a. Start B_{12} injections
    b. Order a CBC
    c. Order a TIBC and serum iron
    d. Start on multivitamins with iron

13. Ms. Z.'s CBC reveals a MCV of 110 and Hgb of 10.2 g/dL. Your next step should be to:

    a. Start B_{12} injections
    b. Order serum iron and TIBC
    c. Order RBC-folate and B_{12} levels
    d. Order an MMA level

14. Which of the following would help in your differential diagnosis?

    a. Patient's history of ice pica
    b. A + Romberg test and distal paresthesias on physical examination
    c. A confirmed diagnosis of sickle cell trait
    d. Family history of iron deficiency

15. The anemias most often associated with pregnancy are:

    a. Folic acid and iron deficiency
    b. Folic acid deficiency and Thalassemia
    c. Iron deficiency and Thalassemia
    d. Thalassemia and B_{12} deficiency

16. Neural tube defects in the fetus have been primarily associated with which type of deficiency in the mother?

    a. Iron
    b. Folic acid
    c. Vitamin B_{12}
    d. Vitamin E

17. Most common causes of megaloblastic, macrocytic anemia are:

    a. Folate and or B_{12} deficiency
    b. Chronic disease
    c. Iron deficiency and infection
    d. Hemolysis of blood cells

18. Patients with iron deficiency anemia should be instructed that:

    a. Return of normal blood values will occur within a week of oral iron supplementation
    b. Iron supplements will need to be taken for the rest of their lives
    c. Taking iron preparations with milk will enhance absorption
    d. Iron preparation may be taken with meals

19. Elderly persons with pernicious anemia should:

    a. Be instructed to increase their dietary intake of foods high in B_{12}
    b. Be told they will not need to return for follow-up for at least a month after initiation of treatment
    c. Be told that oral B_{12} is safer and less expensive than parenteral replacement
    d. Be told that diarrhea can be a transient side effect of B_{12} injections

20. Which of the following would be included in a diet rich in iron?

    a. Peaches, eggs, beef
    b. Cereals, kale, cheese
    c. Red beans, enriched breads, squash
    d. Legumes, green beans, eggs

21. A woman taking folic acid supplements for folic acid deficiency will need to know that:

    a. It will take several months before she will feel better
    b. Folic acid should not be taken with meals and may cause diarrhea
    c. Iron supplements are contraindicated while one is on folic acid
    d. Oral contraceptives, pregnancy, and lactation increase dietary requirements for folic acid

22. In alcoholics with anemia:

    a. Pernicious anemia is more common than folic acid deficiency
    b. Iron deficiency and folic acid deficiency may coexist
    c. Alcohol interferes with iron absorption
    d. Oral vitamin replacement is contraindicated

23. Which statement best characterizes macrocytic anemias?

    a. The underlying problem is usually a RBC deficiency
    b. They are most commonly hereditary
    c. They may produce neurological findings
    d. The pathophysiology includes abnormalities of hemoglobin synthesis

24. In normocytic anemia of chronic disease:

    a. Treatment is purely symptomatic
    b. Long-term supplementation of folic acid and B_{12} is needed
    c. Treatment is focused on the associated disease
    d. Serum iron and TIBC are the most specific and sensitive diagnostic tests

25. Which of the following is true of anemia of chronic disease?
    a. A Hgb of < 9 g/dL confirms the diagnosis
    b. Symptoms associated with the anemia may be masked by the symptoms of the underlying disease
    c. Is manifested by more severe signs than most of the other common anemias
    d. Is never associated with reversible causes

26. Sickle cell anemia is caused by:
    a. Abnormalities in one or more hemoglobin chain
    b. Transposition of glutamic acid on hemoglobin A molecule
    c. Abnormal hemoglobin S in place of hemoglobin A
    d. In utero deficiency of folate

27. The test used to differentiate sickle cell anemia/sickle cell trait is:
    a. Sickle cell preparation
    b. Peripheral smear
    c. Sickledex
    d. Hemoglobin electrophoresis

28. Chronic myelogenous leukemia usually presents with the following:
    a. Increased platelets and leukocytosis
    b. Presence of Reed-Stemberg cells in bone marrow aspirate
    c. Ph[1] chromosome in bone marrow
    d. With typical fatigue, weakness, anorexia, and frequent nosebleeds

29. A 32-year-old male presents in the office with concerns about a painless lump in the area of his collar bone. He says that he feels well, but someone told him that it might be a sign of some kind of cancer. Your best response at this time would be to:
    a. Examine him and tell him to come back in 2 weeks to be reevaluated
    b. Inquire whether he has any cats that might cause cat scratch fever
    c. Work him up for a possibility of infectious mononucleosis
    d. Examine him with referral to physician for possible lymphoma disease workup

30. Diagnosis of Hodgkin's disease is based upon:
    a. Hepatomegaly with fatigue, weight loss, pruritus, and night sweats
    b. Presence of Ph[1] chromosome in lymphoid tissue
    c. Extensive lymphadenopathy with elevated WBC count
    d. Presence of Reed-Sternberg cells in lymph node tissue

Answers

1.	**b**	16.	**b**
2.	**b**	17.	**a**
3.	**b**	18.	**d**
4.	**b**	19.	**d**
5.	**b**	20.	**a**
6.	**a**	21.	**d**
7.	**d**	22.	**b**
8.	**c**	23.	**a**
9.	**a**	24.	**c**
10.	**d**	25.	**b**
11.	**a**	26.	**c**
12.	**b**	27.	**d**
13.	**c**	28.	**c**
14.	**b**	29.	**d**
15.	**a**	30.	**d**

◼ BIBLIOGRAPHY

Amin, N. M. (2003). What's wrong with this picture: Diagnostic images, treatment issues . . . iron deficiency anemia. *Consultant, 40,* 2333, 2335, 2339.

Balducci, L. (2003). Epidemiology of anemia: Information on diagnostic evaluation. *Journal of the American Geriatric Society, 51*(3 supp) 52–59.

Behrens, R. J., & Cymet, T. C. (2000). Sickle cell disorders: Evaluation, treatment, and natural history. *Hospital Physician, 36*(9), 17–18, 21–28.

Bleibel, S. A. (2008). Thalassemia, alpha. Retrieved from http://www.emedicine.com/med/TOPIC2259.htm

Conrad, M. E. (2008). Anemia. Retrieved from http://www.emedicine.com/med/TOPIC132.htm

Gilliland, D. G. (2001). Hematologic malignances. *Current Opinion in Hematology, 8*(1), 189–191.

Goldberg, M. (2001). The diagnostic challenge . . . non-Hodgkin's lymphoma. *Emergency Medicine, 33*(3), 77–78.

Goldman, D. (2000). Test your knowledge: Chronic lymphocytic anemia and its impact on the immune system. *Clinical Journal of Oncology Nursing, 4,* 233–234, 236.

Linker, C. A. & Damon, L. E. (2009). Blood disorders. In S. J. McPhee, & M. A. Papadakis (Eds.), *Current medical diagnosis and treatment* (51st ed.). New York: McGraw-Hill.

McPherson, R. A. & Pincus, M. R. (2007). *Henry's clinical diagnosis and management by laboratory methods* (21st ed.). Philadelphia: W.B. Saunders.

Russel, L. C. (2000). Hereditary hemochromatosis: Should clinicians screen for this common disease? *Journal of the American Academy of Nurse Practitioners, 12,* 273–279.

Streiff, M. B., Smith, B., & Spivak, J. L. (2002). The diagnosis and management of polycythemia vera in the era since the Polycythemia Vera Study Group: A survey of American Society of Hematology members' practice patterns. *Blood, 99,* 1144–1149.

Takeshita, K. (2007). Thalassemia, beta. Retrieved from http://www.emedicine.com/med/TOPIC2260 .htm

Gastrointestinal Disorders

8

Sister Maria Salerno

◘ PEPTIC ULCER DISEASE (PUD)

- Definition—ulceration of the GI mucosa in areas bathed by acid pepsin; stomach, duodenum, and esophagus are common sites

- Etiology/Incidence
  1. Infection with *Helicobacter pylori* leading to imbalance between mucosal protective factors and corrosive effects of acid and pepsin is considered primary cause
  2. Steroidal and nonsteroidal anti-inflammatory drug (NSAID) therapy is the second most common cause
  3. Other causes include processes or factors leading to
     a. Hypersecretion of gastric mucosa
     b. Increased parietal cell mass
     c. Increased secretion of gastrin and hydrochloric acid
     d. Increased gastric emptying time
  4. Precipitating or aggravating factors include
     a. Steroidal and NSAID therapy, particularly aspirin
     b. Physiologic stress—severe trauma, burns, shock
     c. Psychological stress
     d. Alcohol and nicotine use; caffeine, coffee
     e. Presence of alcoholic liver cirrhosis, chronic pancreatitis, chronic lung disease, hyperparathyroidism, rheumatoid arthritis

  5. Lifetime prevalence about 10% for adult population
     a. Duodenal
        (1) 80% are duodenal
        (2) Higher incidence in males
        (3) Without antibiotic treatment 80% recur in year following initial healing
        (4) Incidence decreasing in United States
        (5) Familial disposition—more frequent in persons with type O blood
        (6) Peak incidence between 25 and 55 years of age
     b. Gastric
        (1) Occur with about the same incidence in males and females
        (2) About 5% are malignant
        (3) Peak incidence—age 55–65 years of age; rare < 40 years of age

- Signs and Symptoms
  1. Intermittent epigastric pain—gnawing, burning, boring, nagging
  2. Pain begins 1–3 hours after eating, frequently awakens person at night
  3. Pain relieved by food or antacids, particularly with duodenal ulcer
  4. Food sometimes aggravates pain of gastric ulcer
  5. Weight loss frequent in persons with gastric ulcer
  6. Dyspepsia (bloating, nausea, anorexia, excessive flatulence)

- Differential Diagnosis
  1. History of typical pain-food-relief pattern is most important criterion for diagnosis of duodenal ulcer
  2. History not helpful in distinguishing gastric from duodenal
  3. Rule out other causes of epigastric pain
     a. Pancreatitis
     b. Biliary tract disease
     c. Neoplasms
     d. Liver disease
     e. Gastritis
     f. Pneumonia
     g. Functional problems
     h. Cardiovascular disease, e.g., angina
- Physical Findings
  1. Usually none
  2. Epigastric tenderness in advanced disease
- Diagnostic Tests/Findings
  1. Barium radiograph of the upper GI tract will detect 90% of peptic ulcers—indications include
     a. Diagnosis of atypical cases
     b. Typical presentations with failure to respond to treatment in 3–4 weeks; cases of recurrence
     c. Differentiating gastric from duodenal
     d. Limited accuracy for differentiating malignant from nonmalignant gastric ulcers
     e. Documentation of healing
  2. Endoscopy
     a. Should always be performed when alarm symptoms present
        (1) Dysphagia
        (2) Unplanned weight loss
        (3) GI bleeding
     b. Expensive but more sensitive and specific than barium radiographs; test of choice in most settings
     c. Indicated if clinical symptoms persist despite negative barium studies
     d. Rule out malignancy in gastric ulcers—should be performed if gastric ulcer suspected
        (1) Age of symptom onset > 55 years
        (2) Pain worsened with food
        (3) Typical symptoms do not respond to standard course of therapy
     e. For those with diagnosed or suspected blood loss, perforation, vomiting, early satiety, or weight loss
  3. Stool for occult blood—positive if bleeding is present
  4. CBC
     a. Hgb and Hct may be decreased
     b. With chronic slow bleeding—hypochromic, microcytic anemia is likely
     c. If bleeding is acute—normocytic, normochromic anemia
  5. Tests for *Helicobacter pylori*
     a. Urea breath test
        (1) 95–98% sensitivity and specificity; results comparable to endoscopic biopsy
        (2) Ingested drugs can cause false negatives; perform 4 weeks after last antibacterial treatment; 7 days after use of proton pump inhibitor
     b. Serological tests
        (1) IgA, IgG antibodies, enzyme-linked immunosorbent assay (ELISA)
        (2) Inexpensive; sensitivity and specificity about 95%
        (3) Not useful for follow-up testing because of slow decline after treatment
        (4) High serum lipid levels can interfere with results
     c. Histological evaluation
        (1) Requires endoscopic biopsy
        (2) Invasive and expensive
     d. Fecal antigen test
        (1) Sensitive to reinfection
        (2) Can be used to indicate response to treatment
     e. Culture of biopsy
        (1) Grows slowly and requires selective medium and environment
        (2) Primary use in research
- Management/Treatment
  1. Goals
     a. Relief of symptoms
     b. Healing
     c. Prevention of recurrence
     d. Eradication of bacteria
  2. Nonpharmacological
     a. Stop smoking
     b. Avoid nonsteroidal anti-inflammatory drugs
     c. Reduce stress
     d. Reduce use of alcohol and caffeine (conflicting data, but still recommended until healing is documented)
  3. Pharmacological
     a. Antimicrobials to eradicate *H. pylori*
        (1) Options include
            (a) Preferred treatment in United States is a 10–14 day course of combination antibiotic and antisecretory therapy including amoxicillin, clarithromycin, levofloxacin, tetracycline, metronidazole, and bismuth
            (b) Sequential therapy consisting of a proton pump inhibitor (PPI) and amoxicillin for 5 days followed by a PPI, clarithromycin, and tinidazole

for an additional 5 days as an alternative to treatment failure with initial therapies

  (c) Levofloxacin-based salvage therapy for patients with treatment failure on regimens containing clarithromycin

(2) Bismuth compounds act as topical antimicrobial, complementing antibiotics

(3) Compliance with combination therapies a problem

(4) Acquired resistance of microbe to metronidazole and, to a lesser extent clarithromycin, often occurs with either if given alone

(5) Standard therapy currently least expensive

(6) Side effects of antimicrobial treatment

  (a) Candida

  (b) Rash

  (c) Pseudomembranous colitis

  (d) Photosensitivity

(7) No one "right" regimen

b. Antisecretory therapy (proton pump inhibitors provide faster pain relief and more rapid healing than H_2 receptor antagonists)

(1) Omeprazole or rabeprazole 20 mg per day

(2) Lansoprazole 30 mg per day

(3) Esomeprazole or pantoprazole 40 mg per day

(4) Taken for 4–8 weeks

(5) Should be administered 30 minutes before meals (usually breakfast)

(6) Like H_2 antagonists some may have cytochrome P450 implications

(7) Create less acidic environment suppressing but not eradicating *H. pylori*

(8) Particularly useful in prevention/treatment of NSAID-induced ulceration

(9) Available in parenteral and enteral forms

c. H_2 receptor antagonists

(1) Cimetidine—300 mg orally t.i.d. with meals and at bedtime for 4–6 weeks (more recent studies indicate similar healing with 400 mg b.i.d. or 800 mg at bedtime)

  (a) May be given IV in inpatient settings

  (b) Side effects

    (i) Frequently associated with acute confusional states in elderly or very ill patients

    (ii) Muscular pain; mild, transient diarrhea; impotence; gynecomastia; leukopenia; mildly

elevated creatinine and transaminase levels are rare and tend to be seen only with long-term use

  (c) Interferes with metabolism and increases blood levels of benzodiazepines, lidocaine, metronidazole, phenytoin, theophylline, and warfarin

  (d) Should not be taken within an hour of taking antacids

(2) Ranitidine—150 mg orally b.i.d. or 300 mg orally at bedtime for active PUD; 150 mg orally at bedtime for maintenance

  (a) Also available for IV use

  (b) Side effects—rise in transaminase levels alanine aminotransferase (ALT); dizziness; headache; tachycardia; malaise; constipation; diarrhea; rash; and, rarely, confusion

  (c) No significant drug interactions

  (d) May cause false-positive protein on urinary dip-stick analysis

(3) Famotidine—20 mg orally twice a day or 40 mg at bedtime

  (a) As efficacious as ranitidine

  (b) Least risk of drug interaction

(4) Nizatidine—150 mg orally twice a day or 300 mg at bedtime for up to 8 weeks

  (a) No safer than cimetidine

  (b) More expensive than cimetidine

d. Antacids (used primarily as supplement to antisecretory agents)

(1) Should give dose equivalent to 80–100 mEq acid neutralizing capacity; for most, 30–40 mL given 1 and 3 hours after each meal; see **Table 8-1** for comparison of various antacid preparations

(2) Primarily aluminum-, calcium-, or magnesium-containing agents; sodium bicarbonate very short acting and systemic absorption can cause alkalosis (not recommended)

(3) Length of effect dependent on gastric emptying time; 30 minutes on an empty stomach, longer when taken with meals

(4) Side effects

  (a) Diarrhea with magnesium hydroxide–based agents

  (b) Constipation with aluminum hydroxide-containing agents

  (c) Hypophosphatemia in aluminum-containing agents due to aluminum phosphate binding and decreased GI absorption

■ **Table 8-1** Antacids

Content Comments	Brand Name	Dose Required for 80–100 mEq of Acid-Neutralizing Effect per Dose	mEq of Sodium per Dose
Low Buffering Capacity			
$CaCO_3$ Rebound hyperacidity	Tums Alka II Chooz	8–10 tablets	0.5–0.6
$Al(OH)_3$ Constipating; high sodium	Amphogel	60–75 mL	1.2–1.5
$Al(OH)_3$ and $Mg(OH)_3$ Only for esophageal reflux	Gaviscon	94–118 mL	10.6–13.2
Moderate Buffering Capacity			
$Al(OH)_3$ and $Mg(OH)_3$	Gelusil	35–44 mL	0.23–0.29
Low sodium	Mylanta	32–40 mL	0.20–0.25
	Maalox Plus	30–38 mL	0.36–0.45
	Riopan	30–38 mL	0.08–0.1
High Buffering Capacity			
$Al(OH)_3$ and $Mg(OH)_3$	Geluxil II	17–21 mL	0.2–0.25
Liquid more effective than tablets	Maalox TC	14–18 mL	0.1–0.13
	Mylanta II	16–20 mL	0.15–0.2

Note: Sodium Bicarbonate, Alka Seltzer have a very short duration of action; acid rebound, systemic alkalosis are problems

     (d) Osteopenia with long-term use of agents containing aluminum
     (e) Rebound acid secretion and hypercalcemia with calcium-containing agents
  (5) Drug interactions
     (a) Interfere with taste; absorption of iron, digoxin, and some antibiotics, e.g., tetracyclines
     (b) Interfere with effectiveness of oral contraceptives
 e. Treatment of NSAID-induced ulcers
  (1) Antibiotic therapy not indicated
  (2) Antisecretory therapy with a PPI or histamine 2 receptor antagonists (H_2RA) as described previously
  (3) Discontinue NSAID during acute therapy
  (4) If NSAID must be reintroduced, replace prostaglandin with synthetic option, e.g., misoprostol
  (5) H_2RA along with antisecretory therapy may provide some benefit
 f. Sucralfate (mucosal protectant)—1 g orally q.i.d. on an empty stomach
  (1) No significant side effects
  (2) Drug interaction
     (a) Decreases absorption of digoxin, tetracycline, phenytoin, cimetidine, theophylline, and other drugs
     (b) Antacids interfere with effectiveness and should not be given within 1 hour of sucralfate administration

 g. Treatment with antacids, H_2 receptor antagonists, or sucralfate results in 90–95% cure rate in 8–12 weeks
4. General considerations
 a. Consult with physician regarding
  (1) Additional diagnostic studies for persons with suspected underlying disease or failure to respond to treatment in 2–4 weeks
  (2) Persons with concurrent weight loss
  (3) Persons with indications of peritonitis (rigidity, rebound tenderness, fever)
 b. Refer to physician persons with confirmed or suspected complications
  (1) Bleeding occurs in about 10–15% of persons with PUD
     (a) Immediate medical emergency with possible surgical intervention required
     (b) Signs and symptoms—heartburn, belching, epigastric discomfort, vomiting of bright red or coffee ground liquid
     (c) Sudden relief of epigastric pain may be related to bleeding as blood acts as an acid buffer
     (d) Diarrhea may also be evident; blood is a cathartic
  (2) Perforation occurs in about 5–10% of persons with duodenal ulcers and 2–5% of those with gastric ulcers
     (a) Surgery is the indicated treatment

(b) Signs and symptoms include acute pain, fever, leukocytosis, hypotension, peritoneal irritation

(c) Peritoneal irritation is evidenced by abdominal rigidity, guarding, rebound tenderness, decreased or absent bowel sounds

(3) Gastric outlet (pyloric) obstruction is seen in less than 5% of all patients diagnosed with PUD and is most often associated with duodenal ulceration

(a) Surgical intervention may be indicated

(b) Signs and symptoms include worsening pain; vomiting of undigested food; dehydration; hypokalemia; and metabolic alkalosis

c. Patient education

(1) Disease and therapeutic management

(2) Purpose, dosage, side effects of medications

(3) Diet

(a) No evidence to support need for bland diet or small, frequent meals

(b) Encourage avoidance of known gastric acid stimulants, e.g., coffee, cola, and other caffeine-containing beverages

(c) Avoidance of any foods or beverages that aggravate symptoms

(d) Avoid eating within 3 hours of bedtime to avoid nocturnal stimulation of acid secretion

(4) Stress reduction

(5) Need to report to healthcare provider lack of response to medications, rectal bleeding, weight loss, increased weakness or dizziness, increasing pain

(6) Advise that smoking will delay gastric healing

d. Follow up

(1) In 2–4 weeks to review

(a) Symptom response to medications

(b) GI bleeding

(c) Side or toxic effects of medications

(2) For those with gastric ulcers document healing with upper GI barium radiograph or endoscopy—in 6 weeks for small ulcers; 12 weeks for large; imperative in gastric ulcers; unnecessary in uncomplicated duodenal ulcers

❑ GASTROESOPHAGEAL REFLUX DISEASE

- Definition—a condition that develops when the reflux of stomach contents causes troublesome symptoms and/or complications; symptoms are considered troublesome if they affect a person's well-being after assurance of their benign nature

- Etiology/Incidence
  1. Most often related to inappropriate relaxation of the lower esophageal sphincter (LES), which allows reflux of gastric acid and pepsin into the distal esophagus
     a. Idiopathic
     b. Foods and other agents (see **Table 8-2**)
  2. Inflammation can also be caused by ingestion of caustic agents such as lye or infectious agents such as candida, herpes simplex, or cytomegalovirus, which directly attack esophageal mucosa
  3. Infectious agents most often noted in immunosuppressed individuals, e.g., persons with AIDS or diabetes, and persons receiving chemotherapy
  4. Incidence not known, however, a monthly prevalence rate of heartburn, the major symptom of gastroesophageal reflux disease (GERD), has been estimated to be 40% in adult population

- Signs and Symptoms
  1. Retrosternal aching or burning heartburn (pyrosis) occurring 30–60 minutes after eating; associated with large meals, aggravated by lying down or bending over, and relieved with antacids
  2. Chest heaviness, pressure radiating to neck, jaw, or shoulders

■ **Table 8-2** Foods and Other Substances that Decrease Lower Esophageal Sphincter Tone

Anticholinergics	Alcohol
Benzodiazepines	Caffeine
Calcium channel blockers	Nicotine
Diazepam	Chocolate
Meperidine	Fatty foods
Narcotics	Peppermint
Progesterone	Yellow onions

3. Regurgitation of fluid or food particles
4. Nocturnal aspiration
5. Extraesophageal symptoms may occur but role is less certain
   a   Bronchospasm
   b   Pharyngeal discomfort
   c   Dysphonia
   d   Chronic cough

- Differential Diagnosis
  1. Myocardial infarction/angina
  2. Esophageal spasm
  3. Cholelithiasis
  4. Neoplasms
  5. Chemical or infectious esophagitis
  6. Conditions leading to gastric dysmotility, e.g., scleroderma, diabetes

- Physical Findings—generally insignificant

- Diagnostic Tests/Findings
  1. Not indicated in typical cases that respond to once- or twice-daily PPI therapy
  2. Endoscopy has become standard for documenting the type and extent of tissue damage
     a. Should be initiated at any time that alarm symptoms become present
        (1) Dysphagia
        (2) Unplanned weight loss
        (3) GI bleeding
     b. Is indicated for the evaluation of patients with GERD who do not respond clinically to b.i.d. PPI therapy
  3. Manometry for patients who have not responded to b.i.d. PPI therapy and have normal endoscopic findings
  4. pH monitoring for patients who remain symptomatic on b.i.d. PPI therapy and have normal endoscopic and manometry findings; should be performed only after PPI therapy has been withheld for 7 days

- Management/Treatment
  1. Nonpharmacologic measures should be targeted to specific patient circumstances; no evidence to suggest that across-the-board lifestyle interventions are effective
     a. Weight reduction if obese
     b. Elevation of head of bed if symptoms worse when supine
     c. Avoid large meals and carbonated beverages, particularly 3 hours prior to going to bed if nocturnal symptoms predominate
     d. Limit fats and carbohydrates
     e. Avoid straining at stool
     f. Discontinue agents that decrease lower esophageal sphincter (LES) tone if the patient is using them—nicotine, alcohol, chocolate, caffeine, theophylline, calcium channel blockers, anticholinergics
     g. Antacids—(see Table 8-1)
        (1) May be effective for those with infrequent heartburn; however with a diagnosis of GERD they are not indicated for routine therapy
        (2) 80–100 mEq of neutralizing activity (30 cc for most agents) after meals and at bedtime
        (3) Liquid preferred to tablet forms
  2. Pharmacologic therapy
     a. PPI 30 minutes before breakfast
     b. If unresponse to A.M. therapy, add second PPI 30 minutes before dinner
     c. No evidence that additional therapies, e.g., h.s. H_2RA, promotility agents, improve outcomes—not routinely indicated
     d. PPI clearly superior to H_2RA for GERD management
     e. If unresponsive to b.i.d. PPI, refer to GI for endoscopy
  3. Currently there is no indication for management of extraesophageal symptoms without concomitant pyrosis
  4. Phase IV—surgical intervention reserved for patients with stricture, bleeding, pulmonary aspiration, or severe refractory symptoms
  5. General considerations
     a. Consult with physician regarding persons
        (1) With atypical presentation
        (2) Refractory to simple treatment
        (3) With dysphagia and or weight loss in addition to heartburn
     b. Education
        (1) Mechanism of esophageal reflux and goals of management
        (2) Aggravating factors
        (3) Correction of misconceptions regarding causes (hiatal hernia seldom a cause) and treatment
        (4) Proper use, dosage, side effects of pharmacologic agents

◘ CHOLECYSTITIS

- Definition—acute or chronic inflammation of the gallbladder

- Etiology/Incidence
  1. About 90% related to presence of pigmented or cholesterol calculi, which can vary in diameter from 1 mm to 4 cm; when a stone becomes impacted in the cystic duct, inflammation develops behind the obstruction; if not relieved, pressure builds up in the gallbladder and leads

to distension, ischemic changes, gangrene, and perforation with subsequent abscess formation and less frequently generalized peritonitis
2. Occurs subsequent to bile stasis, bacterial infection, or ischemia
3. Most common form of gallbladder disease; affects more than 20 million Americans
4. Risk factors include age 50–70 years, female over 40 years old, obesity, and Western European descent
5. Pregnancy, sedentary lifestyle, low-fiber diet, use of oral contraceptives or antilipemics also associated with the development of cholecystitis

- Signs and Symptoms
  1. Episodic occurrences of postprandial fullness, heartburn, nausea, flatulence, regurgitation of bitter fluid, vomiting often precipitated by a large or fatty meal
  2. Anorexia (inability to finish an average-size meal)
  3. Recurrent episodes of biliary colic—sudden appearance of severe pain in the epigastrium or right hypochondrium, which subsides relatively slowly (12–18 hours)
     a. Tenderness of the same area may persist for days
     b. Accompanied by vomiting in 75% of the cases
  4. Constant aching pain or pressure in the right upper quadrant or epigastrium that radiates to the back or right shoulder

- Differential Diagnosis
  1. Perforated peptic ulcer
  2. Acute pancreatitis
  3. Appendicitis
  4. Salpingitis
  5. Diverticulitis
  6. Perforated hepatic carcinoma
  7. Liver abscess
  8. Hepatitis
  9. Pneumonia with right-sided pleurisy
  10. Myocardial infarction

- Physical Findings
  1. General appearance—unremarkable between attacks; ill during attack
  2. Vital signs—mild temperature elevation, tachycardia, and increased respiratory rate during acute attack
  3. Integument—mild jaundice occurs in about 20% of cases
  4. Abdomen—guarding, rebound tenderness in right hypochondrium; palpable, tender sausage shaped mass in right upper quadrant (RUQ) during acute attack in 20–30% of cases

5. Positive Murphy's sign—inspiratory arrest secondary to extreme tenderness when subhepatic area is palpated during deep inspiration

- Diagnostic Tests/Findings
  1. CBC—mild leukocytosis with increased bands (shift to the left)
  2. ECG—normal, important in ruling out myocardial infarction as cause of symptoms
  3. Chest radiograph—normal, important in ruling out pneumonia as cause of symptoms
  4. Flat plate radiograph of abdomen—gallstones
  5. Ultrasound (study of choice with 95% sensitivity, 98% specificity for stones)—gallstones, thickened gallbladder wall stones, but not as sensitive in acute cases
  6. Technetium T_c99_m PIPIDA (HIDA) scan—cystic duct occlusion and nonvisualized gallbladder; has high reliability if bilirubin < 5 mg/dL
  7. Alkaline phosphatase—elevated
  8. Serum amylase—elevated, > 1,000 suspect concomitant pancreatitis
  9. Serum aspartate aminotransferase (AST) and serum alanine aminotransferase (ALT) may be transiently elevated
  10. Bilirubin—mildly increased
  11. Old age, lymphoma, malnutrition, and immunosuppression may alter laboratory tests
  12. CT scan has no advantage over ultrasound in diagnosis of acute attack
  13. Oral cholecystography not used for acute attack

- Management/Treatment
  1. Elective cholecystectomy recommended for
     a. Symptomatic patients with radiologic or ultrasound evidence of gallbladder disease
     b. Those at high risk for complications such as those with
        (1) A calcified gall bladder
        (2) Gallstones > 2 cm in diameter
        (3) Diabetes
        (4) Symptoms present for > 48 hours
  2. Conservative treatment for those who are asymptomatic
     a. If on clofibrate (an antilipemic) or oral contraceptives, stop or decrease dosage
     b. Avoid foods that seem to precipitate symptoms, otherwise no need to alter diet or restrict fats
     c. Anticholinergics not helpful
     d. Treat dyspeptic symptoms with antacids (25–50% of patients will respond)
     e. Some patients may be put on a trial of chenodiol 750 mg orally per day
        (1) Best results are obtained in patients with small floating cholesterol stones

(2) Contraindicated in patients with inflammatory bowel disease or peptic ulcer disease

(3) Approximately 50% recurrence rate within 5 years after treatment

(4) Side effects—hepatotoxicity, diarrhea, and increased LDL cholesterol

(5) Expensive

3. Lithotripsy or destruction of stones with extracorporeal shock waves has limited application at present

4. General considerations
   a. Refer all persons with suspected cholecystitis to physician for further evaluation, possible hospitalization, and possible surgery
   b. Patient education
      (1) Disease course, expected outcomes, and treatment
      (2) Changes in symptoms that necessitate contact of health professional, e.g., change in pain pattern or pain accompanied by fever, chills
      (3) Teach purpose, dosage, side effects of medications
      (4) Nutrition
         (a) If fatty foods seem to precipitate symptoms, a low-fat diet may be helpful
         (b) Some research has shown that increased fiber in the diet reduces incidence of gallstone formation
         (c) If obese, a reducing diet is indicated; avoid rapid weight loss and fad diets that may actually increase risk of gallstone formation and precipitate acute symptoms
      (5) Encourage regular physical exercise; sedentary life style is associated with stone formation as well as obesity
   c. Follow up annually and for acute attacks
   d. Complications include empyema, gangrene, and perforation

◘ APPENDICITIS

- Definition—inflammation of the vermiform appendix

- Etiology/Incidence
  1. Obstruction of the appendix with hardened feces (fecalith), stricture, inflammation, foreign body, or neoplasm
  2. Occurs in all age groups, but more common in males between 10 and 30 years of age
  3. Higher mortality rate due to complications in children, adolescents, and person over 55 years of age
  4. One of the leading causes for abdominal surgery

- Signs and Symptoms
  1. Acute onset of periumbilical or epigastric pain that ranges from mildly diffuse to severe
  2. Anorexia, nausea—vomiting not typical; if patient has several episodes of vomiting, consider alternate diagnosis
  3. Shifting of pain to right lower quadrant (McBurney's point) after several hours; aggravated by walking or coughing
  4. Occasional radiation of pain into the ipsilateral testicle or labia
  5. Spasm of abdominal muscles
  6. Constipation usual; diarrhea rare
  7. Elderly clients may present with mild symptoms of unexplained weakness, anorexia, tachycardia, and abdominal distention with little pain
  8. After 24 hours may progress to perforation with sudden cessation of pain and subsequent peritonitis manifested by
     a. Abdominal rigidity
     b. Generalized abdominal tenderness
     c. High fever
     d. Vomiting
     e. Dehydration
     f. Decreased bowel sounds
     g. Shock

- Differential Diagnosis
  1. Gastroenteritis
  2. Pneumonia
  3. Ruptured ovarian cyst
  4. Tubal pregnancy
  5. Acute cholecystitis
  6. Neoplastic perforation of the colon
  7. Renal calculi
  8. Pyelonephritis of the right kidney

- Physical Findings
  1. General appearance—may or may not appear ill
  2. Vital signs—fever 100–102° F
  3. Slight tachycardia related to pain and fever
  4. Abdominal—point and rebound tenderness in RLQ (McBurney's point); decreased or absent bowel sounds
  5. Positive psoas and obturator signs (hip flexion maneuvers that stretch the inflamed peritoneum producing pain)
  6. Rectal/pelvic exams—tenderness in the right perirectal area
  7. Musculoskeletal—abdominal pain (RLQ) with hip extension and with straight leg raise

- Diagnostic Tests/Findings
  1. CBC with differential—leukocytosis with increased band cells (shift to the left); in the elderly shift may be present without leukocytosis
  2. CT scan of the abdomen
     a. Enlarged appendix
     b. Appendiceal wall thickening and enlargement
     c. Periappendiceal fat stranding

- Management/Treatment—all persons with suspected or diagnosed appendicitis should be immediately referred to a physician for hospitalization and surgery. Appendicitis that has progressed to perforation or peritonitis will be associated with longer morbidity and higher mortality

◘ DIVERTICULITIS

- Definition—inflammation of one or more diverticula in the bowel wall with microperforation and abscess formation in the pericolic fat

- Etiology/Incidence
  1. Inflammatory process similar to etiologic agents in appendicitis
  2. Occurs in about 33% of persons with diverticula (estimated to be 5–20% of the adult population)
     a. Incidence increases over age 40
     b. More frequent in females than males
     c. Higher incidence in persons with low-fiber dietary habits
     d. Diverticula found most often in the sigmoid colon but may occur anywhere in the GI tract
  3. Free perforation with signs of peritonitis is rare

- Signs and Symptoms
  1. Acute left lower quadrant pain—steady and severe lasting for several days or crampy and intermittent
  2. Constipation more common than diarrhea
  3. Pain increased with defecation
  4. Flatulence
  5. Nausea
  6. Low-grade fever

- Differential Diagnosis
  1. Appendicitis
  2. Carcinoma of the colon
  3. Crohn's disease
  4. Ischemic colitis
  5. Gynecologic disorders, including
     a. Ectopic pregnancy
     b. Ovarian abscess

- Physical Findings
  1. Vital signs—mild fever, tachycardia
  2. Abdomen—guarding, rebound tenderness, rigidity especially over left lower quadrant (LLQ); if abscess has formed, a tender palpable mass may be noted
  3. Rectal examination—tender painful mass may be present

- Diagnostic Tests/Findings
  1. CBC—mild to moderate leukocytosis
  2. Sedimentation (sed) rate—elevated
  3. Stool guaiac—positive in about 25% of cases
  4. Urine—normal unless colovesicular fistula present then bacteriuria, leukorrhea, hematuria
  5. CT scan of the abdomen and pelvis is preferred diagnostic modality
  6. Colonoscopy after resolution of acute symptoms to confirm diagnosis and rule out other disorders
  7. Plain radiograph film of the abdomen to identify free air, ileus, or obstruction in acute phase
  8. Barium enema may confirm presence of diverticulosis; greatest utility in ruling out other etiologies
  9. Stool for ova/parasites—negative

- Management/Treatment—for most patients with mild disease outpatient treatment will be indicated and includes
  1. Clear liquids for 1–2 days followed by a bland diet once symptoms have subsided
  2. Broad-spectrum antibiotics with anaerobic activity for 7–10 days or until symptoms abate; for example
     a. Amoxicillin/clavulanate potassium 875 mg/125 mg twice a day
     b. Metronidazole 500 mg 3 times a day plus ciprofloxin 500 mg twice a day or trimethoprim-sulfamethoxazole 160/800 mg twice a day
  3. Bed rest to promote colon rest recommended until symptoms subside
  4. Low-fiber diet in acute phase
  5. Bowel rest—clear liquids, slowly advance as tolerated in acute phase
  6. Chronically avoid nuts and seeds in diet
  7. General considerations
     a. Consult with physician regarding hospitalization
        (1) Those who fail to improve in 72 hours
        (2) Those with a temperature > 102° F
        (3) Need for additional testing
        (4) Those in advanced age
     b. Patients with severe disease require hospitalization, antibiotics, bowel rest, and IV

hydration; approximately 20–30% of patients with diverticulitis will require surgical management

   c. Patient education

     (1) Etiology/incidence and usual clinical course of the disease and rationale for recommended treatment

     (2) Instruction on recommended dietary guidelines

       (a) After acute phase, high-fiber diet to include foods such as bran; whole grains; cereals; raw, cooked, or dried fruit; raw vegetables; cooked high-residue vegetables

       (b) High-fiber diet may cause bloating and flatulence during the first 2 weeks of use; this resolves with continued high-fiber intake

     (3) Avoid laxatives, enemas, antidiarrheal agents, and uncooked high-residue foods

     (4) Report fever, bleeding, increasing pain to healthcare provider immediately

     (5) Bulk forming agents such as psyllium hydrophilic muciloid and use of stool softeners such as docusate sodium may help prevent frequent recurrence

   d. Follow up—return visit or phone follow-up in 24–48 hours to verify relief with initiating therapy; and then again after completion of antibiotic therapy

□ VIRAL HEPATITIS

- Definition—inflammation of the liver

- Etiology/Incidence
  1. Type A (infectious)
     a. Infection with hepatitis A virus (HAV), a small RNA enterovirus
        (1) Spread primarily by fecal-oral route; also parenterally
        (2) Found in infected water, food, shellfish
        (3) Intimate contact and poor sanitation and personal hygiene seem to be contributing factors
        (4) Incubation period 2–6 weeks
        (5) Infectivity—2–3 weeks in late incubation and early clinical phase
     b. Common in crowded situations such as low-income housing, school, military, and prison dormitories; can occur in any age group; common in immigrants from underdeveloped countries, school-age children, and young adults
        (1) Self limiting in > 99% of cases
        (2) No carrier state or chronic infection

     (3) Severity increases with age

     (4) In United States seroprevalence of anti-HAV in adults indicates 40–50% have had the disease

  2. Type B (serum)
    a. Infection with hepatitis B virus (HBV), a DNA virus with core and surface components

     (1) HB$_s$Ag (hepatitis B surface antigen) found in serum, saliva, semen, stool, and urine

     (2) Core contains HB$_c$Ag (hepatitis B core antigen) and, sometimes, HB$_e$Ag (secretory form of HB$_c$Ag present only in HB$_s$Ag positive sera); HB$_e$Ag associated with high virus titer and high infectivity

     (3) Incubation period 6 weeks to 6 months

     (4) Transmission by blood, blood products, and other body fluids, such as saliva and semen

     (5) Mother-infant transmission if mother infected during third trimester

     (6) Approximately 10% of infected individuals become chronic carriers

    b. Common in drug addicts, homosexual males, those with multiple sexual partners and densely populated urban neighborhoods; higher-risk individuals include persons exposed to needle punctures and blood products such as IV drug abusers; those on hemodialysis; those requiring blood transfusions or IV chemotherapy; and healthcare personnel such as nurses, laboratory workers, surgeons, and hemodialysis personnel

     (1) Considered to be a sexually transmitted disease

     (2) Accounts for about 40% of acute hepatitis cases/annually

  3. HDV (hepatitis delta virus) incomplete RNA virus
    a. Requires antecedent or simultaneous HBV infection
    b. Common in IV drug users and recipients of multiple transfusions
    c. Concomitant infection usually results in more severe manifestations than HBV alone
    d. Immunity to HBV protects against HDV
    e. Associated with increased risk of hepatic cancer

  4. Hepatitis C
    a. Infection with hepatitis C virus (HCV), an RNA virus
     (1) Incubation variable—2 weeks to 6 months

(2) Chronic liver disease develops in 70%

(3) Related to development of hepatocellular carcinoma in 10%

b. High-risk population—IV drug users, hospital personnel, male homosexuals, those receiving multiple transfusions, intranasal cocaine users, and those with body piercings

5. Type E (enteral non-A)

a. Infection with hepatitis E virus (HEV), a single-stranded RNA virus

(1) Viral particles found in stool of infected persons

(2) Does not progress to chronic liver disease

(3) Incubation—2–9 weeks

(4) Usually mild disease in adults > 15 years

(5) Mortality as high as 10–20% in pregnant woman

b. Rare in the United States

6. Type G (HGV)

a. Infection with a flavivirus

(1) Transmitted percutaneously

(2) Most infections asymptomatic

(3) May result in chronic viremia, but chronic disease rare

b. Risk groups include transfusion recipients, IV drug users

c. Frequent coinfection with HCV

- Signs and Symptoms—clinical manifestations for type A, B, D, and E are similar and can vary from a minor flu-like illness to fatal liver failure; type C does not typically present in an acute state

1. HAV may present with nonspecific or "flu" syndrome

2. HBV clinical course more variable than HAV and associated with extrahepatic manifestations, e.g., urticaria, other rashes, arthritis—acute infection subsides and asymptomatic chronic state may ensue

3. HCV may rarely produce acute flu-like illness that subsides spontaneously; however most cases asymptomatic and discovered via routine screening of high-risk individuals

4. Prodromal phase or preicteric phase in types A and B (lasts approximately 2 weeks)

a. Fatigue, malaise

b. Anorexia

c. Nausea/vomiting

d. Headache

e. Hyperalgia

f. Cough, coryza, pharyngitis

g. Changes in taste with aversion to alcohol and smoking

h. Right upper abdominal pain

i. Weight loss of 2–4 kg

5. Active or icteric phase (lasts 2–6 weeks)

a. Jaundice—sclera and skin (never manifested in some patients); not an indication of severity

b. Dark urine

c. Clay-colored stools; often precedes jaundice

d. Enlarged tender liver

e. Pruritus, urticarial rash more often associated with HBV

6. Posticteric or recovery phase

a. Resolving jaundice, increasing sense of well-being, and decrease in symptomatology

b. Chronic active hepatitis in those with HBV may begin at this point and is manifested by persistence of symptoms

- Differential Diagnosis

1. Infectious mononucleosis

2. Choledocholithiasis

3. Hepatotoxic drugs, e.g., chloramphenicol, acetaminophen, methyldopa

4. Carcinoma of the head of the pancreas

5. Alcoholic cirrhosis

6. History and serological tests assist in differentiating type

- Physical Findings

1. General appearance—mildly ill to generally debilitated

2. Vital signs—mild fever

3. Integumentary—slight jaundice; rash

4. Head, ears, eyes, nose, throat (HEENT)—yellow sclera, lymphadenopathy

5. Abdomen—enlarged, tender liver; splenomegaly (in about 10% of cases); normal bowel sounds

- Diagnostic Tests/Findings

1. CBC with differential—WBC low to normal, lymphocytosis, mild anemia

2. Urinalysis—proteinuria; bilirubinuria

3. Abnormal liver function tests

a. Elevated AST and ALT typically 500–2,000 IU/L

b. Rise 7–10 days before jaundice

c. Begin to fall shortly after onset of jaundice; should return to normal after 6 months

d. Degree of increase does not necessarily parallel disease severity

e. LDH, serum bilirubin, alkaline phosphatase, prothrombin time normal or slightly increased

4. Serology tests—refer to **Table 8-3**

- Management/Treatment

1. Consult with physician regarding patient management

■ **Table 8-3** Serology Tests for Viral Hepatitis

IgM antibody to HAV—appears during acute or early convalescent phase and disappears in about 8 weeks; implies recent infection with HAV

IgG antibody to HAV—implies previous infection with HAV; confers immunity

HB$_s$Ag (hepatitis B surface antigen)—positive throughout the active phase of illness; first test to obtain if acute HBV infection is suspected; will remain positive in asymptomatic carriers and in chronic hepatitis

Anti-HB$_s$ (HB$_s$Ag) (antibody specific to HB$_s$Ag [hepatitis B surface antigen])—positive indication of noninfectious state and recovery, and immunity; appears after HB$_s$Ag disappears

Anti-HB$_c$ (antibody to HB$_c$Ag [hepatitis B core antigen])—present at onset of acute illness; remains present for years and is found in asymptomatic carriers; in many patients there is a period (window) between the disappearance of HB$_s$Ag and the appearance of anti-HB$_s$ antibody, usually during late stages of acute phase or early convalescence; during this period, anti-HB$_c$ will be the only serological marker of the infection; presence of anti-HB$_c$ indicates immunity due to natural infection (not present in immunized individual)

Anti-HDV (antibody to hepatitis D)—marker of co/ or superinfection by hepatitis D in persons with hepatitis B; appears late and is short lived

HB$_e$Ag (protein derived from HBV core)—indicates active viral replication, circulating HBV, and highly infectious sera

Anti-HB$_e$ (antibody to HB$_e$Ag)—appears weeks to months after HB$_e$Ag and HBV are no longer detectable in blood; presence indicates substantially less infectious sera

Anti-HCV (antibody to HCV)—appears 6 months after initial infection, remains elevated indefinitely, considered infectious and capable of transmission

HCV-RNA (hepatitis C RNA)—can detect circulating virus in 1–2 weeks after infection; becoming the gold standard for HCV detection

2. Approach is primarily supportive in uncomplicated cases
   a. Activity/rest
      (1) Rest recommended during active phase
      (2) Resumption of full activities during the recovery period does not appear to prolong illness or cause relapse or development of chronic disease
      (3) Avoidance of activity that might cause trauma to liver or spleen
   b. Adequate fluid and dietary intake
      (1) 3,000 to 4,000 mL fluid per day; high carbohydrate fluids such as fruit juices and carbonated beverages are encouraged but not always well tolerated
      (2) Foods high in protein, carbohydrates, and calories
      (3) Low-fat diet not shown to be beneficial
      (4) Most important to eat whatever is tolerated
   c. Antiemetics may be prescribed 30 minutes before meals to control nausea and vomiting; rectal administration may be better tolerated than oral
   d. Patients with elevated PT may be given vitamin K
   e. Symptomatic relief of pruritus with colloidal baths, soaps, and lotions
   f. Avoid alcohol and other drugs detoxified or metabolized by the liver
   g. Avoid birth control pills and C-17 alpha alkyl-substituted androgenic steroids during acute phase; may increase bilirubin levels
3. For HCV—combination therapy with pegylated interferon and ribavirin; treatment is complex and guidelines change frequently; consultation with a specialist for newly diagnosed cases is recommended
   a. Exact mechanism of action unknown
   b. Combination therapy can get rid of the virus in up to 5 out of 10 persons for genotype 1 and in up to 8 out of 10 persons for genotypes 2 and 3
   c. Most positive response with
      (1) Low serum titer HCV RNA
      (2) Younger age
      (3) Female
      (4) Absence of cirrhosis
   d. No data to date showing better survival rates or inhibition of progress to chronic active hepatitis
4. General considerations
   a. Refer for possible hospitalization and further testing
      (1) Complicated cases
      (2) Severely ill patients
      (3) Persons with signs of fulminating hepatitis or encephalitis
      (4) Dehydrated persons
      (5) Those with a PT > 15 seconds
      (6) Those suspected of having another underlying disease process
      (7) Avoid cephalosporins in those with acute disease or significantly elevated liver function tests (LFTs)

b. Newly diagnosed cases reported to health department
c. Patient education
   (1) Disease course and expected outcomes
   (2) Verify any drug use including over-the-counter medications and vitamin supplements with the healthcare provider until completely recovered
   (3) Maintain proper hygiene; proper hand washing, disposal of all body wastes
       (a) Should not donate blood
       (b) Close personal contacts, family members, and sexual contacts should be evaluated for active disease and may receive immune serum globulin for passive immunity (not useful once disease is clinically evident)
d. Follow up
   (1) Follow weekly for the first 2–3 weeks; monthly thereafter if symptoms subside and LFTs improving

   (2) Closer follow-up in those > 40 years of age
e. Complications
   (1) HBV infection tends to be longer and more severe than HAV
   (2) Carrier states and chronic hepatitis are associated with HBV and HCV, but not with HAV
   (3) Chronic HBV treatment includes recombinant interferon a-2b and direct inhibitors of HBV replication, but treatment rarely produces permanent remission of the disease
   (4) Fulminant liver failure occurs in less than 1% of those with HAV and in about 5% of those with HBV
   (5) Chronic hepatitis can be associated with hepatic cancer
   (6) 70% of patients with hepatitis C will develop chronic hepatitis
f. Prophylaxis—see **Table 8-4**

■ **Table 8-4** Adult Prophylaxis for Viral Hepatitis

Time of Exposure	Agent	Dose	Time
Preexposure			
Hepatitis A Persons traveling to or working in endemic areas; men who have sex with men; drug users; those who work with nonhuman primates with HAV infection or in labs with HAV; persons with chronic liver disease; those with clotting factor disorders; and some food handlers	HA vaccine (preferred over serum)	1 mL IM	2 doses separated by 6–12 months depending on brand; protection begins 4 weeks after first dose; both doses needed for long-term protection
If travel or exposure expected in less than 4 weeks after 1st HAV vaccine dose	Immune serum globulin	0.02 mL/kg once	
Hepatitis B Recommended for healthcare personnel especially laboratory personnel; surgeons; dialysis personnel; also recommended for adolescents in areas with high incidence of HBV, drug abuse, STD, teen pregnancies, and for homosexually active men	HB vaccine × 3	1 mL IM	Usually given in 3 doses; 2nd and 3rd given approximately 1 mo and 6 mo after the 1st dose; need all 3 doses for adequate protection
Postexposure			
Hepatitis A Close contacts; family members; sexual partners	Immune serum globulin	0.02 mL/kg	Once, not more than 2 weeks postexposure
Hepatitis B Percutaneous needle stick or mucosal exposure if unvaccinated and source HB$_s$Ag +	HB immune globulin and HB vaccine × 3	0.06 mL/kg 1 mL IM	Within 24–48 hours of exposure; at same time as HBIg, then at 1 and 6 mo
Sexual exposure	Globulin and HB vaccine × 3	0.6 mL/kg 1 mL IM	Within 14 days of last sexual contact; at same time as HBIg, then at 1 mo and 6 mo

Contact Centers for Disease Control and Prevention hotline for most current and more specific information 1-404-332–4555 or www.cdc.gov

▣ ACUTE GASTROENTERITIS

- Definition—acute inflammation of the gastrointestinal mucosa

- Etiology/Incidence
  1. Commonly due to infectious agents—viruses, bacteria, and parasites (*Giardia*, amoebae)
     a. Exotoxins produced by some organisms, (e.g., *Staphylococcus*) induce hypersecretion or increased peristalsis resulting in diarrhea or vomiting
     b. Bacteria such as *E. coli* and salmonella penetrate and invade the gastric mucosa and lead to diarrhea accompanied by fever and fecal leukocytes
     c. See **Table 8-5** for characteristics of some etiologic agents in gastroenteritis
  2. Among the top 10 leading cause of morbidity in the United States
     a. Occurs universally in all age groups
     b. Epidemic outbreaks of bacterial enteritis occur in groups of persons who have ingested contaminated food
     c. Viral gastroenteritis occurs more frequently in the winter months
     d. Primarily a self-limiting disease (1–2 weeks)
     e. The very young, elderly, and those with concomitant chronic debilitating disease are at higher risk for mortality

- Signs and Symptoms
  1. Abrupt onset of nausea, vomiting
  2. Explosive flatulence
  3. Crampy abdominal pain
  4. Frequent, watery diarrhea
  5. Myalgia
  6. Headache
  7. Fever
  8. Generalized weakness/malaise

- Differential Diagnosis
  1. Acute appendicitis
  2. Cholecystitis
  3. Inflammatory bowel disease, e.g., colitis
  4. Bowel obstruction
  5. Fecal impaction with overflow
  6. Pelvic inflammatory disease

- Physical Findings
  1. General appearance—ill
  2. Vital signs—fever moderate to high 101–102° F in bacterial; up to 103° F in viral
  3. Abdomen—diffuse tenderness; no spasm or rebound tenderness except with salmonella infection; hyperactive bowel sounds; slight distention; absent or hypoactive bowel sounds common with botulism
  4. Neurological—dizziness, difficulty in swallowing and other neurological deficits are indication of botulism and require emergency intervention; with other etiologies findings are expected to be normal

- Diagnostic Tests/Findings
  1. Normally not indicated unless symptoms > 72 hours in duration
  2. CBC—normal indices
  3. Stool guaiac—usually negative in viral infections; positive with invasive bacterial infections
  4. Stool examination—if etiologic agent is an invasive bacteria, leukocytes will be present
  5. Stool culture—diagnostic for bacteria
     a. Done in suspected cases of bacterial infection and food poisoning, and if symptoms do not begin to abate in 72 hours
     b. Special cultures needed for suspected campylobacter, cholera

■ **Table 8-5** Characteristics of Select Etiologic Agents in Gastroenteritis

	Incubation or Onset	Fever	Fecal Leukocytes	Other
E. coli	24–72 hrs	+	+	Common cause of travelers' diarrhea; doxycycline, bismuth subsalicylate used preventively; treatment with rifaximin
Campylobacter	2–5 days	+	+	Erythromycin and tetracycline used in treatment
Staphylococcus	1–6 hrs	-	-	Grows in meats; dairy foods
Shigella/Salmonella	8–24 hrs	+	+	Highly infectious
Botulism	12–36 hrs	-	-	Neuro. signs—diplopia, vertigo, dysphagia; respiratory support may be needed
Giardia lamblia	7–21 days	-	-	Rifaximin used in treatment; cause of travelers' diarrhea

- Management/Treatment
  1. Immediately refer to a physician those with
     a. Dehydration
     b. Rebound tenderness
     c. Severe abdominal pain
     d. Neurological symptoms
     e. Concomitant debilitating illness
  2. Most can be treated for 72 hours without laboratory testing with
     a. Bed rest as needed progressing to regular activity
     b. NPO except for cracked ice while nausea and vomiting are present, then restriction to clear liquids for 24 hours; follow with addition of toast and crackers, proceeding to a bland then regular diet
     c. Antiemetics and antidiarrheals are usually not indicated and may prolong the problem; treatment of salmonella has been noted to prolong the carrier state
     d. Provide for parenteral administration of prescription medications if necessary
  3. General considerations
     a. Consult with physician if major symptoms do not abate in 72 hours; approach may include stool for ova and parasites, specialized stool cultures, and proctosigmoidoscopy
     b. Report bacterial infections and food poisoning to the health department
     c. Routine use of antibiotics is not recommended; consider use in those with
        (1) Symptoms lasting > 3 days
        (2) Impaired immune response
     d. Patient education
        (1) Disease course and expected outcome; symptoms usually resolve in 72 hours but mild diarrhea may persist for a week or 2
        (2) Explain proper food preparation and storage
        (3) Appropriate dosage and side effects of medications
        (4) Proper methods of hygiene including hand washing and disposal of stool and vomit
        (5) Signs of dehydration; neurological involvement that requires contacting healthcare professional
     e. Follow up
        (1) Usually self-limiting; return visit warranted if symptoms (other than mild diarrhea) do not abate in 72 hours or if they worsen
        (2) Diarrhea may continue for 1–2 weeks with salmonella infection

☐ IRRITABLE BOWEL SYNDROME (IBS) (FUNCTIONAL BOWEL SYNDROME)

- Definition—idiopathic clinical syndrome characterized by abdominal pain or discomfort occurring in association with altered bowel habits for at least three days per month for the last three months

- Etiology/Incidence
  1. Disturbance in bowel motor activity thought to include a normal response to severe stress and learned visceral response to stress leading to
     a. Nonpropulsive colonic contractions that lead to constipation
     b. Increased contraction in the small bowel and proximal colon with diminished activity in the distal colon leading to diarrhea
  2. May be influenced by emotional factors
  3. Common GI disorder
     a. Accounts for about 50% of most GI complaints seen by healthcare professionals and a major cause of morbidity in the United States
     b. Onset usually occurs before age 35
     c. Women affected more often than men
     d. More common in those with other functional disorders

- Signs and Symptoms
  1. Aching or cramping periumbilical or lower abdominal pain often precipitated by meals and relieved by defecation; does not awaken patient at night
  2. Pain may radiate to left chest or arm (gas in splenic flexure)
  3. Changes in bowel function
     a. Diarrhea
        (1) 4–6 movements/day
        (2) Small watery stools with clear mucus
        (3) Nocturnal diarrhea (rare)
     b. Constipation with irregular passage of small hard stools
     c. Alternating episodes of diarrhea and constipation
  4. Flatulence
  5. Exaggerated response to and preoccupation with bowel symptoms
  6. Bleeding, weight loss, and nocturnal diarrhea are not characteristic of IBS

- Differential Diagnosis
  1. Inflammatory bowel disorder, e.g., ulcerative colitis
  2. Viral or bacterial gastroenteritis
  3. GI neoplasms
  4. Parasitic infections

5. Lactose deficiency
6. Laxative abuse
7. Side effects of drugs affecting bowel motility
8. Rome III criteria for diagnosis requires three days per month for at least three months of continuous or recurrent abdominal pain or discomfort plus at least two of the following
   a. Improvement with defecation
   b. Change in stool frequency (diarrhea or constipation)
   c. Change in stool form or appearance (loose, watery, mucus, or pellet-like)
   d. Symptom onset at least six months prior to diagnosis

- Physical Findings
  1. General appearance—"worried well," anxious, depressed
  2. Vital signs—normal
  3. Abdomen—mild abdominal tenderness, normal or mildly hyperactive bowel sounds, distension
  4. Rectal examination—normal
  5. Systemic symptoms, e.g., fever and weight loss, are absent

- Diagnostic Tests/Findings
  1. Stool examination—negative for blood, ova, parasite, pathogenic bacteria, and *Giardia*-specific antigen
  2. CBC, thyroid screen, chemical analysis—normal
  3. Barium enema—decreased motility, otherwise normal
  4. Proctosigmoidoscopy—normal

- Management/Treatment
  1. Confer with physician before ordering barium enema or proctosigmoidoscopy
  2. Provide emotional support, reassurance, information on stress reduction
  3. Dietary changes may improve symptoms
     a. High-fiber diet
     b. Avoid lactose-containing and gas-producing foods
     c. Fiber supplement may be indicated in addition to high-fiber diet
  4. Pharmacologic agents
     a. Bulk laxatives—psyllium hydrophilic mucilloid
     b. Narcotics, depressants, and long-term pharmaceutical use to be avoided
     c. Anticholinergics
        (1) Dicyclomine hydrochloride 20-40 mg orally q.i.d. or propantheline 15 mg orally q.i.d.
        (2) Usually given only after nonpharmacologic measures have failed
        (3) Side effects—dry mouth, tachycardia, orthostatic hypotension

        (4) Contraindicated if history of glaucoma, urinary retention, cardiac arrhythmia
        (5) Loperamide or other opiate-derived antidiarrheals are reserved for only very severe cases; potential for abuse in these patients is great
     d. Tricyclic antidepressants
     e. 5-HT$_3$ antagonists and 5-HT$_4$ agonist (suspended from general use but available under certain circumstances via certified providers in extreme cases)
     f. Chloride channel activator (lubiprostone) for IBS-C
     g. Refaximin (non-absorbable antibiotic) not yet approved for IBS but may be appropriate for refractory patients
     h. Probiotic data are conflicting but present a safe, well-tolerated option in refractory patients
     i. Zofran primarily used for management of severe nausea and vomiting
  5. Patient education
     a. Disease course and expected outcomes
     b. Rationale for treatment
     c. High-fiber diet
  6. Planned exercise (may help in stress reduction)
  7. Need for annual rectal examination and sigmoidoscopy after age 40
  8. Some patients may benefit from psychological counseling and/or relaxation techniques

◘ COLORECTAL CANCER

- Definition—malignancy of gastrointestinal tract, primarily colon or rectum

- Etiology/Incidence
  1. Causes remain unclear
  2. Risk factors include history of colonic polyps, breast or female genital tract cancer, chronic inflammatory bowel disorders, positive family history; high-fat, low-fiber, high-caloric diet
  3. Third leading cause of cancer morbidity and mortality in the United States

- Signs and Symptoms—vary by location
  1. Right-sided colon cancer
     a. Usually asymptomatic
     b. Vague or crampy, colicky abdominal pain
     c. Unexplained weight loss, fatigue, weakness
     d. Occult blood in stool
     e. Anemia
  2. Left-sided colon cancer
     a. Alternating constipation with diarrhea
     b. Change in stool caliber (narrow, ribbon-like)
     c. Lower abdominal pain
     d. Red blood in stool
     e. Sensation of incomplete evacuation

3. Rectal cancer
    a. Tenesmus
    b. Rectal bleeding (bright red)
    c. Mucous discharge

- Differential Diagnosis
    1. Diverticular disease
    2. Lymphoma
    3. Irritable bowel syndrome
    4. Inflammatory bowel disease

- Physical Findings
    1. Palpable mass primarily in right colon
    2. Lymphadenopathy
    3. Rectal mass found on rectal examination
    4. Stools positive for occult blood

- Diagnostic Tests/Findings
    1. Colonoscopy—diagnostic study of choice; allows for biopsy of lesions
    2. Barium enema radiograph used much less commonly but may reveal lesions when evaluating other bowel symptoms
    3. Testing of stools for occult blood—effective for early detection, positive findings to be followed with colonoscopy
    4. Carcinoembryonic antigen (CEA) test—often performed, although not specific for colon cancer; normal level of CEA does not exclude possibility of malignancy
    5. CBC can demonstrate an iron deficiency anemia; should be followed with endoscopic assessment in middle-aged and older adults
    6. Chest radiograph may reveal metastases

- Management/Treatment
    1. Referral for surgical excision or resection depending upon the depth of invasion of tumors
    2. Patients with metastatic lesions, noted at the time of diagnosis, have a poor prognosis; palliative treatment is then indicated
    3. Patients with a resection often require a temporary colostomy
    4. General considerations
        a. American Cancer Society recommendations for colon cancer screenings for persons of average risk begin at age 50 and include
            (1) Testing for fecal occult blood annually
            (2) Flexible sigmoidoscopy every 5 years or
            (3) Double-contrast barium enema every 5 years or
            (4) CT colonography (virtual colonoscopy) every 5 years or
            (5) Colonoscopy every 10 years

    b. Monitor for signs of dehydration during colon preps
    c. Instruct patient on possibility of a colostomy after procedure and begin patient teaching on care of colostomy preoperatively
    d. Encourage patient and family to ventilate feelings regarding the diagnosis
    e. Make referrals to pastoral care or mental health liaison as indicated
    f. Refer to community agencies for assistance after discharge, i.e., American Cancer Society, United Ostomy Associations of America

☐ QUESTIONS

Select the best answer.

Questions 1–4 refer to the following scenario.

Mr. P., a 55-year-old Irish male, complains of pain in his chest and stomach for the past 2 weeks. He has been taking Alka Seltzer, which seems to give him temporary relief. The pain is intermittent but has awakened him at night. The pain has a burning quality, and radiates up into his chest. He has hypertension, which is controlled with diuretics.

1. Which of the following would least likely be the cause of his pain?

    a. Coronary artery insufficiency
    b. Diverticulitis
    c. Duodenal ulcer
    d. Esophageal reflux

2. Your next step would be to:

    a. Start Mr. P. on antacids and a proton pump inhibitor
    b. Discontinue his diuretic and switch to another class of antihypertensive
    c. Order an endoscopy
    d. Obtain additional medical history data

3. The fact that Mr. P.'s pain is not increased with activity and is unrelieved by rest makes it less likely that his problem is:

    a. Coronary artery insufficiency
    b. Gastric ulcer
    c. Duodenal ulcer
    d. Esophageal reflux

4. Which fact favors a diagnosis of gastric ulcer in this case?

    a. The patient's gender
    b. The patient's age
    c. The patient's ethnic origin
    d. The use of diuretics

5. Which of the following would be most beneficial in distinguishing a duodenal ulcer from a gastric ulcer?

   a. A history of a confirmed healed duodenal ulcer in the past year
   b. Reported unexplained weight loss in the past 6 months
   c. Pain aggravated by food intake
   d. An endoscopy or upper GI barium radiograph

6. Causative factors for duodenal ulcer include:

   a. High-fat diet
   b. Stress
   c. Use of anti-inflammatory drugs
   d. ETOH ingestion

7. Bleeding from a duodenal ulcer:

   a. Usually causes increased pain
   b. In large amounts can cause diarrhea
   c. Is associated with constipation
   d. Indicates perforation

8. The physical examination of most patients with peptic ulcer disease:

   a. Is noncontributory
   b. Reveals epigastric discomfort to deep palpation
   c. Should be performed after an 8-hour fast
   d. Differentiates gastric from duodenal ulcer

9. A 55-year-old male with a peptic ulcer and mild anemia has a negative stool guaiac. You need to:

   a. Start iron supplementation
   b. Start a proton pump inhibitor and reschedule for return visit in 2–4 weeks
   c. Repeat the stool guaiac
   d. Refer for hematologic work up

10. After 2 weeks of treatment for *H. pylori* ulcer disease, all symptoms of a small nonbleeding duodenal ulcer have abated in your 35-year-old patient. You:

    a. Need to confirm healing with an upper GI barium radiograph or endoscopy
    b. Instruct her that she may discontinue medications
    c. Instruct her to stop all medication and get a urea breath test
    d. Stop these medications and put her on H_2 antagonists

11. A major side effect of cimetidine that would be of special concern when prescribing for an elderly patient is:

    a. Confusion
    b. Decreased digoxin levels
    c. Hypophosphatemia
    d. Osteopenia

Questions 12, 13, and 14 refer to the following scenario.

Mr. J. is an overweight 38 year old who has had intermittent heartburn for several months. He has been taking Tums, which do provide temporary relief. During the past week he has been awakening during the night with a burning sensation in his chest. He is on no medication and has had no other major health problems.

12. Which additional information would lead you to believe that gastroesophageal reflux is the cause of his pain?

    a. The pain seems better when he smokes to relieve his nerves
    b. Constipation has been a chronic problem and he uses over-the-counter laxatives at least weekly
    c. He often awakens at night with coughing and a bad taste in his mouth
    d. Coffee and fried foods never bother him

13. Mr. J. had no weight loss or dysphagia and his physical examination is unremarkable. Your next step would be to:

    a. Order an endoscopic exam
    b. Refer him to a gastroenterologist
    c. Start him on a proton pump inhibitor
    d. Tell him to eat a snack before bedtime

14. If you diagnose GERD, you will tell him:

    a. He probably has a hiatal hernia causing the reflux
    b. He will probably require surgery
    c. He should avoid all fruit juices
    d. Smoking, alcohol, and caffeine can aggravate his problem

15. The standard for documenting tissue damage in gastroesophageal reflux is:

    a. Stool guaiac
    b. Upper GI barium radiograph
    c. Cardiac and abdominal examination
    d. Endoscopy

Questions 16–19 refer to the following scenario.

Mary L. is 26 years old, slightly overweight, and 2 months postpartum. She is complaining of heartburn, flatulence, and anorexia. During her pregnancy she had experienced similar symptoms, but they have become more severe in the last week and she vomited twice. She has an intermittent pain in her right hypochondrium. She also thinks she pulled a shoulder muscle as she has an almost constant dull ache there.

16. Your first step is to:

    a. Order liver function tests
    b. Obtain a more detailed history
    c. Refer her back to her obstetrician
    d. Refer her to a gastroenterologist

17. Mary's physical examination is unremarkable except for RUQ tenderness and a positive Murphy's sign. Which of the following becomes your primary differential diagnosis?

    a. Appendicitis
    b. Salpingitis
    c. Cholecystitis
    d. Diverticulitis

18. Which would be the most helpful diagnostic test at this point?

    a. CBC and liver function studies
    b. Ultrasound
    c. Liver scan
    d. Chest radiograph and ECG

19. Mary's ultrasound is negative, but she remains symptomatic and you still think cholecystitis is likely. What is the next step in your assessment?

    a. Refer for surgical evaluation
    b. Obtain a CT scan of the abdomen with contrast
    c. Obtain a CT scan of the abdomen without contrast
    d. Order a HIDA scan

20. A 22-year-old male student comes to the student health service complaining of generalized abdominal pain and nausea. He had been out with a group of friends the night before and had been eating pizza and drinking beer. He awoke with generalized abdominal pain this morning and took some Alka Seltzer without much effect. The pain has gotten steadily worse throughout the day and he now feels nauseated. He wonders if he might have food poisoning. Examination reveals hypoactive bowel sounds and some tenderness in the RLQ. There is no guarding or rebound tenderness. His temperature is 100° F. The absence of guarding and rebound tenderness:

    a. Suggests a psychogenic cause of his pain
    b. Rules out appendicitis
    c. Makes peritonitis unlikely
    d. Indicates irritable bowel syndrome

21. When a patient has abdominal pain accompanied by several episodes of vomiting:

    a. It is not likely to be a surgical problem
    b. Stopping the vomiting becomes the primary priority
    c. Diarrhea is likely to occur within 6 hours
    d. An antiemetic is contraindicated until the cause is definitively identified

22. Diverticulitis is most often characterized by:

    a. Left lower quadrant discomfort
    b. Bloody diarrhea
    c. Rebound tenderness in the LLQ
    d. Associated vomiting

23. When should a patient with GERD be referred for endoscopy?

    a. At the time of diagnosis
    b. When he is over 55 years old at symptom onset
    c. When he has symptoms despite b.i.d. PPI therapy
    d. When manometry is not consistent with GERD

24. In elderly patients which of the following would not be an expected indication of appendicitis?

    a. Mild fever
    b. Abdominal distention with little pain
    c. Flatulence and hyperactive bowel sounds
    d. Shift to the left without leukocytosis

Questions 25, 26, and 27 refer to the following scenario.

Ms. J is a 29-year-old accountant who comes in complaining of frequent crampy abdominal pain after meals. She is often constipated and takes over-the-counter laxatives, which are followed by a couple of days of diarrhea. She does feel better after having a bowel movement but only temporarily. She has also been embarrassed by flatulence and has noticed some abdominal distention. She has had no weight loss and has not noticed any blood in her stool. This problem has gone on for at least 6 months.

25. Your next step would be to:

    a. Obtain a complete history
    b. Order a barium enema
    c. Order a Bernstein test
    d. Suggest a trial of antispasmodics

26. Which of the following makes diverticulitis an unlikely diagnosis in this patient?

    a. Her age
    b. Frequent constipation
    c. Flatulence
    d. Crampy, intermittent pain

27. Which of the following would not be expected to occur with irritable bowel syndrome?

    a. Anxiety
    b. Nocturnal diarrhea
    c. Pain radiating to the left chest and arm
    d. Bloating

28. Which of the following would be the reason for hospitalizing a patient with acute diverticulitis?

    a. LLQ tenderness
    b. Advanced age
    c. Leukocytosis
    d. Increased pain with defecation

29. Which of the following is not indicated for treatment of acute diverticulitis?

    a. Bed rest
    b. Liquid diet
    c. Antibiotics
    d. High-fiber diet

30. A positive stool guaiac in a person suspected of having diverticulitis is:

    a. Expected in 25–30% cases
    b. An ominous sign indicating need for hospitalization
    c. Often accompanied by more pronounced pain
    d. An indication of pending perforation

31. Bacteriuria in persons with acute diverticulosis may indicate:

    a. Abscess formation
    b. Bowel-bladder fistula
    c. Free perforation into the abdomen
    d. Reason for leukocytosis

32. Ms. S., a 19-year-old college freshman, has just completed exam week. She comes in complaining of fatigue, headache, anorexia, and a runny nose. Symptoms began about 2 weeks ago. She has been taking vitamins and over-the-counter cold preparations but feels worse. "Just the smell" of food makes her nauseated. Her boyfriend had mono about a month ago and she wonders if she might have it. Physical examination reveals cervical lymphadenopathy, a slightly enlarged, tender liver, and enlarged spleen. Which laboratory tests in addition to a CBC, throat culture, and mono spot test would be most helpful in the differential diagnosis at this point?

    a. HAV IgG antibody test
    b. Anti-HB$_s$Ag
    c. Liver enzymes
    d. Stool culture

33. There is no indication in Ms. S.'s history to indicate IV drug abuse or exposure to blood products. Given the duration of her symptoms and a confirmed increase in her liver enzymes, which test would be most helpful in confirming your diagnosis?

    a. IgM antibody to HAV
    b. IgG antibody to HAV
    c. Anti-HDV
    d. Anti-HB$_s$

34. A 30-year-old male with a history of acute hepatitis C over 1 year ago who was treated with interferon still tests anti-HCV positive. He should be considered:

    a. Infectious
    b. Incapable of transmitting the virus
    c. Fully recovered
    d. To have high serum viral levels

35. Infection with HDV requires antecedent or simultaneous infection with:

    a. HAV
    b. HBV
    c. HCV
    d. HGV

36. When jaundice occurs with hepatitis infection it:

    a. Indicates a more severe infection
    b. Increases the risk of acute liver failure
    c. Indicates development of chronic active hepatitis
    d. Usually resolves in 2–6 weeks

37. A normally healthy young adult diagnosed as having salmonella food poisoning should be told:

    a. To take doxycycline 100 mg t.i.d.
    b. That antidiarrheal drugs may decrease his diarrhea temporarily but may also prolong the problem
    c. That he should try to force fluids despite his nausea and vomiting to prevent dehydration
    d. The diarrhea should abate in about 24 hours

38. Which is the next laboratory test to obtain if diarrhea and vomiting persist for more than 48 hours?

    a. Stool guaiac
    b. Sigmoidoscopy
    c. Flat plate of the abdomen
    d. Stool culture and microscopic examination

39. Blurred vision and dizziness in a patient with suspected food poisoning requires:

    a. Gastroenterologic consult
    b. Antibiotic therapy
    c. Immediate hospitalization
    d. Follow up in 24 hours

40. An 18-year-old previously healthy female presents with a case of a sudden onset of nausea, vomiting, generalized crampy abdominal pain followed by explosive diarrhea. The stools are uniformly thin and watery, without blood or pus. Physical exam reveals hyperactive bowel sounds and bilateral lower quadrant tenderness but no guarding or rebound. Rectal exam is negative and she is afebrile. The hypothesis that best explains these findings is:

a. Acute appendicitis
b. Acute salpingitis
c. Acute gastroenteritis
d. Ruptured ovarian cyst

Answers

1. **b**		21. **a**
2. **d**		22. **a**
3. **a**		23. **c**
4. **b**		24. **c**
5. **d**		25. **a**
6. **c**		26. **a**
7. **b**		27. **c**
8. **a**		28. **b**
9. **c**		29. **d**
10. **b**		30. **a**
11. **a**		31. **b**
12. **c**		32. **c**
13. **c**		33. **a**
14. **d**		34. **a**
15. **d**		35. **b**
16. **b**		36. **d**
17. **c**		37. **b**
18. **b**		38. **d**
19. **d**		39. **c**
20. **c**		40. **c**

◘ BIBLIOGRAPHY

The AGA Institute Medical Position Panel. (2008). American Gastroenterological Association Medical Position Statement on the Management of GERD. *Gastroenterology, 135,* 1383–1391.

Boche, S. P., & Kobos, R. (2004). Jaundice in the adult patient. *American Family Physician, 69*(2), 299–304.

Brunton, S. (2004). Irritable bowel syndrome: New perspectives on treatment. *The Female Patient, 29*(4), 15–20.

Chey, W. D., Wong, B. C. Y., & Practice Parameters Committee of the American College of Gastroenterology (ACG). (2007). The American College of Gastroenterology guidelines on the management of *Helicobacter pylori* infection. *American Journal of Gastroenterology, 102,* 1808–1825.

Field, S. (2003). Approaches to diverticular disease. *The Clinical Advisor,* 25–31.

Friedman, L. S. (2012). Liver, biliary tract, and pancreas. In S. J. McPhee, & M. A. Papadakis (Eds.), *Current medical diagnosis and treatment* (51st ed., pp. 644-698.). New York: McGraw-Hill.

Lin, K. W., & Kirchner, J. T. (2004). Hepatitis B. *American Family Physician, 69*(1), 75–82.

McQuaid, K. R. (2012). Gastrointestinal disorders. In S. J. McPhee, & M. A. Papadakis (Eds.), *Current medical diagnosis and treatment* (51st ed., pp. 546–643). New York: McGraw-Hill.

National Institutes of Health. (2006). *Chronic hepatitis C: Current disease management.* NIH publication no. 07-4230. Bethesda, MD: Author. Retrieved from http ://digestive.niddk.nih.gov/ddiseases/pubs/chronic hepc/

Rayburn, N., & Rayburn, D. J. (2002). Inflammatory bowel disease: Symptoms in the bowel and beyond. *The Nurse Practitioner, 27*(11), 13–29.

Salzman, H., & Lillie, D. (2005). Diverticular disease: Diagnosis and treatment. *American Family Physician, 72,* 1229–1234, 1241–1242.

Sherman, C. (2007). Dyspepsia guidelines emphasize *H. pylori. The Clinical Advisor, 69,* 73–74.

Talley, N. J., & Spiller, R. (2002). Irritable bowel syndrome: A little understood organic bowel disease? *Lancet, 360,* 555–564.

Trowbridge, R. L., Rutkowski, N. K., & Shojania, K. (2003). Does this patient have acute cholecystitis? *Journal of the American Medical Association, 289*(1), 80–86.

U.S. Preventive Services Task Force. (2006). *The Guide to Clinical Preventive Services: Recommendations of the United States Preventive Services Task Force.* Retrieved from http://www.ahrq.gov/clinic/pocketgd.pdf

Vakil, N., van Zanten, S. V., Kahrilas, P., Dent, J., Jones, R. (2006). The Montreal definition and classification of gastroesophageal reflux disease: A global evidence-based consensus. *American Journal of Gastroenterology, 101,* 1900–1920.

Viera, A. J., Hoag, S., & Shaughnessy, J. (2002). Management of irritable bowel syndrome. *American Family Physician, 66*(10), 1867–1874.

Yoshida, E. M. (2003). Abnormal liver function tests: What to do for the patient. *Consultant, 43*(4), 505–513.

9

Endocrine Disorders

Sister Maria Salerno

◘ DIABETES MELLITUS (DM)

- Definition—metabolic disorder of carbohydrate, fat, and protein metabolism characterized by abnormally high blood glucose levels due to inadequate or absent insulin production and/or impaired insulin action

- Etiology/Incidence
  1. Type 1—immune mediated (formerly insulin-dependent [IDDM] type I, juvenile-onset, ketosis-prone)
     a. Genetic susceptibility (HLA-DR3 gene) with environmental exposure to virus or other infectious processes leading to abnormal autoimmune response and destruction of insulin-producing pancreatic beta cells is suspected
        (1) Family history of autoimmune disorders
        (2) Islet cell antibodies
        (3) Insulin autoantibodies
        (4) Absence of C-peptide
     b. Occurs more often in those < 20 years of age; those with European ancestry
     c. 10–15% of diabetics are of this type
     d. < 10% of patients with type 1 diabetes are idiopathic; no immune component appreciated
  2. Type 2 (formerly type II, non-insulin-dependent [NIDDM] adult or maturity onset, ketosis-resistant)—may range from predominantly insulin resistant with relative insulin deficiency as a result of insulin resistance secondary to impaired peripheral insulin receptors (obese type) to predominantly insulin secretory defect (nonobese type); most patients have both features at time of diagnosis
     a. Obese type 2
        (1) Intracellular fat accumulation results in distended cell membranes with change in insulin receptor morphology
        (2) Insulin resistance as a result of altered insulin receptor morphology in target cells
        (3) Post cell receptor defect impairing glucose transport into the cells
        (4) Hyperinsulinemia results; precedes hyperglycemia by years
        (5) Eventual beta cell burnout results in decreased insulin production; hyperglycemia ensues
        (6) Most type 2 diabetes is of this type
     b. Nonobese type 2
        (1) Beta cells lose responsiveness to insulinogenic stimuli, e.g., glucose, glucagon
        (2) Decreased beta cell production of insulin leads to hyperglycemia
        (3) Insulin receptor abnormalities not a problem initially
     c. No specific human leukocyte antigen (HLA) or islet cell antibodies
     d. Risk factors include
        (1) Family history of diabetes
        (2) Being previously identified as glucose intolerant

(3) African-American, Asian American, Hispanic American, Native American, or Pacific Islander race

(4) Age ≥ 45

(5) Physical inactivity/obesity

(6) Having given birth to an infant weighing ≥ 9 lbs

(7) Metabolic syndrome

3. Diabetes associated with certain conditions or syndromes

  a. Includes endocrinopathy, infection, drug/chemically induced

  b. Genetic syndromes

4. Impaired fasting glucose (IFG)

  a. Glucose levels fall between normal and overt diabetes

  b. May worsen over time, remain unchanged, or revert to normal

5. Gestational diabetes mellitus (GDM)

6. About 8 million diagnosed cases and estimated 8 million undiagnosed; after thyroid disease and obesity most common metabolic disorder encountered in primary care settings; third leading cause of death in United States

- Signs and Symptoms

1. Type 1

  a. Usually sudden and severe in onset

  b. Early

    (1) Polyuria

    (2) Polydipsia

    (3) Polyphagia

    (4) Weight loss with normal or increased appetite

    (5) Blurred vision

    (6) Fatigue/weakness

    (7) Nausea/vomiting

  c. With advanced disease and long-term complications

    (1) Loss of appetite

    (2) Bloating

    (3) Dehydration

    (4) Decreased level of consciousness

    (5) Neurogenic and microvascular changes

      (a) Paresthesias

      (b) Progressive visual impairment

      (c) Cold extremities

      (d) Decreased or absent pedal pulses

      (e) Constipation, nocturnal diarrhea

      (f) Nocturia, neurogenic bladder, uremia, impotence

2. Type 2

  a. Onset more insidious

  b. Early disease typically not noticed; discovered incidentally

  c. With advanced disease and long-term complications

(1) Similar to type 1, but macrovascular changes more prominent than microvascular

  (a) Atherosclerosis

  (b) Vascular insufficiency

  (c) Coronary heart disease

  (d) Recurrent vaginal or genital infection, fungus

  (e) Poor wound healing, skin rashes

  (f) Target organ damage to include microalbuminuria, cardiac hypertrophy, retinopathy

(2) Hyperosmolar, nonketotic syndrome (HNS)

- Differential Diagnosis

1. Pancreatitis

2. Cushing's syndrome

3. Pheochromocytoma

4. Acromegaly

5. Cirrhosis

6. Secondary effects of drug therapy

  a. Oral contraceptives

  b. Corticosteroids

  c. Thiazides

  d. Phenytoin

- Physical Findings

1. Type 1

  a. Early

    (1) Thin, decreased weight

    (2) Ill appearance

    (3) Orthostatic hypotension

    (4) Volume contraction

    (5) Paresthesias

    (6) Mental status changes as diabetic ketoacidosis (DKA) occurs

  b. With more advanced disease

    (1) Skin—ulcerations of feet and legs, "shin spots" over tibial bones; loss of hair over lower legs and toes

    (2) Eyes—retinopathy, including microaneurysms; yellow hard or fluffy "cotton wool" exudates; neovascularization, cataracts, glaucoma

    (3) Cardiovascular—diminished or absent pedal pulses; decreased capillary filling, pretibial edema, cool extremities

    (4) Neurologic—sensory loss, absent knee and ankle jerks, deficits in extraocular movements

2. Type 2

  a. Early

    (1) Usually obese

    (2) Hypertension

  b. With advanced disease similar to type 1

- Diagnostic Tests/Findings
  1. Plasma blood sugar—criteria for confirmation
     a. The diagnosis of diabetes will be made if FBS ≥ 126 mg/dL and is ≥ 126 mg/dL on repeat testing *or*
     b. HgbA$_{1c}$ > 6.5%
     c. Random plasma glucose (RPG) level is ≥ 200 mg/dL and
        (1) Symptoms of polydipsia, polyuria, and weight loss are present *or*
        (2) On a subsequent day the FBS is ≥ 126 mg/dL or oral glucose tolerance test (OGTT) glucose level at 2 hours is ≥ 200 mg/dL
     d. It is advised that the OGTT not be used routinely
     e. If fasting glucose level are ≥ 100 mg/dL but < 126 mg/dL, a diagnosis of "prediabetes" is made
     f. Pregnant women should be screened for gestational diabetes at 24–28 weeks gestation with a 50-g glucose load
        (1) A 1-hour glucose level < 140 mg/dL is negative
        (2) A 1-hour glucose level > 200 mg/dL is diagnostic
        (3) A 1-hour glucose level between 140 mg/dL and 200 mg/dL requires confirmation by a 100-g OGTT—the diagnosis is confirmed if two of four values meet or exceed recommended cutoff points
            (a) Fasting 105 mg/dL
            (b) 1-hour 190 mg/dL
            (c) 2-hour 165 mg/dL
            (d) 3-hour 145 mg/dL
        (4) Those with known risk factors such as race/ethnicity do not need the screening level 50-g exam but should receive the diagnostic 100-g exam at the 24–28 week point
  2. Urinalysis—presence of glucose, acetone (in type 1), and, in advanced stages, protein
  3. Blood urea nitrogen and urine creatinine— elevated in acute dehydration and with renal involvement
  4. Serum cholesterol and triglyceride levels— often elevated especially in type 2
  5. Electrocardiogram and chest radiography—for coronary and pulmonary pathology
  6. Hemoglobin A$_{1c}$—predominately used as a measure of glycemic control; indicates average plasma glucose level for previous 60–90 days; tested every 3–6 months, < 7% considered good control
  7. Glycated serum protein (GSP), serum fructosamine
     a. Index of glycemic status over past 1–2 weeks
     b. Clinical utility still under study; best used for those with hemoglobinopathies that render HgbA$_{1c}$ inaccurate

- Management/Treatment
  1. Goals of therapy are to attain best possible metabolic control while avoiding potential side effects—see **Table 9-1**
  2. Unless acutely ill treatment can be instituted on an outpatient basis
  3. Consult physician for
     a. Newly diagnosed
     b. Anyone refractory to treatment
     c. Anyone with a blood sugar > 400 mg/dL
  4. Give consideration to work schedule, lifestyle, economic, social, and cultural aspects in management approach, e.g., persons who are homeless, persons working a night shift
  5. Diet along with exercise is cornerstone of therapy
     a. Refer newly diagnosed to registered dietician and annually or semiannually for follow-up
     b. Consistent dietary schedule; ideally three meals and three snacks; especially important for persons on insulin

■ **Table 9-1** Glycemic Control for Diabetics

Glycemic Index	Target	Non-Diabetic	Therapeutic Action Suggested
Fasting and preprandial glucose (mg/dL)	80–120	< 115	< 80
			> 140
Bedtime glucose (mg/dL)	100–140	< 120	> 160
			< 100
HbA$_{1c}$ (%)	< 7	< 6	> 8

c. Avoid refined carbohydrates and simple sugars

d. Total carbohydrate intake should be 50–60% of total caloric intake

e. Limit fats to 20–30% of total calories; saturated at < 8–9%

f. Increase fiber to 25 g/1,000 calories

g. Moderate protein intake, 0.8 g/kg/day or 20% of total caloric intake

h. Total caloric intake to maintain or achieve ideal body weight (IBW)

   (1) Calculation of IBW

      (a) Females—allow 100 lbs for first 5 feet of height plus 5 lbs for each additional inch of height

      (b) Males—allow 106 lbs for first 5 feet of height and add 6 lbs for each additional inch of height

      (c) Small frame subtract 10%

      (d) Large frame add 10%

   (2) Caloric requirement

      (a) Multiply IBW by 10 = baseline calories

      (b) Add $3 \times$ IBW if activity level is sedentary (most fall in this category); $5 \times$ IBW if moderate; and $10 \times$ IBW if strenuous

      (c) IBW = 125 lbs

          $125 \times 10 = 1,250$ (baseline calories)

          $125 \times 3 = 375$ (activity calories)

          $1250 + 375 = 1625$ (total calories needed per day)

      (d) In type 2—obese, where weight reduction is primary treatment, subtract 500 calories from the total number needed per day

6. Exercise

a. Planned daily exercise is an essential component for all diabetics, at least 30 minutes 5 days weekly of moderately intense exercise or 20 minutes 2 days weekly of vigorously intense exercise

b. Older persons with diabetes may be limited in types of exercise due to other concurrent problems such as arthritis, retinopathy

c. Diminishes need for insulin by enhancing oxidation of sugar and facilitating absorption of insulin from injection sites

d. Those on insulin should be instructed to inject insulin furthest from site of intensive exercise, e.g., abdomen rather than arms or thighs

e. Additional carbohydrate should be ingested prior to exercise

f. Contributes to weight and lipid control, reduces risks of CVD, improves insulin action

7. Examples of oral pharmacologic agents

a. Beta cell stimulants (secretagogues)

   (1) Sulfonylureas

      (a) First generation potent with long duration of action, increased risk of hypoglycemia, especially in the elderly

      (b) Contraindicated in pregnancy, for those with sulfa allergy, gestational, or type 1 diabetes, or in ketoacidosis

      (c) Few side effects, but special precautions in those with renal, liver, or cardiovascular disease

      (d) Risk of hypoglycemia and weight gain

   (2) Meglitinides cause brief but rapid pulse of insulin secretion

      (a) Fast acting

      (b) Taken just before each meal

   (3) D-phenylalanine derivatives

      (a) Nateglinide

      (b) Fast acting

      (c) Taken 1–30 minutes before each meal

b. Insulin-resistance reducers

   (1) Biguanide (metformin) 1.5–2.5 g daily in divided doses

      (a) Increases peripheral insulin sensitivity and inhibits hepatic gluconeogenesis

      (b) Causes moderate weight loss

      (c) Improved lipid profile regardless of glycemic effect

      (d) Low risk of hypoglycemia

      (e) Side effects of flatulence, diarrhea; metallic taste minimized by taking with meals and increasing doses more slowly

      (f) Contraindicated in renal, liver, or advanced cardiovascular disease (cannot be used if serum creatinine level is > 1.5 μ/dL in males and above 1.4 μ/dL in females)

      (g) Rare incidence of lactic acidosis; check pharmacology reference for precautions

   (2) Thiazolidinediones (pioglitazone, rosiglitazone)

      (a) Used for type 2 diabetes as monotherapy or in combination with insulin, metformin, or a sulfonylurea

      (b) Pioglitazone 15–45 mg/day; rosiglitazone 4–8 mg/day (refer to pharmacology reference for details on dosing)

    (c) Monitor liver function every 2 months for first 12 months and periodically thereafter

    (d) Increased risk of hypoglycemia with combination therapy

    (e) May induce postmenopausal ovulation/risk of unintended pregnancy

    (f) May cause or potentiate congestive heart failure or myocardial infarction

    (g) Potential for multiple drug interactions

    (h) Adverse reactions include upper respiratory infections, sinusitis, headache, pharyngitis, anemia, and edema

  c. Alpha-glucosidase inhibitor (acarbose and miglitol)

    (1) Lowers postprandial blood glucose levels

    (2) Low risk of hypoglycemia or weight gain

    (3) Somewhat less efficacious than sulfonylureas or biguanides

    (4) Flatulence, bloating, diarrhea frequent but abate with continued use

  d. Incretin mimetics (exentide and liraglutide)

    (1) Stimulates glucose-dependent insulin secretion and lowers glucagon concentrations during periods of hyperglycemia

    (2) Inhibits postprandial glucagon release

    (3) Slows gastric emptying

    (4) 40% incidence of nausea; high dropout rate due to this effect

    (5) Used as adjunct to sulfonylurea or metformin

    (6) Maximal $HgbA_{1c}$ reduction 1–2%

    (7) Used for type 2 only; intact beta cell function required

  e. Amylin analogs (pramlintide)

    (1) Modulates gastric emptying

    (2) Used in both type 1 and type 2 diabetes when response to therapy is inadequate

    (3) Contraindicated in gastroparesis

    (4) Strict warning about hypoglycemia; diet requirements include 250 kcal meal with 30 g carbohydrate

  f. Dipeptidyl peptidase-4 (DPP-4) inhibitors (sitagliptin, saxagliptin, linagliptin)

    (1) Incretin stimulates synthesis and release of insulin from beta cells

    (2) This drug increases endogenous incretin by blocking inactivating enzyme DPP-4

    (3) Maximal $HgbA_{1c}$ reduction 0.4–0.6%

    (4) Does not cause hypoglycemia

  g. Administer angiotensin-converting enzyme inhibitor (ACEI) if not contraindicated

    (1) Drug of choice to treat hypertension in those with DM

    (2) Shown to prevent progression of nephropathy even in normotensives with type 2 DM

8. Insulin (categorized as basal or bolus based on duration of action) (see **Table 9-2**)

  a. Indicated

    (1) Confirmed or suspected type 1 or gestational diabetes

    (2) Type 2 dietary and/or oral agent management fails to control glucose levels, or in times of stress

    (3) For those for whom oral agents are contraindicated

  b. Some may need more than three injections per day and or need to use an insulin pump to maintain control

  c. Weight gain and need for frequent glucose monitoring can be problems

  d. Purity

    (1) Standard beef or pork—> 10 but < 25 parts per million (ppm) proinsulin (immunogenic agent)

    (2) Purified beef or pork—< 10 ppm proinsulin

    (3) Human synthetic < 10 ppm proinsulin

    (4) Beef more antigenic than pork species; human insulin least antigenic of all

  e. Insulin replacement and augmentation

    (1) No medical contraindications to insulin use and glycemic control can be obtained with exogenous insulin replacement

    (2) Replacement therapy is indicated with glucose toxicity (fasting plasma glucose [FPG]) > 250 mg per dL with ketosis, weight loss; pregnant or planning pregnancy and in poor control; during acute illness, infection, or cardiovascular disease

      (a) Basal bolus mealtime insulin, start with 0.5 units/kg per day

      (b) Consider twice-daily administration of mixed dose insulin if patient has set routine of meals and activity; needs a simpler regimen, or has economic constraints

        (i) Amount of regular insulin normally should not exceed 50% of insulin given at any time

(ii) Do not mix lente or ultra-lente with regular; zinc in lente precipitates regular, decreasing effective proportion of regular and increasing that of the lente

(iii) Do not mix lente with velosulin short acting (Nordisk); phosphate buffer increases concentration of unmodified soluble insulin and diminishes effect of intermediate acting preparation

(iv) Regular insulin should be drawn up first if mixing regular and NPH in same syringe

(v) Do not mix glargine with other insulins and do not use syringes that have been used with other insulins to draw up glargine

(c) Consider more intensive therapy for those with irregular schedule or unstable medical condition, able to adjust insulin doses, and able to monitor and correct hypoglycemia

(3) Augmentation is initiated when an individual cannot achieve an A_{1c} equal to or < 7 with diet, exercise, and oral medications insulin

(a) 0.15 mg/kg per day of NPH at bedtime or twice daily, or glargine once daily. Monitoring is done weekly and dosage adjusted based on FPG until glycemic control is achieved. Goal is FPG of 80–130 mg/dL

(b) If FPG is in range but A_{1c} is still > 7% and postprandial glucose levels are > 180 mg/dL, move to replacement therapy as outlined previously

(i) Preprandial plasma glucose goal is less than 140 mg/dL

(ii) Adjust one insulin dosage at a time and adjust dosage by no more than 2–5 units every 2–3 days

(4) Once daily regimen is established, urine and self-monitored plasma glucose levels are tested 3–4 times a day as indicated by the insulin schedule and severity of the disease

(a) Daily dose requirement decreases with progressive renal failure

(b) Control is assessed at 3- to 6-month intervals; glycosylated Hgb, which reflects average glucose levels of the preceding 8–12 weeks, may be helpful

9. Patient education—should begin at time of diagnosis and will extend over several weeks

a. Cause and general management of diabetes

b. Importance of diet and weight control

c. Self-monitoring of blood and urine glucose

■ **Table 9-2**   Insulins

Type	Onset	Peak (Hours)	Duration (Hours)
BOLUS/MEALTIME			
Ultra Short Acting aspart (NovoLog, Novo Nordisk)	5–10 minutes	1–3	4–6
lispro (Humalog)	<15 minutes	0.5–1.5	4–6
Short Acting regular (Humulin R, Novalin R)	30 minutes	2–3	6–10
BASAL INSULINS			
Intermediate NPH (Humulin N, Novolin N)	2–4 hours	4–10	14–18
Lente	3–4 hours	4–12	16–20
Long Acting ultralente	6–10 hours	peakless	20–24
Glargine	1–6 hours	peakless	24
PREMIXED			
%NPH/regular 70/30 50/50	30–60 minutes	dual	14–18
75% NPL/25% lispro (Humalog 75/25)	<15 minutes	dual	14–18
70% NPH/30% aspart (NovoLog 70/30)	5–10 minutes	dual	14–18

Note: Pork, beef-pork, and human synthetic insulin available in rapid, intermediate, and long acting. Onset and duration values are highly variable among individuals and may vary within patients depending on the site of injection and tissue blood flow among other factors. Duration also depends on dose size and is increased in renal failure.

NPH = neutral protamine Hagedorn; NPL = neutral protamine lispro

d. Administration of insulin, dosing, action, side effects, and site rotation

e. Administration of oral hypoglycemic agents, dosing, action, and side effects

f. Potential alteration in glucose metabolism with acute illness, exercise, and emotional stress

g. Test for and significance of ketonuria

h. Recognition and treatment of hypoglycemia

i. Proper leg and foot care

j. Sick-day guidelines

k. Guidelines for economizing with repeated use of needles and splitting glucose test strips

10. Complications

a. Hypoglycemia
   (1) Causes
       (a) Insulin overdosage
       (b) Omission or delay of meals
       (c) Heavy exercise
       (d) Errors in injection technique
       (e) Renal failure
       (f) Weight loss
       (g) Development of hepatitis, pituitary or adrenal insufficiency, or other conditions that cause hypoglycemia
       (h) Drugs that affect insulin metabolism/action; see **Table 9-3**
   (2) Symptoms
       (a) Weakness
       (b) Sweating
       (c) Shakiness
       (d) Tremors
       (e) Nervousness
       (f) Headache
       (g) Dizziness
       (h) Hunger
       (i) Irritability
       (j) Convulsions, confusion, coma
       (k) Tachycardia, palpitations

b. Somogyi phenomenon
   (1) Cause—morning rebound hyperglycemia; occurs in response to nocturnal hypoglycemia with excessive insulin administration
   (2) Clues—erratic plasma glucose and urine ketone values; symptoms of nocturnal hypoglycemia (night sweats, nightmares, low serum glucose 2–3 A.M.), weight gain in presence of heavy glycosuria
   (3) Treatment—reduce insulin dose 10–20%
   (4) Distinguish from *dawn phenomenon*, which is early morning fasting hyperglycemia without nocturnal hypoglycemia; thought to be related to circadian rhythm secretion of growth hormone and treated by evening or bedtime dose of insulin

c. Lipodystrophy
   (1) Atrophy—subcutaneous fat atrophy at insulin injection sites
       (a) Cause—impurities in the insulin, possible autoimmune mechanism
       (b) Treatment—switch to purified insulin, inject directly into atrophic areas

■ **Table 9-3** Medication Effect on Insulin Metabolism/Action

Medication	Action
Alcohol	Decreased half-life of sulfonylureas in alcoholics, can cause severe hypoglycemia in those on hypoglycemics
Beta-adrenergic	Inhibit insulin secretion; block most hypoglycemia symptoms; prolong effect of insulin
Calcium channel blockers	Inhibit insulin secretion
Diazoxide	Inhibits insulin secretion
Glucocorticoids	Insulin antagonism
Nicotinic acid	Insulin resistance
Oral contraceptives	Insulin resistance
Phenytoin	Inhibits insulin secretion
Sympathomimetics	Insulin antagonism; inhibit insulin secretion
Thiazide diuretics	Inhibit insulin secretion
MAO inhibitors	Increase effects of antidiabetic agents
Salicylates	Increase effects of antidiabetic agents
Coumarin	Increase effects of sulfonylureas
Phenylbutazone	Increase effects of sulfonylureas

(2) Hypertrophy—overgrowth of subcutaneous tissue
  (a) Cause—growth promoting effects of insulin; improper rotation of injection sites
  (b) Treatment—prevent by proper rotation of injection sites

d. Insulin allergy
  (1) Rare and usually localized
  (2) Treatment—change to human synthetic insulin
  (3) Localized allergies may be treated with antihistamines or corticosteroid; consultation required

e. Insulin resistance requiring more than 200 units per day
  (1) Rare and even less common with increased use of human insulins
  (2) Cause—overproduction of insulin-binding immunoglobulins
  (3) Treatment—change to less immunogenic pork or human synthetic insulins
  (4) May require glucocorticoid treatment; consultation required

f. Diabetic ketoacidosis (DKA)—hyperglycemia with ketonuria and disruption of the fluid, electrolyte, and pH balance leading to coma and even death; marked by hyperglycemia, metabolic acidosis, and ketonemia; sometimes presenting signs in undiagnosed type 1
  (1) Cause—infection, trauma, myocardial infarction, other severe stress, and noncompliance with therapeutic regimen
  (2) Treatment—emergency fluid replacement, insulin therapy, sodium bicarbonate therapy, and close monitoring of blood chemistries

g. Hyperosmolar nonketotic syndrome—severe hyperglycemia, hyperosmolarity, and dehydration in the absence of ketoacidosis, which may lead to coma; most often occurs in elderly on oral hypoglycemics and those with undiagnosed type 2
  (1) Precipitating factors—calcium channel blockers, corticosteroids, thiazide diuretics, propranolol, phenytoin
  (2) Treatment—similar to ketoacidosis, but need less insulin and more fluid replacement
  (3) Prognosis is poor in elderly, particularly those with concurrent renal disease, hypertension, or congestive heart failure

11. Follow-up
  a. Well-controlled patients—minimum every 3–4 months
  b. Yearly ECG, chest radiograph, creatinine, urinalysis with microprotein analysis, lipid profile, physical examination including fundoscopic, full neurologic examination
  c. Annual ophthalmologic examination by ophthalmologist
  d. Skin inspection, feet inspection, fundoscopic, and evaluation of glycemic control by fasting or postprandial plasma glucose measurements at each visit
  e. Hemoglobin A_{1c} every 3–6 months

12. Referrals to local support groups and identification of local chapters of the American Diabetes Association for information, support, and publications

13. Routinely screen all $\geq$45 years of age, if negative repeat every 3 years or earlier if risk factors are present

◘ THYROTOXICOSIS

- Definition—a metabolic state characterized by symptomatic circulating thyroid hormone excess; common due to hyperthyroidism, which is a state of excessive secretory activity of the thyroid gland (Graves' disease), or a state of circulating thyroid hormone excess produced by excess exogenous or endogenous thyroid hormone in the presence of a normally functioning gland (subacute thyroiditis, exogenous thyroid hormone administration)

- Etiology/Incidence
  1. Causes
     a. Autoimmune response (Graves' disease accounts for more than 85% of cases)
     b. Subacute thyroiditis—normal gland releases its hormone stores in a burst following glandular insult, e.g., viral inflammation
     c. Toxic multinodular goiter; toxic uninodular goiter (autonomous thyroid adenoma)
     d. Metastatic follicular thyroid carcinoma
     e. Thyrotoxicosis factitia
     f. Thyroid stimulating hormone (TSH) secreting pituitary tumor (secondary hyperthyroidism)
     g. Human chorionic gonadotropin (hCG) secreting tumors (choriocarcinoma, hydatidiform mole)
     h. Testicular embryonal carcinoma
  2. One of the most common endocrine disorders
  3. Highest incidence in women between 20 and 40 years of age

- Signs and Symptoms
  1. Most frequent
     a. Anxiety
     b. Diaphoresis

    c.   Fatigue
    d.   Hypersensitivity to heat
    e.   Nervousness
    f.   Palpitations
    g.   Weight loss
    h.   Insomnia, nightmares

2. Frequent
   a. Dyspnea
   b. Weakness
   c. Increased appetite
   d. Eye complaints, e.g., difficulty focusing
   e. Swelling of legs
   f. Hyperdefecation without diarrhea, hyperactive bowel sounds
   g. Diarrhea
   h. Oligomenorrhea or amenorrhea
   i. Tremors
   j. Angina

3. Infrequent
   a. Anorexia
   b. Constipation
   c. Weight gain
   d. Signs of pseudobulbar palsy

4. Elderly patients may present with few signs or symptoms noted in younger patients (apathetic hyperthyroidism); may present with cardiovascular problems unresponsive to digitalis, quinidine, or diuretics
   a. Atrial fibrillation
   b. Angina
   c. Congestive heart failure

- Differential Diagnosis
  1. Anxiety neurosis, especially in menopause
  2. Other diseases associated with hypermetabolism, e.g., pheochromocytoma and acromegaly
  3. Myasthenia gravis (causes the same ophthalmoplegic signs)
  4. Orbital tumors, which can cause exophthalmos
  5. Psychosis

- Physical Findings
  1. General—thin, muscle wasting may be evident; nervous; quick motions
  2. Vital signs—tachycardia, irregular pulse, widened pulse pressure
  3. Integumentary—skin moist, velvety, may show increased pigmentation or vitiligo; hair thin, fine; spider angiomas and gynecomastia may be evident
  4. Eyes—prominent; appear to "stare;" lid lag; lack of accommodation, chemosis; proptosis (exophthalmos)
  5. Neck—enlarged thyroid gland (goiter) smooth or nodular, symmetric or asymmetric; thyroid bruit or thrill; absence of signs does not rule out hyperthyroidism

6. Cardiovascular—tachycardia, paroxysmal atrial fibrillation, harsh pulmonary systolic murmur, congestive failure, possible enlargement
7. Neurologic—hyperactive reflexes; fine tremors of fingers, tongue; mental changes ranging from mild exhilaration to delirium; in elderly, apathy, lethargy, and severe depression may be manifested
8. Lymphatic—lymphadenopathy and splenomegaly may be present

- Diagnostic Tests/Findings (see **Table 9-4** for list of thyroid function tests)
  1. TSH assay best test for thyroid dysfunction—decreased in hyperthyroidism
  2. Free thyroxine index (FT_4I) usually elevated; order if normal and clinical impression is strong for hyperthyroidism
  3. T_3 radioimmunoassay (T_3, RIA)—elevated with a normal T_4 in early hyperthyroidism and T_3 toxicosis
  4. T_4 level elevated in later stages
  5. TSI present

- Management/Treatment
  1. Refer for hospitalization for suspected "thyroid storm"
     a. High fever
     b. Severe agitation
     c. Confusion
     d. Cardiovascular collapse
     e. Malignant exophthalmus
     f. Difficulty in breathing due to enlarged or tender thyroid gland
  2. Obtain physician consult for clients suspected of/or newly diagnosed with hyperthyroidism for treatment, which may include
     a. Propranolol 10–60 mg orally every 6 hours to control symptoms
     b. Radioactive iodine (^{131}I)
        (1) In United States preferred treatment
        (2) Therapeutic dose is 80–120 mCi administered in doses of 5–15 mCi based on estimated weight of the thyroid gland
        (3) Most become euthyroid after 6–8 weeks
        (4) Hypothyroidism is frequent and can occur anytime after radioactive iodine therapy
        (5) Contraindicated in pregnancy
     c. Antithyroid drugs—indicated for initial control of thyrotoxicosis especially in pregnant women, those not wanting to take ^{131}I, or in preparation for surgical removal; effective in patients with small goiters

■ Table 9-4   Thyroid Assessment Tests

Thyroxine (T_4)	Major hormone secreted by the thyroid gland
T_4 (RIA-serum)	By radioimmunoassay (RIA); normal adult is 5–12 µg/dL
Free Thyroxine Index (FT$_4$I)	Unaffected by TBG and is a better reflection of the true index hormonal status; serum T_4 and T_3 resin uptake (T_3, RU) used to calculate this index; normal adults 0.9–2.2 ng/dL
T_3 Resin Uptake (T_3RU)	Indirect measure of T_4 levels by assessing T_4 binding sites; may be thought of as the reciprocal of the T_4 RIA; in hyperthyroidism there is a high T_3 resin uptake; in hypothyroidism the T_3 is low; normal adult is 25–35%
T_3 RIA (Serum)	Direct measure of triiodothyronine (T_3) thyroid hormone; helpful in diagnosing thyrotoxicosis when T_4 is normal; in hypothyroidism T_3 often normal; T_4 more helpful; normal adult is 80–200 ng/dL (RIA)
Antithyroid Peroxidase Antibody (Anti-TPO) (Serum)	Mediate antibody-dependent thyroid cell destruction; when present in a patient with elevated TSH and normal T_4, suggests early disease; may be elevated in 10% asymptomatic individuals (nl < 1 IU/mL)
Thyroid Stimulating Immune Globulins (TSI)	Autoantibodies frequently present in Graves' disease; stimulate TSH receptors, accelerating function of the gland independent of the pituitary-thyroid gland feedback loop; normal range < 130% activity, although persons with Graves' disease usually at < 2%
Thyroid Stimulating Hormone (TSH)	Direct measure of TSH secreted from the anterior pituitary in response to thyroid-releasing hormone (TRH); normal adult is 2–5.4 µU/mL < 10 µU/mL (RIA); most sensitive indicator of thyroid hormone function
TSH Immunoradiometric Assay (IRMA)	Newer assay replacing TSH (RIA); normal adult is 0.5–5.0 µU/mL; more sensitive to suppressed TSH in hyperthyroidism
Radioactive Iodine Uptake (RAIU)	Used primarily to detect hyperthyroidism etiology; radioactive iodine given orally or intravenously; the thyroid is scanned at three different intervals to determine iodine uptake of the thyroid gland; an elevated RAIU indicates hyperthyroidism; normal adult is 2 hr, 1–13%; 6 hr, 2–25%; 24 hr, 15–45%

(1) Propylthiouracil (PTU)—usual dose 300–400 mg/day in divided doses
  (a) Preferred for use in pregnant women
  (b) During pregnancy dose kept < 200 mg/day
(2) Methimazole (MMI)—15–60 mg/day orally in three divided doses
(3) Side effects
  (a) Dermatitis
  (b) Nausea
  (c) Agranulocytosis (most serious)
  (d) Hypothyroidism, which can cause a TSH-stimulated increase in goiter size
3. Patient education
  a. Medication is to be taken for about 2 years and not abruptly discontinued
  b. At first sign of infection or fever drug should be stopped and healthcare professional contacted
  c. Therapeutic effect of medication is not usually evident for about 3 weeks
4. Surgery
  a. Not used as frequently now

  b. Indicated for children, adolescents, pregnant women unable to tolerate PTU, adults nonresponsive to thiourea treatment who refuse RAI
  c. Usually rendered euthyroid with drugs preoperatively
5. General considerations
  a. Client education
    (1) Rationale for treatment; dosage and side effects of medications; takes at least 3 weeks before antithyroid medications become effective
    (2) Instructions regarding nutritional needs: high-carbohydrate, high-calorie diet until medication takes effect; avoidance of stimulants such as caffeine
    (3) Symptoms of "thyroid storm"
    (4) Symptoms of hypothyroidism
  b. Follow-up
    (1) Periodic examinations until euthyroid
    (2) All patients who have been treated for hyperthyroidism should be periodically checked for hypothyroidism, which may occur anytime during treatment

◻ ADULT HYPOTHYROIDISM (MYXEDEMA)

- Definition—decreased or deficient thyroid hormone—primary (glandular dysfunction) or secondary (pituitary insufficiency); occurs in all age groups

- Etiology/Incidence
  1. Major classifications
     a. Primary—caused by damage to the hormone-producing capabilities of the thyroid gland itself
        (1) Most common cause in adults is autoimmune thyroiditis (Hashimoto's, or chronic lymphocytic)
        (2) Can also be caused by ablation of the gland by surgery, medication, radiation, and goitrogens (thiocyanates, rutabagas, lithium carbonate)
        (3) More common than secondary
     b. Secondary—often related to destructive lesions of the pituitary gland as with chromophobe adenoma or postpartum necrosis (Sheehan's syndrome); frequently associated with signs of adrenal and gonadal disorders
     c. Tertiary—TRH deficiency arising in the hypothalamus; sometimes grouped with secondary
  2. Occurs in all age groups; more prevalent in women and those
     a. With a history of thyroiditis
     b. With previously treated hyperthyroidism (all modalities)
     c. Being treated with lithium or para-aminosalicylic acid
     d. With coexistent autoimmune disorders (e.g., rheumatoid arthritis, lupus, pernicious anemia)

- Signs and Symptoms
  1. Most frequent
     a. Cold intolerance
     b. Coarse skin
     c. Decreased sweating
     d. Dry skin
     e. Lethargy
     f. Swelling of eyelids
  2. Frequent
     a. Anemia (normocytic, normochromic, microcytic, or macrocytic)
     b. Anorexia
     c. Coarse hair
     d. Cold skin
     e. Constipation
     f. Hair loss
     g. Hoarseness or aphonia, thick tongue
     h. Hyperlipidemia including hypercholesterolemia
     i. Leg edema
     j. Menorrhagia
     k. Memory impairment
     l. Swelling of face
     m. Paresthesias
     n. Weight change

- Differential Diagnosis
  1. Rule out coexisting autoimmune disease or secondary hypothyroidism
  2. Nephrotic syndrome
  3. Chronic renal disease

- Physical Findings
  1. Vital signs—bradycardia, mild hypotension, or diastolic hypertension
  2. Edema of hands, face, eyelids
  3. Integumentary—dry, scaly skin with carotenemic tone; brittle nails; alopecia; puffy eyelids; temporal thinning of the eyebrows; generalized hair loss, nonpitting edema
  4. ENT—enlarged tongue, possible hearing decrease, thyroid often enlarged
  5. Cardiovascular—bradycardia, decreased intensity of heart tones, cardiac enlargement (myxedemic heart may be related to pericardial effusion)
  6. Respiratory—pleural effusion
  7. Abdominal—ascites, decreased bowel sounds
  8. Neuromuscular—slow or delayed deep tendon reflexes, cerebellar ataxia, dementia (myxedema madness, manifested with hallucinations, paranoid ideation, and hyperactive delirium), pseudomyotonia, carpal tunnel syndrome

- Diagnostic Tests/Findings (see **Table 9-5**)
  1. TSH elevated in primary hypothyroidism
  2. Free thyroxine index (FTI) or T_4; if low a TSH is helpful in determining etiology
  3. TSH elevated in primary hypothyroidism
  4. If T_4 is normal and TSH is elevated, may be mild hypothyroidism
  5. Thyrotropin releasing hormone (TRH) stimulation done if low TSH with low T_4 or low FTI; may indicate secondary hypothyroidism
  6. CBC—may demonstrate anemia

- Management/Treatment
  1. Refer for immediate hospitalization any client suspected of developing myxedemic coma—severe hypothyroidism associated with hypothermia, decreased mentation, hypoventilation, respiratory acidosis, relative hypotension, hyponatremia, hypoglycemia

■ **Table 9-5** Laboratory Values in Hypothyroidism

Type	TSH	FT$_4$	FT$_3$
Primary	High	Low	Low
Subclinical	High	Normal	Normal
Secondary (pituitary deficiency) TSH	Low	Low	Low

TSH = thyroid stimulating hormone, T$_4$ = thyroxine, T$_3$ = triiodothyronine

2. Obtain physician consultation for clients with suspected or newly diagnosed hypothyroidism for further testing and/or initiation of treatment, which would include administration of synthetic T$_4$ (levothyroxine)
   a. Average replacement dose of T$_4$ is thyroxine 1.6 mcg/kg/day day in healthy, non-elderly adults
   b. Replacement at 1.0 mcg/kg/day for those > 50 years of age or with known ischemic heart disease without angina
   c. Dosage begins with ½ projected replacement, increased every 4-6 weeks as tolerated until clinically euthyroid
      (1) 70 kg, 45-year-old female would have projected dose of 70 × 1.6 mcg (112 mcg or 1.12 mg
      (2) Begin at 50 mcg/day, increase every four weeks by 25% until clinically euthyroid
   d. Patients with coexisting adrenal insufficiency, coronary insufficiency, or angina require particular care
   e. Initial effects of replacement not usually perceptible for at least 2 weeks after initiation of therapy and are initially demonstrated by decreased facial edema and increased urination
3. On follow-up visits, after replacement therapy has been instituted
   a. Check cardiopulmonary status; if pulse is > 100/minute consider need to reduce dose
   b. Monitor for symptoms or signs of too vigorous therapy, side effects, and toxic effects of replacement therapy; ask about dyspnea, orthopnea, angina, palpitations, nervousness, insomnia
   c. Be alert to concomitant use of opiates, barbiturates, other central nervous system depressants, digitalis, and insulin; persons with hypothyroidism are particularly sensitive to these agents; as they become euthyroid dosages may have to be increased
4. Monitor control of clinical symptoms and periodically monitor serum FTI and TSH; persistently high TSH or low FTI may indicate under-replacement; a high T$_4$ and low TSH

with symptoms of hyperthyroidism usually indicates over-replacement
5. Patient education
   a. Nature and chronicity of the disease and the need for lifelong treatment
   b. Rationale for treatment—dosage, side effects, and toxic effects of treatment
   c. Teach signs of hyperthyroidism
   d. Management of symptoms of hypothyroidism until abatement with replacement therapy
      (1) Fatigue
      (2) Dry skin
      (3) Constipation (increased fiber, fluids)

▣ THYROID NODULE

- Definition—discrete enlargements within the thyroid gland

- Etiology unknown but nodules are common
  1. Palpable in 5–10% of U.S. population
  2. Majority are benign
  3. Risk of nodule malignancy less than 10% in most adults
     a. Men have a higher incidence than women
     b. Papillary and follicular carcinoma are most common types of malignancy
        (1) Papillary tends to spread within the thyroid gland or to cervical lymphatics
           (a) Twice as common in women as men
           (b) Accounts for 80% of thyroid malignancies in adults < 40
        (2) Follicular accounts for approximately 20% of all thyroid cancers
           (a) Incidence somewhat higher in older individuals
           (b) Usually slow growing but more aggressive than papillary; can spread rapidly to lymph nodes and to distant sites via the blood stream, often to lung, bone, brain, or liver
           (c) More aggressive in the elderly
     c. Medullary and anaplastic carcinoma are rarer but tend to metastasize very early; anaplastic carcinoma, because of high invasiveness and early metastasis, results

in death in weeks or months regardless of treatment modality

   d. Risk of carcinoma is increased with a history of radiation exposure, particularly during childhood, to the head or neck for acne, tonsils, adenoids; the risk is also increased in those with a family history of thyroid cancer—this is especially true for medullary carcinoma

- Signs and Symptoms
  1. Thyroid mass
  2. Expanding goiter or nodule, which is hard and/or tender
  3. Hoarseness or dysphagia

- Differential Diagnosis—distinguish from non-neoplastic enlargements, e.g., cystic nodules, multinodular goiters

- Physical Findings
  1. Single hard thyroid nodule (or multiple nodules) fixed to overlying tissue
  2. Regional lymphadenopathy

- Diagnostic Tests/Findings
  1. FTI—usually normal; if elevated chances of malignancy are decreased
  2. RAI scan—nonfunctioning (cold) nodule
  3. Ultrasonography—if cystic, rarely malignant
  4. Thyrocalcitonin—increased in medullary carcinoma
  5. Biopsy (open or needle)—positive cytology if malignant

- Management/Treatment
  1. Treatment may include
     a. Excision of the nodule (complete thyroidectomy in the case of medullary carcinoma) and regional lymph nodes
     b. Ablation of metastasis with large doses of radioactive iodine
     c. Suppression of thyroid function with L-thyroxine
     d. Chemotherapy for anaplastic carcinoma (thyroid suppression and radioactive ablation of metastasis are not effective in medullary thyroid carcinoma)
  2. Client education related to diagnostic tests
  3. Follow-up for detection of metastasis, recurrence, and subsequent treatment is usually on an annual basis

▫ CUSHING'S SYNDROME (HYPERCORTISOLISM)

- Definition—a constellation of clinical abnormalities due to an excess of corticosteroids

- Etiology/Incidence
  1. Excessive or prolonged administration of glucocorticoids (most common)
  2. Excessive pituitary adrenocorticotropic hormone (ACTH) secretion (Cushing's disease)
  3. Secretion of ACTH by a nonpituitary tumor (ectopic tumor), e.g., carcinoma of the lung or other malignant growths
  4. Tumors within the adrenal cortex—adenomas or carcinoma
  5. Cushing's disease and primary adrenal tumors more common in females
  6. Ectopic corticotropin production more common in males

- Signs and Symptoms
  1. Central obesity with slender extremities
  2. Full face
  3. Muscular weakness
  4. Back pain
  5. Mental changes
  6. Thin fragile skin
  7. Poor wound healing
  8. Acne
  9. Menstrual disorders

- Differential Diagnosis
  1. Hypercortisolism due to alcoholism
  2. Hypercortisolism due to depression

- Physical Findings
  1. Moon face with facial plethora
  2. Hirsutism
  3. Skin—thin and atrophic
  4. Purplish-red striae on abdomen, breasts, or buttocks
  5. Truncal obesity with wasting of limbs
  6. Prominent supraclavicular and dorsal cervical fat pads ("buffalo hump")
  7. Hypertension

- Diagnostic Tests/Findings
  1. Dexamethasone test (most reliable for distinguishing among causes of Cushing's syndrome)
  2. Urinary cortisol—elevated
  3. Plasma cortisol—evening cortisol levels and 24-hour total levels are elevated
  4. MRI, CT, and ultrasonographic imaging for identification of pituitary tumor, nonpituitary ACTH-producing neoplasms
  5. Blood glucose—increased
  6. Hypokalemia but not hypernatremia

- Management/Treatment
  1. Treatment of choice for Cushing's disease—surgery
  2. Adrenal tumors or hyperplasia—removal

3. If surgery is contraindicated, radiation and drug therapy (used to control cortisol excess) may be used, which includes ketoconazole 400–500 mg b.i.d.; metyrapone 2 g per day; aminoglutethimide 1 g per day
4. When surgery and aggressive medical management not options, controlling consequences is indicated
   a. Replace K+
   b. Control hypertension
   c. Control hyperglycemia
   d. Aggressive management of wounds and rashes
5. For Cushing's syndrome due to prolonged administration of steroids
   a. Discontinuation of therapy gradually
   b. Reduction of steroid dose
   c. Changing to an alternate-day schedule

☐ ADDISON'S DISEASE (PRIMARY ADRENOCORTICAL INSUFFICIENCY)

- Definition—an insidious, usually progressive disease due to destruction of the adrenal cortex
  1. Primary—due to destruction of adrenal cortex
  2. Secondary—lack of corticotropin stimulation

- Etiology/Incidence
  1. Idiopathic autoimmune destruction of adrenal tissue (over 80%); two to three times more common in females; usually diagnosed between ages 30–50 years
  2. Tuberculosis—second most frequent cause (common cause in underdeveloped countries)
  3. Acquired immunodeficiency syndrome (AIDS)—becoming a more frequent cause
  4. Less common—hemorrhage, fungal infections, antineoplastic chemotherapy, abrupt withdrawal of exogenous steroids
  5. Primarily a rare disease

- Signs and Symptoms
  1. Chronic primary adrenocortical insufficiency—develops gradually
     a. Weakness and fatigue, orthostatic hypotension may be early symptoms
     b. Anorexia, weight loss
     c. Tan appearance to the skin
     d. Gastrointestinal symptoms
  2. Acute adrenocortical insufficiency—seen more often in patients without previous diagnosis or those with a diagnosis who are exposed to stress with related increased requirement for glucocorticoids; symptoms of chronic are exaggerated, especially profound hypotension
  3. Most dangerous feature of Addison's disease is hypotension, which may cause shock,

especially during stress AND is nonresponsive to usual treatment; requires glucocorticoid replacement

- Differential Diagnosis
  1. Antidiuretic hormone (ADH) syndrome
  2. Salt-losing nephritis
  3. Hemochromatosis

- Physical Findings
  1. Hyperpigmentation of skin
  2. Hypotension
  3. Black freckles over forehead, face, neck, and shoulders
  4. Areas of vitiligo
  5. Bluish-black discolorations of the areolae and of the mucous membranes of the lips, mouth, rectum, vagina

- Diagnostic Tests/Findings
  1. Sodium levels—low (< 130 mEq/L; normal 135–145 mEq/L)
  2. Potassium levels—high (> 5 mEq/L; normal 3.5–5 mEq/L)
  3. BUN—elevated
  4. Plasma renin level—increased
  5. ACTH plasma levels—increased
  6. Ratio of serum sodium to potassium (< 30:1)
  7. Low fasting blood glucose (< 50 mg/dL; normal 60–115 mg/dL)
  8. Hematocrit—elevated
  9. WBC—low
  10. Eosinophils—increased

- Management/Treatment
  1. In acute crisis referral with hospitalization
  2. Chronic
     a. Lifetime of treatment
     b. Cortisol 15–20 mg orally every A.M.; 5–10 mg 4–6 P.M.
     c. Fludrocortisone acetate 0.05–0.3 mg daily or every other day if insufficient sodium retention with cortisol alone; frequently needed in times of physiologic crises, e.g., acute systemic illness, operation
        (1) When fludrocortisone therapy has been initiated, monitor closely for symptoms of sodium and fluid retention
        (2) Discontinue as able when patient recovers from physiologic crisis
     d. Monitor weight, blood pressure, and electrolytes
  3. General considerations
     a. Education regarding increasing cortisol during times of stress
     b. Education regarding carrying an identification bracelet or card

c. Salt additives for excess heat or humidity
d. Prognosis is excellent with continued substitution therapy

❑ QUESTIONS

Select the best answer.

Questions 1 and 2 refer to the following scenario:

Mrs. O. is a 46-year-old female whose hypertension has been controlled with hydrochlorothiazide 50 mg every day for the past 3 years. She is 5′ 8″ and weighs 220 lbs. Although no other abnormal physical findings were noted, blood work done as part of her routine annual physical examination reveals a fasting blood glucose of 230 mg/dL. Other abnormal laboratory tests included elevated serum cholesterol (250) and triglyceride level (170), a K^+ of 3.4, and 4^+ glycosuria.

1. You should then:
   a. Discontinue her hydrochlorothiazide
   b. Order a glucose tolerance test
   c. Repeat a fasting glucose
   d. Start insulin therapy

2. Mrs. O. is about how many pounds over her ideal body weight?
   a. 80
   b. 105
   c. 140
   d. 154

3. Persons with type 2 diabetes:
   a. Tend to have peripheral muscle loss
   b. Account for less than 10% of persons with diabetes
   c. Tend to be obese and hypertensive
   d. Have early symptoms similar to persons with type 1 diabetes

4. The pathophysiology of type 2 diabetes frequently includes:
   a. Insulin receptor abnormalities
   b. Islet cell antibody development
   c. Activation of a genetic predisposition
   d. Beta cell insensitivity to insulinogenic stimuli

5. You are managing the primary care needs of a patient with difficult-to-control type 2 diabetes. He is under the care of an endocrinologist and recently started taking pramlintide. Patient education should reinforce the potential for:
   a. Renal dysfunction with contrast dye
   b. Development of hypoglycemia
   c. Significant nausea in the first weeks of therapy
   d. Headache and upper respiratory symptoms

6. Which of the following is not a diagnostic criterion for diabetes mellitus?
   a. $HgbA_{1c} > 6.5\%$
   b. The presence of islet cell antibodies
   c. FPG > 126 mg/dL on two separate occasions
   d. CPG > 200 mg/dL along with classic symptoms

7. Dietary recommendations for persons with diabetes do not include:
   a. Strict carbohydrate restriction
   b. Limiting fats and cholesterol
   c. Limiting protein intake
   d. Eating meals at regular intervals

8. Indications for starting a person with diabetes on oral hypoglycemics include:
   a. Allergy to sulfa drugs
   b. Pregnancy in type 2 diabetes controlled by diet
   c. Diagnosis of type 2 diabetes
   d. Failure to control hyperglycemia with diet in a patient with type 2 diabetes

9. A person with type 2 diabetes has had good control of his blood glucose with oral agents. He is in for a routine 3-month check. He had a complete work up 6 months ago. Which of the following is LEAST likely to be done at this visit?
   a. Urinalysis
   b. Foot examination
   c. Fundoscopic examination
   d. ECG

10. Mr. P. is on 30 units of NPH and 5 units of regular insulin each morning and 15 units of NPH each evening to control his type 1 diabetes. His blood glucose levels for the past 3 days have been:

Fasting	Before Lunch	Before Supper	At h.s.
200–250	95–110	110–120	95–130

He should be instructed to:
   a. Add 2 units of NPH to his P.M. dose
   b. Add 2 units NPH before breakfast
   c. Add 2 units of regular insulin to his P.M. dose
   d. Do nothing

11. Hemoglobin A_{1c} gives an indication of glucose control over the past:
   a. Week
   b. 4–6 weeks
   c. Month
   d. 60–90 days

12. When treating diabetes the goal for hemoglobin A_{1c} (normal 4–6%) is:
   a. < 6%
   b. < 7%
   c. < 8%
   d. < 10%

13. Which of the following is an adverse effect of sulfonylureas?

    a. Increased blood pressure
    b. Weight loss
    c. Gastrointestinal distress
    d. Hypoglycemia

14. In addition to controlling glucose levels metformin may also:

    a. Cause weight loss
    b. Increase total cholesterol levels
    c. Increase triglyceride levels
    d. Be likely to cause hypoglycemia

15. Synthetic human insulin:

    a. Causes more antibody formation
    b. Contains more impurities than purified pork insulin
    c. Is least antigenic of all insulins
    d. Has a more rapid action onset than pork counterparts

Questions 16, 17, and 18 refer to the following scenario:

Mr. J. is a 50-year-old male with type 2 diabetes who has been on insulin for the past 6 months. He reports that his fasting blood glucose levels have been running above 200 mg/dL but they have been great during the rest of the day. His evening dose of NPH insulin has been increased three times in the last 2 weeks with no improvement in the fasting values. Currently he is on 30 units NPH—4 units regular in the morning and 18 units NPH/4 units regular before supper. This is his most recent glucose pattern:

B	L	S	h.s.
250–280	130–144	120–132	100–120

16. If he has fairly good dietary compliance, you should instruct him to:

    a. Increase the evening NPH by 2 more units
    b. Check his blood glucose between 2 and 3 A.M. for the next 2 days
    c. Increase the morning dose of regular insulin by 2 units
    d. Increase the morning dose of NPH insulin by 2 units

17. High fasting glucose after a nocturnal hypoglycemia in a person with diabetes otherwise in good control with insulin would indicate:

    a. Dawn phenomenon
    b. Somogyi effect
    c. Insulin allergy
    d. Lipodystrophy

18. Which action would counteract this problem?

    a. Increase morning dose of NPH
    b. Use human insulin instead of pork insulin
    c. Decrease evening NPH insulin dose
    d. Increase morning dose of regular insulin

19. What is the best option to assess long-term glycemic control in a patient with diabetes who also has sickle cell anemia?

    a. Have the patient keep a log of FPG
    b. Assess serum fructosamine
    c. Subtract 3% from the measured $HgbA_{1c}$
    d. Measure glycosylated fatty acids

20. Ms. W. is a 34-year-old who is seeking care because of increased irritability, weight loss "despite a great appetite," and diarrhea (not watery but 2–3 stools a day). She feels exhausted but can't seem to sleep and states she "feels like I could jump out of my skin." If excess thyroid hormone is the problem, which of the following might be noted?

    a. Yellowing skin
    b. Fine tremor
    c. Delayed tendon reflex
    d. Sinus bradycardia

21. Graves' disease is caused by:

    a. Viral infection
    b. Use of lithium
    c. An autoimmune response
    d. Excessive ingestion of thyroid hormone

22. In Graves' disease you would expect:

    a. TSH to be decreased
    b. Anti-TPO to be increased
    c. TSI to be decreased
    d. T_4 to be decreased

23. Upon initial diagnosis of Graves' disease, which medication should be ordered immediately for symptom control?

    a. PTU
    b. Cytomel
    c. ^{131}I
    d. Propranolol

24. The most serious side effect of both PTU and methimazole is:

    a. Skin rash
    b. Diarrhea
    c. Agranulocytosis
    d. Hepatitis

25. The best guide to adequacy of the dosage of antithyroid medication in thyrotoxicosis is:

    a. Thyroid antibodies
    b. T_3 (RIA)
    c. TSH
    d. T_4

26. Sally G. is a 44-year-old who thinks she is beginning menopause because her menstrual periods have become irregular. Her major complaint is a lack of energy and weight gain. Physical examination reveals dry skin, thinning hair, a puffy facial appearance, and an enlarged, nontender thyroid. Her BP is 130/92 with a heart rate of 60. These findings are consistent with:

    a. Graves' disease
    b. Hypothyroidism
    c. Plummer's disease
    d. Thyrotoxicosis

27. Which of the following findings would be consistent with a hypothyroid state?

    a. Hyperactive bowel sounds and fine tremor
    b. Oligomenorrhea and constipation
    c. Edema and heat intolerance
    d. Dry skin and weight gain

28. Ms. H. is diagnosed with hypothyroidism and is placed on levothyroxine 0.05 mg per day. After a week she calls to tell you she hasn't seen any improvement and wants to discontinue her medication. Your best response would be to:

    a. Add propranolol to her regimen
    b. Change to desiccated thyroid
    c. Increase her dosage 0.125 mg/day
    d. Encourage her to take this dose for at least another week

29. Ms. L. is a 50-year-old female who has been diagnosed as having primary myxedema. An initial dose of 0.1 mg/day of levothyroxine has been prescribed. Patient education would include which of the following?

    a. Discussion of the chronicity of the disease and the lifelong medication use
    b. That it will take 6 months to a year for her fatigue to disappear
    c. Avoidance of foods causing increased peristalsis
    d. Explanation that after 2 years of therapy this medication may not be needed

30. Your 57-year-old patient has been on prednisone for her rheumatoid arthritis. She has the typical "moon face," excess weight in her torso area, and is complaining that she bruises easily when she bumps herself. As her primary care provider the best action would be to:

    a. Discontinue her prednisone immediately
    b. Add a NSAID to her treatment regimen
    c. Convert to an alternate-day schedule
    d. Discontinue prednisone immediately and start on naproxen 250 mg b.i.d.

31. Skin changes in Addison's disease include:

    a. Circumoral pallor
    b. Maculopapular eruptions associated with stress
    c. Hyperpigmentation
    d. Facial plethora and hirsutism

Answers

1. **c**		17. **b**
2. **a**		18. **c**
3. **c**		19. **c**
4. **a**		20. **b**
5. **b**		21. **c**
6. **b**		22. **a**
7. **a**		23. **d**
8. **d**		24. **c**
9. **d**		25. **c**
10. **a**		26. **b**
11. **d**		27. **d**
12. **b**		28. **d**
13. **d**		29. **a**
14. **a**		30. **c**
15. **c**		31. **c**
16. **b**		

❑ BIBLIOGRAPHY

American Diabetic Association. (2009). Summary of the revisions for the 2009 Clinical Practice Recommendations. *Diabetes Care, 32*(supp 1).

Bernstein, G. (2002). The diabetes epidemic: Keys to prevention. Guide to therapy. *Consultant, 42*(6), 753–761.

Berra, K. (2003). Treatment options for patients with "Metabolic Syndrome." *Journal of the American Academy of Nurse Practitioners, 15*(8), 361–370.

Blackwell, J. (2004). Clinical practice guidelines: Evaluation and treatment of hyperthyroidism and hypothyroidism. *Journal of the American Academy of Nurse Practitioners, 16*, 422–425.

Dushay, J., & Abrahamson, M. J. (2005). Insulin resistance and type 2 diabetes: A comprehensive review. Retrieved from http://www.medscape.com/viewprogram/3942

Fatourechi, V. (2004). Subclinical hyperthyroidism: When to treat, when to watch? *Consultant, 44*(4), 533–539.

Felicetta, J. V. (2002). Thyroid disease in the elderly: When to suspect, when to treat. *Consultant, 13*(42), 1597–1606.

Kirk Jr., L. F., Hash, R. B., Katner, H. P., & Jones, T. (2000). Cushing's disease: Clinical manifestations and diagnostic evaluation. *American Family Physician, 62*, 1119–1133.

Kutschman, R. F., & Hadley, S. (2004). Diagnosing and treating the metabolic syndrome. *The American Journal of Nurse Practitioners, 8*(2), 9–18.

Li, T-M. (2002). Hypothyroidism in elderly people. *Geriatric Nursing, 23*(2), 88–98.

Liotta, E. A., & Brough, A. (2007). Addison's disease. Retrieved from http://www.emedicine.com/derm/TOPIC 761.htm

Mayfield, J. A., & White, R. D. (2004). Insulin therapy for type 2 diabetes: Rescue, augmentation, and replacement of beta-cell function. *American Family Physician, 70*(3), 489–500.

Streetman, D. D., & Khanderia, U. (2004). Diagnosis and treatment of Graves' disease. *The American Journal for Nurse Practitioners, 8*(1), 27–40.

Whittemore, R., Bak, P. S., Melkus, G. D., & Grey, M. (2003). Promoting lifestyle changes in the prevention and management of type 2 diabetes. *Journal of the American Academy of Nurse Practitioners, 15*(8), 341–350.

10

Genitourinary and Gynecological Disorders

Pamela A. Shuler

Mary D. Knudtson

◻ ACQUIRED IMMUNODEFICIENCY SYNDROME (AIDS)

- Definition—secondary immunodeficiency syndrome resulting from human immunodeficiency virus (HIV) infection and characterized by opportunistic infections, neurologic dysfunction, malignancies, systemic wasting, and a variety of other disorders

- Etiology/Incidence
  1. HIV invades, multiplies within one or more types of susceptible cells; circulating CD4$^+$ lymphocytes, macrophages, and monocytes are most commonly affected, destroying the host's immune system
  2. Median time from HIV infection to AIDS is 10 years
  3. Estimated 1,106,400 cases in the United States; 21% undiagnosed
  4. Estimated 36,000 people are newly infected in the United States annually
  5. Most diagnoses are made in persons 30–39 years old
  6. HIV is transmitted through direct contact with bodily fluids (blood, semen, vaginal secretions) and breast milk
  7. Major routes of HIV transmission
     a. Sexual intercourse (homosexual and heterosexual)
     b. Needle sharing (IV drug users)
     c. Reusing needles for medical purposes (e.g., in developing countries)
     d. Transfusions of contaminated blood and blood products
     e. Needle stick, open wound, and mucous membrane exposure to healthcare workers (0.4% incidence according to the Centers for Disease Control and Prevention [CDC])
     f. Injection with previously used unsterilized needle (acupuncture, tattooing, medical injection)
     g. Pregnancy (mother to unborn fetus)
     h. Breastfeeding (mother to infant)
  8. Trends
     a. 15% increase in newly reported cases in 34 states from 2004 to 2007
     b. Increase in number of newly infected men who have sex with men
     c. African-Americans and Hispanics are disproportionately represented
     d. One in four new HIV infections occur in people younger than 20
     e. Sexual contact leading mode of transmission for women who have sex with men

- Signs and Symptoms—CDC classification
  1. Asymptomatic HIV infection (may last > 10 years)—HIV antibody is detectable in at least 95% of people within 3 months of infection
  2. Acute HIV infection
     a. 2–8 weeks after infection 30–40% may have acute viremia symptoms
        (1) High fever, lymphadenopathy, rash, aseptic meningitis, fatigue, myalgias, arthralgias

(2) Usually mistaken for flu or mono-nucleosis

b. Months to years before AIDS—may have chronic fatigue, weight loss, night sweats, persistent dermatitis, shingles, persistent diarrhea, oral candidiasis, hairy leukopla-kia, chronic vaginal candidiasis, tubercu-losis, cognitive changes

3. Persistent generalized lymphadenopathy (PGL)

a. Palpable lymph node enlargement (two sites other than inguinal)

b. No concurrent illness to explain lymph-adenopathy

4. HIV diseases that contribute to progression of AIDS

a. *Pneumocystis jiroveci* pneumonia, Kaposi's sarcoma, cytomegalovirus, and/or other opportunistic infections/cancers

b. Encephalopathy

c. Wasting syndrome (involuntary weight loss greater than 10% of baseline body weight, plus either chronic diarrhea or chronic weakness and documented fever)

- Differential Diagnosis
  1. Cancer
  2. Tuberculosis
  3. Enterocolitis
  4. Endocrine diseases
  5. Primary cytomegalovirus infection
  6. Drug reaction
  7. Epstein-Barr virus (mononucleosis)
  8. Viral hepatitis
  9. Secondary syphilis

- Physical Findings—variable, depending upon in-fection stage

- Diagnostic Tests/Findings
  1. Informed consent with pretest counseling re-quired prior to HIV testing
  2. Posttest counseling also required
  3. Rapid HIV testing
     a. Oral Quick Rapid HIV-1 antibody test
        (1) Oral fluids, serum, or whole blood tested
        (2) Results in 20–60 minutes
        (3) Sensitivity—99.6%, specificity—100%
        (4) Clinical laboratory improvement amendments (CLIA)—waived
     b. Reveal HIV-1 antibody test
        (1) Serum or plasma tested
        (2) More laboratory dependent
        (3) Results in minutes
        (4) Sensitivity—99.8%, specificity—serum 99.1%, plasma 98.6%
        (5) CLIA—moderate complexity

4. Most commonly used initial blood tests for an-tibody detection

a. Enzyme immunoassay (EIA) (screening test)

b. Western blot or immunofluorescent an-tibody test—confirmatory blood tests for HIV-specific antibody profile

c. Some individuals may not generate an an-tibody response for up to 36 months

5. Detection/quantification of HIV

a. HIV-1 p24 antigen used to diagnose infec-tion before antibodies measurable

b. Qualitative polymerase chain reaction (PCR) circulating cells or plasma—can use in early disease instead of p24

c. Quantitative viral RNA levels—used to decide when to initiate treatment, as a prognostic indicator, and as a basis for evaluating response to treatment

d. CD4+ count used to assess magnitude of disease and to monitor effectiveness of treatment

6. Additional recommended tests if HIV positive

a. HIV viral load test

b. Toxoplasma antibody test

c. Tests for hepatitis A, B, and C viral markers

d. Purified protein derivative (PPD)

e. Chest radiograph

f. Venereal disease research laboratory (VDRL) or RPR

g. Complete blood count (CBC)

h. Fasting blood glucose

i. Fasting lipid panel

j. Pap testing in females

k. Anal pap testing in males

l. Viral genotype

- Management/Treatment—All STD treatment regimens throughout this chapter based on *2011 Guidelines for the Use of Antiretroviral Agents in HIV-1 Infected Adults and Adolescents*, published by CDC. Treatment of HIV and AIDS changing rap-idly; recommendations may have changed due to new or better treatment options; consult with spe-cialist or expert in AIDS care for latest information

  1. All adults in the United States should be screened

  2. No cure or vaccination for HIV infection at present

  3. New treatment regimens are constantly evolving

  4. Treatment of HIV and opportunistic infections, malignancies, and prophylaxis against oppor-tunistic infections continue to evolve rapidly; basic guidelines include

     a. Therapy for opportunistic infections and malignancies

(1) Conditions include *P. jiroveci* pneumonia, toxoplasmosis, cryptococcus, lymphoma, cytomegalovirus, esophageal candidiasis, herpes simplex and zoster, Kaposi's sarcoma

(2) Medications include antibiotics, antifungals, and corticosteroids

b. Antiretroviral treatment (CDC, 2011); treatment of HIV changes very rapidly, consultation with a specialist is recommended

  (1) Recommended treatment—combination drug treatment known as antiretroviral therapy (ART)

  (2) Antiretroviral therapy is based upon disease progression risk

    (a) Option 1—treat any patient with CD4$^+$ count < 350 cells regardless of the presence or absence of opportunistic infection; treatment is also recommended for those with counts between 350 and 500 cells

    (b) Option 2—treat any patient with an AIDS-defining illness regardless of CD4$^+$ count

    (c) Option 3—treat all pregnant patients regardless of CD4$^+$ count or presence/absence of opportunistic infection

  (3) Medications

    (a) Three classes of therapy for treatment-naive patients—nucleoside reverse transcriptase inhibitors (NRTI), non-nucleoside reverse transcriptase inhibitors (NNRTI), protease inhibitors (PI); there are currently four combination options recommended for treatment-naive patients (CDC, 2011)

    (b) Additional classes of therapy for patients not responding to initial treatments—fusion inhibitors, integrase inhibitors

    (c) Viral load monitoring—measure viral RNA every 3–4 months, more frequently if

      (i) Noncompliance suspected

      (ii) CD4$^+$ count drops

      (iii) Clinical symptoms appear

      (iv) Drug adjustments are made (measure at 4–8 weeks then again at 3–4 weeks to document drug effect)

    (d) Initial therapy regimens—important to determine if patient can be compliant with regimen; complicated schedules are extremely difficult to adhere to; viral replication accelerates immediately with noncompliance

    (e) ART therapies combine three or more HIV drugs

    (f) ART therapies recommended for the treatment-naive patient include

      (i) Efavirenz/tenofovir/emtricitabine (Atripla)

      (ii) Ritonavir-boosted atazanavir + tenofovir/emtricitabine

      (iii) Ritonavir-boosted darunavir + tenofovir/emtricitabine

      (iv) Raltegravir + tenofovir/emtricitabine

c. Prophylaxis of opportunistic infections

  (1) *P. jiroveci* pneumonia (begin when CD4$^+$ count < 350)

    (a) Trimethoprim-sulfamethoxazole (TMP/SMX), 1 double-strength tablet daily or 3 times a week

    (b) Dapsone 100 mg per day or aerosolized pentamidine 300 mg monthly if unable to tolerate TMP/SMX

  (2) *Mycobacterium tuberculosis*

    (a) Isoniazid—10 mg/kg/day up to 300 mg plus pyridoxine 50 mg daily for 1 year

    (b) All patients with positive PPD reaction (5 mm of induration or greater) without positive chest radiography should receive prophylactic treatment

  (3) Toxoplasmosis—begin when CD4+ count < 100— TMP/SMX 1 double strength tablet orally 3 times per week or daily

  (4) *Mycobacterium avium* complex—begin when CD4$^+$ count < 50

    (a) Clarithromycin 500 mg orally b.i.d., or

    (b) Azithromycin 500 mg orally 3 times a week, or

    (c) Rifabutin 150 mg orally b.i.d.

d. Indications to change treatment regimens

  (1) Immunologic failure

    (a) CD4+ count falls below baseline

    (b) CD4+ count does not rise > 50 cells after 1 year of therapy

  (2) Virologic failure

    (a) Viral load remains > 400 copies after 6 months of therapy or 50 copies after 1 year

    (b) Viral rebound—viral load rises after initial suppression

    (c) Any reproducible threefold increase in viral load after starting therapy

(3) Clinical failure
  (a) Clinical deterioration despite CD4+ or viral load trends
  (b) Occurrence of HIV-related infection
  (c) Intolerance of adverse effects
  (d) Emergence of resistance
e. Recommended immunizations for HIV infected persons
  (1) Pneumococcal vaccination
  (2) Annual influenza vaccination
  (3) Three-dose schedule of hepatitis B vaccine for those who lack immunity
  (4) Tetanus-diptheria booster
  (5) Inactivated polio virus vaccine (IPV)
  (6) Measles, mumps, rubella vaccine
5. Thorough psychosocial evaluation to include
  a. Signs of severe psychologic distress
  b. Behavioral factors related to risk for transmitting HIV
  c. Information concerning partners who should be notified of possible HIV exposure
6. Discuss therapeutic and diagnostic plans
7. Educate regarding prevention, transmission, and treatment of the disease
8. Emphasize importance of behavioral measures to protect and enhance the immune system
  a. No tobacco, street drugs, alcohol use
  b. Nutritious diet
  c. Stress management, imagery
  d. Exercise as tolerated
  e. Decrease exposure to infectious agents since HIV virus is spread when immune system is activated
9. Encourage continued "safer sex" practices and/or abstinence
10. Assist patient, as appropriate, in meeting physical, psychological, social, cultural, environmental, and spiritual needs
11. Report AIDS cases to local health department

▣ GONORRHEA (UNCOMPLICATED GONOCOCCAL INFECTIONS)

- Definition—a sexually transmitted bacterial infection that produces urethritis in men and cervicitis in women

- Etiology/Incidence
  1. Causative organism is *Neisseria gonorrhoeae*, a gram-negative diplococcus
  2. Approximately 300,000 infectious new cases reported annually
  3. Greatest incidence in the 15- to 30-year-old-age group
  4. Incubation period usually 3–10 days

5. Spectrum of infection—cervicitis, urethritis, salpingitis, proctitis, PID, pharyngitis, conjunctivitis, arthritis
6. A leading cause of female infertility in the United States

- Signs and Symptoms
  1. Female
     a. Often asymptomatic
     b. Dysuria, urinary frequency, urgency with a purulent urethral discharge
     c. Vaginal discharge
     d. Cervicitis
     e. Pelvic pain
     f. Abnormal menstrual bleeding
     g. Pharyngitis
     h. Septic arthritis
     i. Rash—petechial or pustular skin lesions
  2. Male
     a. One-quarter are asymptomatic
     b. Dysuria (urethra most common site in male), frequency
     c. Copious penile discharge (serous/milky to yellow with blood-tinge)
     d. Testicular pain
     e. Pharyngitis
     f. Septic arthritis
     g. Rash—petechial or pustular skin lesions
     h. Proctitis—common in homosexual males

- Differential Diagnosis
  1. Nongonococcal cervicitis, vaginitis, urethritis, or epididymitis
  2. Reiter's syndrome (chlamydia)
  3. Pelvic inflammatory disease (PID)
  4. Proctitis (other origin)
  5. Nongonococcal pharyngitis or arthritis

- Physical Findings
  1. Female
     a. Purulent discharge from cervix (primary site in women of reproductive age)
     b. Inflammation of Bartholin's glands
     c. Evidence of PID (untreated infection)
  2. Male
     a. Evidence of urethritis, prostatitis
     b. Evidence of epididymitis (with untreated infection)
     c. Copious purulent discharge

- Diagnostic Tests/Findings
  1. Female tests
     a. Gram stain of endocervical discharge in women shows WBC with gram negative intracellular diplococci; sensitivity only 40–70% in women; greater than 90% in men

b. Wet prep of purulent cervical discharge may show polymorphonuclear leukocytes (WBC) > 10/HPF

c. Culture material from endocervix and other suspect sites on to Thayer-Martin or Transgrow media to confirm diagnosis

d. DNA probe—sensitivity comparable to culture, 2-hour turnaround time, only one specimen needed for chlamydia and *N. gonorrhoea*

e. Urine-based ligase chain reaction—highly sensitive and specific in men and women

2. Male tests

a. Gram stain of urethral discharge smear shows gram-negative diplococci and WBC

b. Culture of urethra and other suspect sites

c. DNA probe

3. Test for concomitant infection from other STD including HIV, syphilis, and chlamydia

4. Test partners

- Management/Treatment

1. Evaluate and treat all contacts for *N. gonorrhoeae* and chlamydia; evaluate and treat other partners of contacts, since patients infected with *N. gonorrhoeae* often are coinfected with chlamydia, dual presumptive therapy should be considered for patients who may not return for test results and for those with signs/symptoms suggestive of a dual diagnosis

2. Quinolone-resistant *N. gonorrhoeae* is recognized nationally; quinolone options no longer recommended for treatment

3. Recommended treatment regimens for uncomplicated gonococcal infections of the cervix, urethra, and rectum—cefixime 400 mg orally in a single dose or ceftriaxone 125 mg IM in a single dose PLUS azithromycin 1 g orally in a single dose or doxycycline 100 mg orally twice a day for 7 days if chlamydial infection is not ruled out

4. Alternative regimens for uncomplicated gonococcal infections of the cervix, urethra, and rectum—spectinomycin 2 g IM in a single dose, or ceftizoxime 500 mg IM in a single dose, or cefoxitin 2 g IM in a single dose plus probenecid 1 g orally, or cefotaxime 500 mg IM in a single dose PLUS azithromycin 1 g orally in a single dose or doxycycline 100 mg orally twice a day for 7 days if chlamydial infection is not ruled out

5. Recommended treatment regimens for uncomplicated gonococcal infections of the pharynx—ceftriaxone 125 mg IM in a single dose PLUS azithromycin 1 g orally in a single dose or doxycycline 100 mg orally twice a day for 7 days if chlamydial infection is not ruled out

6. Recommended treatment regimens for uncomplicated gonococcal infections during pregnancy—one of the recommended or alternate cephalosporins should be used, or a single, 2-g dose of spectinomycin IM PLUS erythromycin base 500 mg orally 4 times a day for 7 days, or amoxicillin 500 mg orally 3 times daily for 7 days for presumptive or diagnosed chlamydia during pregnancy; tetracyclines should not be used during pregnancy

7. Test of cure not essential; repeat culture if symptoms persist or recur

8. Discuss therapeutic and diagnostic plans

9. Emphasize importance of complete treatment

10. Avoid sexual intercourse until patient and partner(s) cured

11. Educate regarding prevention, transmission, and treatment of the disease; encourage continued use of condoms

12. Report cases to health department

13. Can cause disseminated infection, acute arthritis, hepatitis, or endocarditis

◘ GENITAL CHLAMYDIAL INFECTION

- Definition—a sexually transmitted disease that produces urethritis in men and cervicitis in women

- Etiology/Incidence

1. Causative organism is *Chlamydia trachomatis*

2. Over 1.2 million new cases occur annually

3. The most common bacterial sexually transmitted disease in United States

4. A leading cause of female infertility and ectopic pregnancy in United States

5. Incubation period 7–21 days

6. Screening for high-risk individuals recommended—sexually active adolescents and young adults, multiple partners, history of previous or current STD

- Signs and Symptoms

1. Female

a. Often asymptomatic

b. Dysuria

c. Mucopurulent vaginal discharge/spotting

d. Lower abdominal/pelvic pain

e. Dyspareunia

f. Dysmenorrhea, menstrual irregularity

g. Infertility

h. Enlarged, tender inguinal lymph nodes

i. Friable cervix

2. Male

a. Often asymptomatic

b. Urethral discharge (any color)

c. Dysuria

d. Testicular pain/swelling

e.   Enlarged, tender inguinal lymph nodes
f.   Rectal pain, bleeding, and diarrhea

- Differential Diagnosis
  1.   Gonococcal cervicitis
  2.   Urethritis
  3.   Proctitis
  4.   PID
  5.   Urinary tract infection
  6.   Epididymitis
  7.   Prostatitis from other infective agent
  8.   Vaginitis

- Physical Findings
  1.   Female
      a.   Mucopurulent urethral and/or cervical discharge
      b.   Hypertropic, eroded, and friable cervix (maybe)
      c.   Evidence of PID (advanced infection)
  2.   Male
      a.   Thin, white urethral discharge; markedly less purulent and copious as gonococcal infection
      b.   Evidence of prostatitis
      c.   Evidence of epididymitis (untreated infection)

- Diagnostic Tests/Findings
  1.   Female
      a.   Wet prep or gram stain shows WBC > 10/HPF
      b.   Most common tests—EIA and direct fluorescence assay (DFA) *or* lipase chain reaction (LCR) for confirmation
      c.   Other tests include tissue culture, DNA hybridization, and PCR
  2.   Male
      a.   Gram stain or wet prep shows WBC > 10/HPF
      b.   Same indirect antigen-detection tests
  3.   Test for concomitant infection from other STD in patient (HIV, gonorrhea, syphilis, trichomonas)
  4.   Test partners

- Management/Treatment
  1.   Evaluate and treat all contacts and partners of contacts
  2.   Recommended treatment regimens for uncomplicated Chlamydial infections—azithromycin 1 g orally in a single dose, or doxycycline 100 mg orally twice a day for 7 days
  3.   Alternative regimens for uncomplicated chlamydial infections—erythromycin base 500 mg orally 4 times a day for 7 days, or erythromycin ethylsuccinate 800 mg orally 4 times a day for 7 days, or ofloxacin 300 mg orally twice a day for 7 days, or levofloxacin 500 mg orally for 7 days
  4.   Recommended treatment regimens for uncomplicated chlamydial infections during pregnancy—erythromycin base 500 mg orally 4 times a day for 7 days, or amoxicillin 500 mg orally 3 times daily for 7 days
  5.   Alternative treatment regimens for uncomplicated chlamydial infections during pregnancy—erythromycin base 250 mg orally 4 times a day for 14 days, or erythromycin ethylsuccinate 800 mg orally 4 times a day for 7 days, or erythromycin ethylsuccinate 400 mg orally 4 times a day for 14 days, or azithromycin 1 g orally, single dose
  6.   Test-of-cure not recommended UNLESS patient was treated with erythromycin, is pregnant, has persistent symptoms or reinfection suspected (wait > 3 weeks after treatment for repeat testing preferably by culture)
  7.   Discuss therapeutic and diagnostic plans
  8.   Emphasize importance of complete treatment
  9.   Avoid sexual intercourse until patient and partner(s) complete treatment
  10.   Educate regarding prevention, transmission, and treatment of the disease; encourage continued use of condoms
  11.   Report cases to health department

◻ SYPHILIS

- Definition—complex infectious disease that can affect almost any organ or tissue in the body and mimics many diseases

- Etiology/Incidence
  1.   Causative organism is *Treponema pallidum*, a spirochete
  2.   Transmission primarily occurs through minor skin or mucosal lesions during sexual encounters; genital and extragenital areas may be inoculated
  3.   Can be transmitted via placenta (after 10th week) from mother to fetus (congenital rate—1 in 10,000 pregnancies)
  4.   Incidence has declined since 1990s; approximately 14,000 cases (primary and secondary types) reported in United States annually in 2009
  5.   Risk of contraction—30–50% (partner-primary syphilis)

- Signs and Symptoms
  1.   Primary
      a.   Painless chancre
      b.   Regional lymphadenopathy

2. Secondary
   a. Skin rash—especially palmar, plantar, and oral mucosa
   b. Malaise, anorexia
   c. Alopecia
   d. Arthralgias/myalgias/flu-like symptoms
   e. Other symptoms depending on affected organs
   f. Generalized lymphadenopathy
   g. Low-grade fever
   h. Condylomata lata
3. Latent
   a. May be asymptomatic
   b. Integumentary, ocular, cardiovascular, gastrointestinal, respiratory, or neurological manifestations may be present
4. Neurosyphilis
   a. May occur during any stage of syphilis
   b. Optic, auditory, cranial nerve and/or meningeal symptoms are most common

- Differential Diagnosis
  1. Primary
     a. Herpes genitalis
     b. Chancroid
     c. Neoplasm
     d. Lymphogranuloma venereum (LGV)
     e. Granuloma inguinale
  2. Secondary
     a. Conditions associated with rash or other presenting symptoms, e.g., flu, mononucleosis, pityriasis rosea, drug eruptions
     b. Infectious hepatitis
  3. Latent
     a. Neoplasms of skin, liver, lung, stomach, or brain
     b. Other forms
        (1) Meningitis
        (2) Cardiovascular disorders
        (3) CNS disorders
        (4) Arthritis
        (5) Primary neurologic lesions

- Physical Findings
  1. Neurological signs may be present at any stage
  2. Primary
     a. Indurated ulcer (chancre) on
        (1) Genitals
        (2) Mouth
        (3) Rectum
        (4) Nipple
     b. Regional lymphadenopathy
  3. Secondary
     a. Low-grade fever
     b. Highly variable skin rash (including palms and soles)
     c. Mucous patches

d. Evidence or manifestations of condyloma latum
e. Generalized lymphadenopathy
f. Evidence of meningitis, iritis, hepatitis, glomerulonephritis
4. Latent
   a. May have no clinical signs of infection
   b. Granulomatous lesions (gummas)—skin, mucous membranes, bone
   c. Leukoplakia
   d. Evidence of periostitis, osteitis, or arthritis
   e. Gummatous infiltrates in larynx, trachea, pulmonary parenchyma, stomach and/or liver
   f. Diminished coronary circulation
   g. Acute myocardial infarction
   h. Cardiac insufficiency
   i. Aortic aneurysm
   j. Meningitis
   k. Hemiparesis
   l. Hemiplegia
   m. Tabes dorsalis
   n. General paresis

- Diagnostic Tests/Findings
  1. Early syphilis—primary, secondary, or latent syphilis of less than 1 year's duration
     a. Definitive methods
        (1) Darkfield microscopy
        (2) Direct fluorescent antibody tests of lesion exudate or tissue
     b. Presumptive methods (neither test alone is sufficient for diagnosis)
        (1) Treponemal serologic tests
           (a) Fluorescent treponemal antibody absorption (FTA-ABS) test
           (b) Microhemagglutination assay for antibody to *T. pallidum* (MHA-TP)
           (c) Tests/titers should be reported as positive or negative and used to confirm nontreponemal tests
           (d) FTA-ABS or MHA-TP confirmation tests positive in 85–95% of primary and in 100% of secondary cases
        (2) Nontreponemal serologic tests
           (a) Venereal Disease Research Laboratory (VDRL)
           (b) Rapid plasma reagin (RPR)
  2. Latent syphilis of more than 1 year's duration and cardiovascular syphilis
     a. VDRL or RPR test (+ in 75% of cases)
     b. FTA-ABS or MHA-TP confirmation test (+ in 98% of cases)
     c. Lumbar puncture with tests on cerebrospinal fluid (CSF)

3. Neurosyphilis (occurs at any stage)
   a. Treponemal and nontreponemal serologic test results dependent upon stage of disease
   b. CSF examinations as above
4. Test for concomitant infection from other STD in patient and contacts
   a. HIV
   b. Gonorrhea
   c. Chlamydia
5. Test partners

- Management/Treatment
  1. Pregnant patients allergic to penicillin should be treated with penicillin after desensitization for all stages
  2. Penicillin alternative treatment for all stages of syphilis except neurosyphilis
  3. Early syphilis and persons exposed within last 90 days
     a. Treat all partners
     b. First choice—benzathine penicillin G, 2.4 million units IM once
     c. Penicillin allergy—doxycycline 100 mg orally b.i.d. for 2 weeks or tetracycline 500 mg orally q.i.d. for 2 weeks
  4. Late latent cases and cardiovascular syphilis (normal CSF examination)
     a. First choice—benzathine penicillin G, 2.4 million units IM weekly for 3 weeks
     b. Penicillin allergy—doxycycline 100 mg orally b.i.d. for 4 weeks or tetracycline 500 mg orally q.i.d. for 4 weeks
  5. Neurosyphilis
     a. First choice—18–24 million units aqueous crystalline penicillin G daily, administered as 3–4 million units IV every 4 hours for 10–14 days
     b. Alternate regimen if compliance assured —2.4 million units procaine penicillin IM daily, plus probenecid 500 mg orally q.i.d., both for 10–14 days
  6. Posttreatment follow-up
     a. Primary and secondary baseline RPR or VDRL at time of treatment and repeated every 3 months; titer should fall fourfold in 3 months, eightfold in 6 months, and become negative within 2 years (MHA-TP and FTA-ABS will be positive for lifetime)
     b. Latent—RPR or VDRL repeated at 6-month and 12-month intervals; titer should fall fourfold in 12–24 months
     c. Neurosyphilis—CSF examination every 6 months until normal
  7. Discuss therapeutic and diagnostic plans
  8. Emphasize importance of complete treatment

9. Avoid sexual intercourse until patient and partner(s) cured
10. Educate regarding prevention, transmission, and treatment of the disease; encourage continued use of condoms
11. Report cases to health department
12. All patients with syphilis should be tested for HIV infection

☐ HERPES GENITALIS

- Definition—a viral STD that produces recurrent, painful genital lesions and has no cure

- Etiology/Incidence
  1. Caused by herpes simplex virus (HSV) types 1 (5–15%) and 2 (85–95%)
  2. Initial (primary) and recurrent infections affect approximately 40 million people annually
  3. Duration of initial infection—10–14 days; recurrent 7–10 days; viral shedding (without clinical symptoms) occurs during latency (interval between outbreaks)
  4. Virus resides in presacral ganglia during latency
  5. Can lead to neuralgia, meningitis, ascending myelitis, urethral strictures, and lymphatic suppuration
  6. Infection during pregnancy can lead to spontaneous abortion or fetal morbidity/mortality; risk for transmission to neonate appears highest among women with first episode near time of delivery
  7. Incubation period 2–21 days after exposure

- Signs and Symptoms
  1. First clinical episode occurs in all persons within 6 weeks of contracting infection
     a. Fever/chills
     b. Malaise
     c. Headache
     d. Dysuria
     e. Vaginal discharge, abnormal bleeding
     f. Dyspareunia
     g. Lymph nodes tender, enlarged, firm
     h. Painful genital vesicles that appear in groups on an erythematous base, then rupture and become painful ulcers before resolution—mean duration 12 days
     i. Prodrome frequently absent
  2. Recurrent episodes
     a. Characterized by a prodrome of tingling, burning, or other neuropathic symptoms for 1 or more days
     b. Grouped vesicles that rupture into less painful ulcers; mean duration 4.5 days

    c.   Severity of outbreak typically less than initial presentation unless immune compromise is present

- Differential Diagnosis
  1. Syphilis
  2. Lymphogranuloma venereum
  3. Gonorrhea
  4. Chlamydia
  5. Chancroid
  6. Vaginitis
  7. Herpes zoster
  8. Condyloma latum
  9. Erythema multiforme
  10. Neoplasm (especially cervical)

- Physical Findings
  1. Fever—first episode
  2. Single or multiple vesicles surrounded by inflammation/edema on external genitalia, penis, scrotum, anus, vagina, or cervix (75%); vesicles spontaneously rupture and form painful, erythematous ulcers, scab over, and heal
  3. Cervix may appear diffusely inflamed, edematous with large punched-out ulcers or a granulomatous-appearing tumor-like mass covered with gray exudate
  4. Profuse, watery vaginal discharge often present and may be only sign
  5. Regional lymphadenopathy may be present

- Diagnostic Tests/Findings
  1. Tzanck stain—identification of multinucleated giant cells with intranuclear inclusions in a cytologic smear
  2. Identification of HSV virus(es) from tissue (vulvar, vaginal, cervical) cultures, antigen test, DNA probe, or PCR assay
  3. Serologic tests for HSV types 1 and 2 antibodies are also available
  4. IgM and IgG markers distinguish recent from remote infection
  5. Test for concomitant infection of other STD in patient and contacts
     a. HIV
     b. Syphilis
     c. Condylomata acuminata
     d. Gonorrhea
     e. Chlamydia
     f. Chancroid

- Management/Treatment
  1. Symptomatic treatment—drying and antipruritic agents and topical anesthetic agents
  2. Chemotherapeutic agents—acyclovir (available in topical, oral, and intravenous formulation), famciclovir, or valacyclovir

    a.   Topical therapy—minimal benefit except may be useful for immunocompromised patients, use is discouraged

    b.   Oral therapy
       (1) First clinical episode of genital herpes
          (a) Acyclovir 400 mg orally 3 times a day for 7–10 days, or
          (b) Acyclovir 200 mg orally 5 times a day for 7–10 days, or
          (c) Famciclovir 250 mg orally 3 times a day for 7–10 days, or
          (d) Valacyclovir 1 g orally twice a day for 7–10 days
       (2) Episodic recurrent genital herpes
          (a) Acyclovir 400 mg orally 3 times a day for 5 days, or
          (b) Acyclovir 200 mg orally 5 times a day for 5 days, or
          (c) Acyclovir 800 mg orally twice a day for 5 days, or
          (d) Famciclovir 125 mg orally twice a day for 5 days, or
          (e) Valacyclovir 500 mg orally twice a day for 3–5 days, or
          (f) Valacyclovir 1.0 g orally once a day for 5 days
          (g) One-day regimens of famciclovir and valacyclovir available if taken at the beginning of prodrome before vesicles erupt
       (3) Suppressive therapy for recurrent genital herpes
          (a) Acyclovir 400 mg orally twice a day, or
          (b) Famciclovir 250 mg orally twice a day, or
          (c) Valacyclovir 500 mg orally once a day, or
          (d) Valacyclovir 1.0 g orally once a day

    c.   Intravenous therapy
       (1) Used in severe disease and when complications necessitate hospitalization
       (2) Acyclovir 5–10 mg/kg IV every 8 hours for 2–7 days followed by oral antiviral therapy to complete at least 10 days total therapy

    d.   Acyclovir is eliminated by the kidneys; hydration is particularly important

    e.   Safety of systemic treatment has not been established during pregnancy

3. Discuss therapeutic and diagnostic plans
4. Avoid sexual intercourse when lesions present; encourage continued use of condoms
5. Educate regarding prevention, transmission, and treatment of the disease and dangers during pregnancy
6. Up to 80% may have viral shedding during asymptomatic periods

◘ GENITAL WARTS (CONDYLOMATA ACUMINATA)

- Definition—sexually transmitted warty growths appearing on any part of the genitalia

- Etiology/Incidence
  1. More than 40 types of human papillomavirus (HPV) cause genital warts; visible genital warts usually are caused by types 6 or 11; types 16, 18, 31, 33, 35, are predominately detected in high-grade neoplastic lesions and cervical cancer
  2. HPV increases risk of penile, vulvar, and cervical cancers
  3. Greatest incidence in the 15- to 25-year-old age group; correlated with multiple sex partners, early coitus, and lack of contraceptive barrier methods
  4. Approximately 6 million new cases each year
  5. Approximately 20 million people currently infected in the United States
  6. The most common symptomatic viral STD in the United States; highly contagious

- Signs and Symptoms
  1. Painless, pruritic, or burning warts on external genitalia (male and female)
  2. Possibly—dyspareunia, dysuria, bleeding

- Differential Diagnosis
  1. Condyloma latum
  2. Neoplasm
  3. Granuloma inguinale
  4. Moles
  5. Molluscum contagiosum

- Physical Findings
  1. Single or multiple soft, fleshy, papillary, or sessile, painless keratinized growths (may be multilobulated papules and quite large) around anus, vulvovaginal area, penis, urethra, perineum, or oral cavity
  2. In women, similar lesions may appear in vagina/on cervix; vaginal discharge from coexisting infection(s) may be present; men may have lesions in urethra
  3. May have no signs since flat warts are visible only by colposcopy

- Diagnostic Tests/Findings
  1. Tissue sample (biopsy) for detection of viral DNA is available, but expense limits clinical utility
  2. Biopsies may be taken to rule out dysplasia and carcinoma
  3. Pap smear may indicate HPV infection on cervix; see section on dysplasia

4. Test for concomitant infection of other STD
   a. HIV
   b. Gonorrhea
   c. Syphilis—RPR or VDRL to rule out Condyloma latum
   d. Chlamydia

- Management/Treatment
  1. Prevention
     a. Condoms may lower risk; however HPV can be shed into areas not covered by condoms
     b. HPV vaccination
        (1) Gardasil indicated for females and males aged 9–26
            (a) Prevents four HPV types
                (i) Types 16 and 18, which cause 70% of cervical cancers
                (ii) Types 6 and 11, which cause 90% of genital warts
                (iii) No effect on HPV-related disease
            (b) May be given to sexually active girls/women and those who already have HPV infection as most not infected with all four types
            (c) Should not be given in pregnancy
            (d) Should not be given in the setting of moderate or severe illness
            (e) Given as a series of 3 IM injections at baseline, 2 months, and 6 months
        (2) Cervarix indicated for females and males aged 9–25
            (a) Prevents two HPV types
                (i) Types 16 and 18, which cause 70% of cervical cancers
                (ii) No effect on HPV-related disease
            (b) May be given to sexually active girls/women and those who already have HPV infection as most not infected with all four types
            (c) Should not be given in pregnancy
            (d) Should not be given in the setting of moderate or severe illness
            (e) Given as a series of 3 IM injections at baseline, 2 months, and 6 months
  2. New treatment regimens are evolving to ameliorate symptoms; no current methods are curative
     a. Small vulvar and perianal warts
        (1) Self-treatment with podofilox 0.5% solution or gel—apply with cotton tip applicator b.i.d. for 3 days followed by no treatment for 4 days; cycle can be

repeated 4 times (caution with podophyllin use concerning size of treatment area)

    (2) 80–90% solution of trichloroacetic acid (TCA) or tincture of podophyllin weekly for 6 weeks (patient must wash off podophyllin in 4 hours); protect surrounding skin with petroleum jelly

    (3) TCA is preferred since it is more effective, not absorbed, and can be used during pregnancy and on penis; treatment may be slightly more painful than podophyllin; immediate application of sodium bicarbonate paste following treatment will decrease pain

    (4) Self-treatment with imiquimod 5% cream applied at bedtime 3 times a week for 16 weeks; wash off 6–10 hours after application

    (5) Surgical removal with tangential scissor or shave excision, curettage, or electrosurgery

    (6) Intralesional interferon

    (7) Cryotherapy with liquid nitrogen

  b. Large warts (> 2 cm), vulvar/vaginal warts

    (1) CO_2 laser

    (2) Electrodesiccation, electrocautery, cryocautery, Leep, intralesional interferon

3. NO MORE THAN ⅓ OF LESION ENCIRCLING AN ORIFICE SHOULD BE TREATED AT SINGLE VISIT

4. Cervical warts—see section on dysplasia

5. Discuss therapeutic and diagnostic plans

6. Educate regarding prevention, transmission, and treatment of the disease; encourage continued use of condoms

7. Emphasize importance of follow-up particularly if Pap abnormal

8. Discuss possible chronicity

  a. Treatment may not be successful

  b. High recurrence rate due to dormant and asymptomatic viral shedding

  c. Individuals who smoke have more difficulty with recurrence

  d. Smoking is HPV cofactor for cervical cancer

◻ PELVIC INFLAMMATORY DISEASE (PID)

- Definition—infection of the upper genital tract, including the endometrium, oviducts, ovaries, uterine wall/serosa, broad ligaments, and pelvic peritoneum

- Etiology/Incidence
  1. A disease of polymicrobial infection caused by a variety of aerobic and anaerobic bacteria including *N. gonorrhoeae*, *C. trachomatis*, group B streptococcus, *Escherichia coli*, bacteroides, *Mycoplasma hominis*, and *Ureaplasma urealyticum*
  2. Clinical PID is usually a polymicrobial infection
  3. More than 1 million episodes occur annually
  4. Most prevalent serious infection for women 16–25 years of age
  5. After initial infection, women more susceptible to reinfection, ectopic pregnancy, and infertility
  6. Oral contraceptives and barrier methods with spermicide provide significant protection
  7. Depot-medroxyprogesterone acetate and Norplant cause changes in cervical mucosa, which provide some protection from PID
  8. Annual costs of PID and its sequelae is $4.2 billion

- Signs and Symptoms
  1. Symptoms may be mild, atypical, subtle, or absent
  2. Fever/chills
  3. Nausea/vomiting
  4. Dysuria
  5. Vaginal discharge
  6. Dysmenorrhea
  7. Abnormal menstrual bleeding
  8. Lower abdominal/pelvic pain (usually < 1 week duration)
  9. Dyspareunia
  10. Infertility

- Differential Diagnosis
  1. Appendicitis
  2. Ectopic pregnancy
  3. Septic abortion
  4. Hemorrhagic or ruptured ovarian cysts or tumors
  5. Twisted ovarian cyst
  6. Degeneration of a myoma
  7. Enteritis

- Physical Findings and Diagnostic Tests/Findings (clinical criteria for diagnosing PID)
  1. Minimum criteria—empiric treatment required if both are present
     a. Uterine/adnexal tenderness
     b. Cervical wall motion tenderness
  2. Additional criteria to enhance specificity of diagnosis
     a. Laboratory documentation of cervical infection with *C. trachomatis* or *N. gonorrhoeae*
     b. Oral temperature > 38.3° C or 101° F
     c. Abnormal cervical or vaginal mucopurulent discharge

d. White blood cells on saline microscopy of vaginal secretions

e. Elevated erythrocyte sedimentation rate and/or C-reactive protein

3. Definitive criteria for diagnosis—warranted in select cases

    a. Histopathologic evidence of endometritis on endometrial biopsy

    b. Tubo-ovarian abscess on sonography or other radiologic tests

    c. Laparoscopic abnormalities consistent with PID

- Management/Treatment

1. Resolution of symptoms and preservation of tubal function are the primary goals in management of PID; ideally all patients are hospitalized; however, for economic and practical reasons many are treated as outpatients

2. Hospitalization is highly recommended if

    a. Diagnosis is uncertain and surgical emergencies (i.e., appendicitis) cannot be excluded

    b. Tubo-ovarian abscess is suspected

    c. Patient is pregnant

    d. Severe illness, e.g., nausea and vomiting precludes outpatient treatment

    e. Patient unable to follow or tolerate outpatient regimen

    f. Patient has failed to clinically respond to outpatient treatment

3. Outpatient treatment

    a. Recommended treatment for PID—ceftriaxone 250 mg IM in a single dose plus doxycycline 100 mg orally twice a day for 14 days WITH or WITHOUT metronidazole 500 mg orally twice a day for 14 days

    b. Alternative treatments—cefoxitin 2 g IM in a single dose and probenecid 1 g orally administered concurrently in a single dose, PLUS doxycycline 100 mg orally twice a day for 14 days WITH or WITHOUT metronidazole 500 mg orally twice a day for 14 days

    c. Alternative treatment—other parenteral third-generation cephalosporin PLUS doxycycline 100 mg orally twice a day for 14 days WITH or WITHOUT metronidazole 500 mg orally twice a day for 14 days

4. Follow-up appointment in 72 hours; should be substantially improved, if not hospitalization usually required

5. Some clinicians advocate test-of-cure 4–6 weeks posttreatment

6. Test and treat partners

7. Discuss therapeutic and diagnostic plans

8. Emphasize importance of complete treatment

9. Avoid sexual intercourse until patient and partner(s) cured

10. Education regarding prevention, transmission, and treatment of the disease; encourage continued use of condoms

11. Discuss fertility issues as appropriate

◻ VULVOVAGINITIS

- Definition—inflammation and infection of the vulva/vagina

- Etiology/Incidence

1. Commonly caused by *Trichomonas vaginalis* (a motile protozoan), bacterial vaginosis (a polymicrobial bacterial vaginal infection), or *Candida albicans* (a fungi or yeast)

2. Trichomonas—transmitted through intercourse, can infect the lower urinary tract in men and women

3. Bacterial vaginosis (BV)—the most frequently diagnosed symptomatic vaginitis in the United States; unclear whether BV results from sexually transmitted pathogen, but incidence is higher in those who are sexually active; should be treated in pregnant women since the infection has been associated with premature rupture of membranes, preterm labor, and preterm birth

4. Vulvovaginal candidiasis (VVC)—occurs in close to 40–75% of women; is not considered to be an STD; is predisposed by pregnancy, diabetes, use of broad-spectrum antibiotics or corticosteroids; heat, moisture, and occlusive clothing also increase risk; VVC has been divided into two categories

    a. Uncomplicated VVC—sporadic or infrequent vulvovaginal candidiasis or mild-to-moderate vulvovaginal candidiasis is likely to be *C. albicans* in nonimmunocompromised women

    b. Complicated VVC—recurrent vulvovaginal candidiasis (four or more episodes of symptomatic VVC in 1 year) or severe vulvovaginal candidiasis or nonalbicans candidiasis, or women with uncontrolled diabetes, debilitation, or immunosuppression in those who are pregnant

5. Several types of vaginitis may coexist

- Signs and Symptoms

1. Trichomoniasis

    a. Malodorous yellow-green discharge with pruritus

    b. Dyspareunia

    c. Dysuria (male partners may also have dysuria)

2. Bacterial vaginosis
   a. Malodorous, white ("fishy") discharge
   b. Spotting
   c. 50% of patients are asymptomatic
3. Candida vaginitis
   a. Thick, "cottage cheese" discharge with pruritus
   b. Erythema of vagina and vulva

- Differential Diagnosis
  1. Chlamydia
  2. Gonorrhea
  3. Herpes genitalis
  4. Condylomata acuminata
  5. Allergy, contact dermatitis
  6. Atrophic vaginitis

- Physical Findings
  1. Trichomoniasis
     a. Diffuse vaginal erythema
     b. Intensely inflamed lesions on cervix and vaginal mucosa—"strawberry patches"
     c. Discharge
        (1) Ranges from white/watery to green, thick, and frothy
        (2) Vaginal pH—higher than 4.5
  2. Bacterial vaginosis
     a. Watery, grayish, or white homogenous discharge, fishy odor
     b. Discharge slightly adherent to vaginal walls
  3. Candida vaginitis
     a. White, "cottage-cheese" discharge
     b. Marked vulvovaginal erythema/edema with intense pruritus

- Diagnostic Tests/Findings
  1. Wet prep microscopic examination of vaginal secretions viewed on low or high power
     a. Trichomoniasis—discharge mixed with saline will show motile trichomonas on microscopic examination
     b. Bacterial vaginosis—discharge mixed with saline will show clue cells on microscopic examination; amine-like odor present when discharge alkalinized with 10–20% potassium hydroxide (KOH) "whiff test"; vaginal pH of 4–5 or more
     c. Candida vaginitis—discharge mixed with 10% KOH will show branched and budding pseudohyphae on microscopic examination
  2. Test for concomitant infection from other STD
     a. HIV
     b. Syphilis
     c. Condylomata acuminata
     d. Gonorrhea
     e. Chlamydia

- Management/Treatment
  1. Trichomoniasis
     a. Recommended treatment—metronidazole 2 g orally as a single dose, alternative treatment metronidazole 500 mg b.i.d. for 7 days; treat partner
     b. Treatment during pregnancy—2 g of metronidazole in single dose
     c. Caution patient to avoid alcohol during metronidazole therapy due to possible disulfiram-like reaction
  2. Bacterial vaginosis
     a. Recommended treatment
        (1) Clindamycin cream 2%, 1 full applicator 5 g intravaginally at bedtime for 7 days
        (2) Metronidazole 500 mg orally b.i.d. for 7 days, or
        (3) Metronidazole gel 0.75%, 1 full applicator (5 g) intravaginally q.d. or b.i.d. for 5 days
     b. Alternative treatment
        (1) Clindamycin 300 mg orally b.i.d. for 7 days (safe during pregnancy)
        (2) Metronidazole 2 g orally in a single dose
        (3) Clindamycin ovules 100 g intravaginally at bedtime for 3 days
     c. Treatment during pregnancy
        (1) Metronidazole 250 mg orally 3 times a day for 7 days
        (2) Clindamycin 300 mg orally twice a day for 7 days
  3. Vulvovaginal candidiasis
     a. Recommended regimens for uncomplicated VVC
        (1) Intravaginal agents—variety of intravaginal antifungal agents available over the counter in single dose, 3-, 5-, 7-, or 14-day regimens
        (2) Oral agent—fluconazole 150-mg oral tablet, 1 tablet in single dose
        (3) Return for follow-up if symptoms recur within 2 months—need to consider underlying cause of recurrent susceptibility to fungal infection
        (4) Intravaginal creams and suppositories are oil-based and may weaken latex condoms and diaphragms
     b. Recommended regimens for complicated VVC
        (1) Recurrent VVC—7–14 days of topical azole therapy or a 150-mg oral dose of fluconazole repeated 3 days later
           (a) Maintenance regimens include clotrimazole (500-mg dose vaginal suppositories once weekly), or

ketoconazole (100-mg dose once daily), or fluconazole (100- to 150-mg dose once weekly), or itraconazole (400-mg dose once monthly or 100-mg dose once daily)

(b) Maintenance regimens usually continue for 6 months

(c) Patients receiving long-term treatment with ketoconazole should be monitored for hepatic toxicity

(2) Severe VVC (i.e., extensive vulvar erythema, edema, excoriation, and fissure formation)—7–14 days of topical azole or 150 mg of fluconazole in two sequential doses (second dose 72 hours after initial dose) is recommended

(3) Nonalbicans VVC—7–14 days of treatment with a nonfluconazole azole drug is recommended

(i) For recurrence—600 mg of boric acid in a gelatin capsule is recommended, administered vaginally once daily for 2 weeks; referral to a specialist is advised

(4) Pregnancy—only topical azole therapies, applied vaginally for 7 days

4. Discuss therapeutic and diagnostic plans
5. Avoid sexual intercourse until patient and partner(s) cured
6. Education regarding prevention, transmission, and treatment of the disease; encourage continued use of condoms
7. Emphasize importance of treating BV, trichomoniasis, and infections during pregnancy
8. Education regarding dangers of douching and incidence of infection
9. Education regarding PID; association with bacterial vaginosis

◘ LOWER URINARY TRACT INFECTION (LUTI, CYSTITIS: ACUTE, UNCOMPLICATED)

- Definition—inflammation and infection of the urinary bladder; urethra may be involved

- Etiology/Incidence
  1. Most common causative organisms—*E. coli* (women) and *Proteus* species (men)
  2. More common in women than men; urological evaluation required for men with UTI
  3. 30–40% of women will experience at least one UTI
  4. Contributing factors in women
     a. Sexual intercourse; diaphragm use
     b. Pregnancy

c. Diabetes
d. Catheterization
e. Instrumentation
f. Retaining urine in bladder despite urge to void

5. Contributing factors in men
   a. Residual urine (prostatic enlargement)
   b. Neuropathic bladder
   c. Calculi
   d. Prostatitis
   e. Catheterization
   f. Instrumentation

- Signs and Symptoms
  1. Dysuria, frequency, urgency
  2. Lower abdominal discomfort
  3. Suprapubic discomfort
  4. Foul smelling urine

- Differential Diagnosis
  1. Vaginitis (females)
  2. Prostatitis (males)
  3. Gonorrhea
  4. Chlamydia infection
  5. Renal calculi
  6. Pyelonephritis
  7. Epididymitis

- Physical Findings
  1. Urinary meatus may be erythematous/edematous
  2. Negative costovertebral angle tenderness
  3. Negative pelvic or prostate examination; women may experience discomfort when bladder palpated during pelvic examination
  4. May have suprapubic tenderness on palpation

- Diagnostic Tests/Findings
  1. Pyuria—> 10 WBC/HPF
  2. Complete urinalysis (clean catch) with culture and sensitivity testing
     a. Bacteria count over 100,000 organisms per mL in fresh "clean catch" midstream specimen is reliable indicator of active urinary tract infection; women with acute cystitis may have more than 10^3 but less than 10^5 per mL in midstream urine cultures
     b. Leukocyte esterase dipstick test—positive
     c. Urine dipstick positive for protein, blood, nitrites suggestive of UTI

- Management/Treatment for Women (men need urological referral)
  1. Single-dose regimens—fosfomycin tromethamine 3-g single dose

2. Three-day regimen examples (uncomplicated lower tract infection, e.g., women < 65 years old who are not pregnant)
   a. TMP/SMX DS tablet b.i.d.
   b. Fluoroquinolones in cases of TMP/SMX resistance or allergy
      (1) Ciprofloxacin 250 mg b.i.d.
      (2) Norfloxacin 400 mg b.i.d.
      (3) Ofloxacin 200 mg b.i.d.
      (4) Levofloxacin 250 mg daily
3. 7- to 10-day regimen examples (for complicated infection, e.g., men, women > 65 years of age)
   a. TMP/SMX 1 DS tablet b.i.d.
   b. Nitrofurantoin 100 mg q.i.d.
   c. Fluoroquinolones in cases of TMP/SMX resistance
      (1) Norfloxacin 400 mg b.i.d.
      (2) Ciprofloxacin 250–500 mg b.i.d.
      (3) Levofloxacin 250 mg daily
4. Treatment during pregnancy—nitrofurantoin 100 mg b.i.d. for 7–10 days or amoxicillin 500 mg orally t.i.d. for 7–14 days; cephalosporin 500 mg q.i.d. for 7–14 days
5. Consider adding phenazopyridine hydrochloride 200 mg orally t.i.d. for 2 days for discomfort associated with urinary tract irritation (caution patient of orange/red tinge to urine)
6. Consider possibility of urethritis from chlamydia if failure of short-course therapy in sexually active women
7. Increase water and decrease carbonated drink intake
8. Encourage frequent voids; do not hold urine in bladder
9. Patient education regarding perineal hygiene, front-to-back wiping
10. Repeat urinalysis with culture and sensitivity after medication regimen completed if still symptomatic
11. Discuss therapeutic and diagnostic plans
12. Advise return appointment if symptoms increase or no improvement
13. Emphasize importance of complete treatment

◘ ACUTE PYELONEPHRITIS (UPPER UTI)

- Definition—an acute bacterial infection of the upper urinary tract (kidney and renal pelvis); usually results from an ascending infection

- Etiology/Incidence
  1. *E. coli* (gram negative) accounts for 80% of infections; *Staphylococcus saprophyticus* and *Streptococcus faecalis* (gram positive) account for 5–10%
  2. If urologic abnormalities or calculi present, the following organisms may cause infection—Enterobacter, Proteus, Klebsiella, Serratia, and Pseudomonas
  3. Majority of infections occur in young women; rare occurrence in men under age 50 years
  4. Most commonly occurs in patients who are pregnant or have disruptive urinary flow, neurogenic bladder dysfunction, or vesicoureteral reflux
  5. May follow incomplete treatment of lower urinary tract infection

- Signs and Symptoms—usually develop rapidly over a few hours
  1. Shaking chills
  2. Malaise, generalized muscle tenderness
  3. Nausea, vomiting, and diarrhea
  4. Flank/back pain (unilateral or bilateral)
  5. Abdominal pain
  6. Dysuria, frequency, or urgency (may be absent)

- Differential Diagnosis
  1. Cystitis
  2. Prostatitis
  3. Musculoskeletal back pain
  4. Appendicitis
  5. Diverticulitis
  6. Pelvic inflammatory disease
  7. Ectopic pregnancy

- Physical Findings
  1. Fever, tachycardia
  2. Costovertebral angle pain (unilateral or bilateral) upon percussion
  3. Peritoneal signs are usually absent
  4. Patient may appear very ill

- Diagnostic Tests/Findings
  1. Microscopic urinalysis
     a. 5–10 WBC/HPF
     b. Occasional erythrocytes
     c. White cell casts may be present
     d. Mild proteinuria
  2. Urine culture—> 100,000 bacteria per mL of urine; sensitivity testing should be done
  3. Gram stain of uncentrifuged urine—one bacterium per oil-immersion correlates with 100,000 bacteria per mL of urine or more
  4. CBC—leukocytosis with left shift
  5. Elevated ESR
  6. BUN and creatinine usually normal
  7. Electrolytes may be abnormal if dehydrated

- Management/Treatment
  1. Outpatient therapy—if compliant/reliable with immediate access to healthcare services, if condition worsens, and if not elderly or pregnant

a. Antibiotics may include fluoroquinolones for 7-day regimen as treatment of choice; alternative regimens include TMP/SMX, first-generation cephalosporins, or amoxicillin/clavulanate, for 14-day course
   b. Resistance to amoxicillin is 30%, therefore should not be used as sole therapy
   c. Follow-up within 24 hours
   d. Hydration measures
2. Inpatient therapy
   a. Patients who are pregnant, have underlying illness, have decreased renal reserve, very toxic (high fever, hypotensive, etc.), or unable to tolerate oral therapy should be hospitalized for parenteral antibiotics
   b. IV antimicrobial therapy is based upon culture and sensitivity report
   c. IV hydration is also required
3. Repeat urine culture 2 weeks after completed course of antibiotics
4. Discuss therapeutic and diagnostic plans
5. Emphasize importance of complete treatment and follow-up appointments
6. Instructions regarding no sexual intercourse until treatment completed
7. Education regarding emergency signs and symptoms if managed as outpatient
8. Second episode of acute pyelonephritis requires urologic consultation or workup

◨ ACUTE BACTERIAL PROSTATITIS

- Definition—inflammation/infection of the prostate gland

- Etiology/Incidence
  1. *E. coli* or other gram-negative bacteria are common causative agents
  2. Occasionally acute urinary retention develops, requiring urgent hospitalization; suprapubic drainage may be necessary; URINARY CATHETERIZATION SHOULD BE AVOIDED
  3. Absence of zinc in prostatic fluid can predispose patient to infection
  4. Young adult men may be more prone to nonbacterial prostatitis or prostatosis
     a. WBC are present in expressed prostatic secretions, but no organisms are cultured
     b. Causative agents include mycoplasma, ureaplasma, gonorrhea, and chlamydia—sexually transmitted organisms more likely in men < 35 years of age

- Signs and Symptoms
  1. Fever/chills, malaise, myalgias
  2. Low back pain
  3. Dysuria, urgency, nocturia, frequency
  4. Perineal pain increased with defecation

- Differential Diagnosis
  1. Acute/chronic bacterial cystitis (urinary retention)
  2. Chronic prostatitis
  3. Nonbacterial prostatitis
  4. Prostatodynia
  5. Prostatic or seminal vesicle abscesses
  6. Benign prostatic hypertrophy
  7. Prostatic cancer
  8. Epididymitis
  9. Acute diverticulitis

- Physical Findings
  1. Fever
  2. Prostate—edematous, firm or "boggy," warm and tender; AVOID VIGOROUS MASSAGE, CAN LEAD TO BACTEREMIA

- Diagnostic Tests/Findings
  1. Urine cultures—positive
  2. Prostatic secretions—expressed prostatic secretions (EPS), WBC > 20 cells/HPF is abnormal
  3. Diagnosis is best made by performing simultaneous quantitative bacterial cultures of urethral urine, bladder urine, and EPS, the three glass test
  4. Patient often treated based only on physical findings and urine culture

- Management/Treatment
  1. Patients who appear septic and/or have urinary retention should be hospitalized
  2. Outpatient treatment
     a. First choice if age > 35 years is TMP/SMX double-strength tablet b.i.d. for 4–6 weeks; if age < 35 years doxycycline 100 mg orally b.i.d. for 10 days plus ceftriaxone 250 mg IM 1 time or ofloxacin 400 mg once then 300 mg b.i.d. for 10 days
     b. Alternative choices are carbenicillin 2 tablets orally q.i.d. for 2–4 weeks or ciprofloxacin 500 mg orally b.i.d. for 2–4 weeks
  3. Bed rest
  4. Sitz bath t.i.d. for 30 minutes
  5. Follow-up appointment 48–72 hours
  6. Discuss therapeutic and diagnostic plans
  7. Avoid sexual intercourse until acute phase resolved; encourage continued use of condoms if multiple partners
  8. Education regarding signs/symptoms of urinary retention and epididymitis
  9. Emphasize importance of follow-up appointments

◘ CHRONIC BACTERIAL PROSTATITIS

- Definition—chronic inflammation/infection of prostate gland

- Etiology/Incidence
    1. Causative organisms are *E. coli*; enterobacter organisms, *Proteus* species, *C. trachomatis* — sexually transmitted organisms more likely in men < 35 years of age
    2. Often associated with urethritis or infection of lower urinary tract
    3. One of the most common causes of recurrent urinary tract infection in men

- Signs and Symptoms
    1. Symptoms similar to, but milder than, acute bacterial prostatitis
    2. Hallmark of disease is relapsing UTI due to same pathogen found in prostatic secretions
    3. Urinary frequency, dysuria, decreased flow, hesitancy, dribbling
    4. Vague lower abdominal pain
    5. Lumbar and perineal pain
    6. Fever and urethral discharge uncommon
    7. May experience swelling and severe tenderness of scrotum

- Differential Diagnosis—same as acute bacterial prostatitis

- Physical Findings
    1. May involve scrotal contents, producing intense local discomfort, swelling, erythema, and severe tenderness to palpation
    2. Prostate may be tender, irregularly indurated, or boggy

- Diagnostic Tests/Findings—diagnosis made by examination of EPS and quantitative bacterial cultures
    1. EPS—abnormal if greater than 10 WBC/HPF
    2. More than 1 or 2 lipid-laden macrophages/HPF—abnormal
    3. EPS culture—positive

- Management/Treatment
    1. Often difficult to treat
    2. Usual antibiotics—TMP/SMX, doxycycline, ciprofloxacin, levofloxacin, norfloxacin for 12 weeks
    3. Sitz baths, prostatic massage
    4. Regular ejaculation through intercourse and/or masturbation
    5. Avoid over-the-counter decongestants if urinary outlet symptoms

◘ EPIDIDYMITIS

- Definition—an acute intrascrotal infection

- Etiology/Incidence
    1. Caused by infection from bladder urine, the prostate, or an ascending urethral infection
    2. Common affliction of men 35 years and younger; chlamydia usual causative organism for this population (*N. gonorrhoeae* far less common)
    3. Infection in men > 35 years usually arises from bladder bacteriuria secondary to coliform organisms or following instrumentation, catheterization, or surgery (prostatectomy)
    4. "Sterile" epididymitis associated with vigorous physical activity is caused by vasal reflux of sterile urine, which leads to a chemical inflammation of the epididymis
    5. Epididymitis in boys may indicate underlying congenital anatomic abnormalities (i.e., ectopic ureter, posterior urethral valve)
    6. Condition is usually unilateral
    7. Epididymitis may be complicated by development of testicular necrosis, testicular atrophy, or infertility

- Signs and Symptoms
    1. Painful, scrotal swelling (pain may radiate up the spermatic cord into the lower abdomen)
    2. Sensation of scrotal heaviness
    3. Symptoms of prostatitis or UTI may be present
    4. Systemic symptoms may develop—fever, chills, and malaise

- Differential Diagnosis
    1. Mumps
    2. Testicular torsion
    3. Testicular abscess
    4. Tumor of testicle with or without hemorrhage
    5. Hydrocele
    6. Trauma
    7. Infarction

- Physical Findings
    1. Enlarged, tender indurated epididymis
    2. Urethral discharge may be present
    3. Massaging prostate may exacerbate epididymitis
    4. Pain relieved with scrotal elevation (Prehn's sign)
    5. Cremasteric reflex present

- Diagnostic Tests/Findings
    1. Men
        a. STD testing (chlamydia, gonorrhea, and syphilis)
        b. Culture and gram-stained smear of uncentrifuged urine

   c. Scrotal ultrasonography if condition initially severe or if fever continues while on antibiotics (rule out abscess)

   d. CBC—may show increased white blood cell count with left shift

   e. Pyuria

2. Boys—require more extensive workup; refer for consult

   a. Intravenous urography

   b. Cystourethroscopy

   c. Voiding cystourethrography

   d. Scrotal ultrasonography (with or without Doppler imaging)

   e. Radionuclide scanning

   f. Surgical exploration may be required

- Management/Treatment

1. Physician referral or consult required if

   a. Patient is a child

   b. Systemic symptoms of infection (leukocytosis, fever) present in adults; patient should be hospitalized for parenteral antibiotics

   c. Possible torsion of testes

2. Outpatient therapy

   a. Antibiotic therapy based on patient's age and symptoms

     (1) Adult < 35 years of age—first choice is ceftriaxone 250 mg IM in a single dose plus doxycycline 100 mg orally b.i.d.; alternative choice for men 17 years of age or older if no gonococcal or chlamydial infection is ofloxacin 200–400 mg orally b.i.d. for 10 days or levofloxacin 500 mg orally once daily for 10 days

     (2) Adult > 35 years of age—TMP/SMX 1 double-strength tablet orally b.i.d. or ciprofloxacin 250–500 mg orally b.i.d. for 10 days; or levofloxacin 250–500 mg daily for 10 days; treat for 4 weeks if underlying prostatitis present

   b. Scrotal elevation, support, and bed rest

   c. Analgesics—nonsteroidal anti-inflammatory agents

   d. Ice (early), heat (late)

   e. Spermatic cord block with lidocaine may be used

3. Follow up within 48 hours if symptoms persist or worsen

4. If STD present or suspected, instruct patient to refer sex partners for evaluation and treatment

5. Discuss therapeutic and diagnostic plans

6. Emphasize importance of complete treatment

7. Avoid sexual intercourse until course of antibiotics completed

8. Inform patient that swelling and discomfort may persist for weeks or months after eradication of infecting organism; epididymis may remain enlarged or indurated indefinitely

9. Educate regarding prevention, transmission, and treatment of sexually transmitted disease (if causative agent); encourage continued use of condoms

10. Encourage patient to discuss concerns and/or fears

◘ BENIGN PROSTATIC HYPERPLASIA (BPH)

- Definition—progressive, benign hyperplasia of prostate gland tissue

- Etiology/Incidence

1. Cause is uncertain

2. Approximately 50% of men have BPH by age 60; incidence increases to 90% by age 85

3. The most common cause of bladder outlet obstruction in males > 50 years

4. Symptoms are attributed to mechanical obstruction of the urethra by the enlarged prostate gland

- Signs and Symptoms

1. May be asymptomatic

2. Frequency, urgency, urge incontinence

3. Nocturia, dysuria

4. Weak urinary stream, dribbling, hesitancy

5. Sensation of full bladder immediately after voiding

6. Retention

7. Urinary tract infection may be first indicator of BPH-induced urinary retention

- Differential Diagnosis

1. Urethral stricture

2. Prostate or bladder cancer

3. Neurogenic bladder

4. Bladder calculus

5. Acute or chronic prostatitis

6. Bladder neck contracture

7. Medications that affect micturition

- Physical Findings

1. Abdomen—may have distended bladder secondary to retention

2. Prostate (patient should void prior to examination)

   a. Nontender with asymmetrical or symmetrical enlargement; gross enlargement atypical

   b. Consistency is smooth and rubbery (consistency of a pencil eraser)

   c. Distinct nodules (spheroids) may be present—differentiation between BPH nodules and cancerous ones is based on induration or firmness of gland; may require biopsy

   d. Blunting of the central sulcus

- Diagnostic Tests/Findings
    1. Urinalysis—typically normal; may be secondary indices of infection
    2. Urinary flow rate—voided volume and peak urinary flow rate (uroflowmetry) tests prostatic obstruction
    3. Abdominal ultrasound—rules out associated upper tract pathology
    4. Serum creatinine and BUN—normal
    5. Prostate-specific antigen (PSA) levels should be normal

- Management/Treatment
    1. Observation
    2. Urology consult required for pharmacologic, mechanical, or surgical treatments
    3. Pharmacologic—drugs selected that reduce bulk and/or tone of gland
        a. Alpha adrenergic antagonists
            (1) Terazosin—1 mg orally at bedtime, increase up to 10 mg at bedtime
            (2) Prazosin—1 mg orally b.i.d. to t.i.d.; increase up to 6–15 mg per day
            (3) Doxazosin—1 mg orally every day up to 16 mg if required
            (4) Tamsulosin—0.4 mg orally daily; alpha antagonist activity specific to prostate
        b. 5-alpha reductase inhibitors
            (1) Finasteride—5 mg orally daily
                (a) Pregnancy category X
                (b) Must not be handled by pregnant women or those trying to become pregnant
            (2) Dutasteride—0.5 mg orally daily
                (a) Same precautions for pregnant women as finasteride
                (b) Patients should not donate blood until > 6 months after last dose
        c. Dutasteride/tamsulosin combination (Jalyn)
            (1) Fixed dose combination of alpha blocker and 5-alpha reductase inhibitors
            (2) Same precautions as each medication individually
    4. Mechanical—balloon dilation of prostatic urethra
    5. Surgery—indications
        a. Acute urinary retention (urgent urology referral)
        b. Gross hematuria
        c. Epididymitis (especially if recurrent)
        d. Recurrent urinary tract infections
        e. Renal failure from obstruction
        f. Intolerable chronic symptoms
    6. Discuss therapeutic and diagnostic plans
    7. Educate regarding signs/symptoms of urinary retention, renal failure, and epididymitis

    8. Emphasize importance of follow-up appointments
    9. Avoid caffeine and alcohol to decrease bladder irritation
    10. Avoid decongestants, antihistamines, tricyclic antidepressants, anticholinergics

■ PROSTATE CANCER

- Definition—a malignant neoplasm of the prostate gland

- Etiology/Incidence
    1. Etiology is unknown; environmental factors may be involved; adenocarcinoma is most common type
    2. Most common malignancy in American men and second most common cause of cancer deaths in men over 65
    3. The relative survival rates have improved over the past 30 years (due to increased awareness and early detection, rather than improved therapy)
    4. May be associated with high-fat diet
    5. Risk factors—family history, age, African-American

- Signs and Symptoms
    1. Many patients are asymptomatic
    2. Symptoms may mimic BPH with frequency, dribbling, nocturia, hesitancy
    3. Occasionally bone pain from metastases (advanced stage)
    4. Occasionally symptoms of uremia due to urethral obstructions (advanced stage)

- Differential Diagnosis
    1. BPH, urethral stricture
    2. Bladder cancer
    3. Neurogenic bladder
    4. Bladder calculus
    5. Acute/chronic prostatitis
    6. Bladder neck contracture
    7. Medications that affect micturition

- Physical Findings
    1. May present with lymphadenopathy, signs of uremia, or urinary retention with distended bladder
    2. More common physical findings are confined to prostate—on rectal examination prostate feels harder than normal and normal boundaries of gland may be obscured; nodules may be present
    3. Prostate may have asymmetric enlargement

- Diagnostic Tests/Findings (performed by consultant physician)
    1. Transperineal or transrectal needle biopsy of prostate—diagnostic accuracy rate > 90%

2. PSA levels between 4 and 10 ng/mL may indicate BPH, levels > 10 ng/mL are suggestive of carcinoma; false negatives occur
3. Transrectal ultrasound can aid in identification of solid nodules and is used to guide biopsy
4. Other tests such as bone scans may be conducted

- Management/Treatment
  1. Consult/referral required
  2. Treatment predicated largely on stage of tumor; accurate staging is therefore essential
  3. Methods of treatment include surgery, radiation, hormonal therapy
  4. Assistance as appropriate in meeting physical, psychological, social, cultural, environmental, and spiritual needs
  5. Emphasize importance of follow-up appointments

◻ FIBROCYSTIC BREAST CHANGES

- Definition—benign breast condition characterized by increased growth of fibrous tissue, proliferation of the ductal epithelial lining, and/or formation of cysts

- Etiology/Incidence
  1. Cause is unknown, estrogen dependency is suspected; condition occurs clinically in 50% and histologically in 90% of women
  2. Three types of fibrocystic changes have been identified
     a. Nonproliferative lesions—most common type; no increased risk of breast cancer
     b. Proliferative lesions without atypia—minimal increased risk of breast cancer
     c. Cellular atypia—fivefold increased risk of breast cancer
  3. May be related to dietary intake of methylxanthines, e.g., coffee, chocolate (inconclusive)

- Signs and Symptoms (more pronounced premenstrually)
  1. Cyclic breast tenderness, engorgement, increased density, increased nodularity, enlargement of cystic lump(s)
  2. Nipple discharge may be present
  3. Symptoms of discomfort decrease after menopause

- Differential Diagnosis
  1. Fibroadenosis/Fibroadenoma
  2. Fat necrosis
  3. Carcinoma (especially in women > 40 years)
  4. Breast cysts

- Physical Findings
  1. Skin and contour usually normal
  2. Mass or thickened area present
     a. Location—upper outer quadrant or any area
     b. Size—varies
     c. Shape—round, oval, or nodular
     d. Mobility—mobile
     e. Consistency—soft to firm (depends on tension of fluid within cysts)
     f. Number—solitary or multiple (may give impression of "beads on a string")
     g. Nipple—clear/serous discharge may be present (rare)
     h. Signs and symptoms may fluctuate with the menstrual cycle

- Diagnostic Tests/Findings
  1. Fine needle aspiration (FNA)—fluid should return if cyst
  2. Excisional biopsy (most definitive test)—no cancer cells
  3. Mammography—negative (for women > 35 years)
  4. Ultrasound—distinguishes cyst vs. solid mass

- Management/Treatment
  1. Warm compresses applied t.i.d.; supportive brassiere
  2. Low-salt diet; diuretics may also be given premenstrually
  3. Elimination of dietary methylxanthines (coffee, tea, colas, chocolate) (inconclusive) and tobacco use
  4. Vitamin E—400–600 international units orally daily
  5. Vitamin B_6—50–100 mg daily
  6. Evening primrose oil 1,000 mg/day (Pizzomo & Murray, 1999)
  7. Hormonal and antihormonal therapy are controversial; the following agents may be used in severe cases
     a. Oral contraceptives—low estrogen with relatively high progesterone
     b. Danazol
     c. Bromocriptine
     d. Tamoxifen
  8. Surgical excision is controversial
  9. Discussion of diagnostic and therapeutic plans
  10. Reassurance of low risk for malignancy
  11. Instruction and demonstration of breast self-examination
  12. Encouragement to report any new mass that does not resolve following menstruation
  13. At follow-up, assess for progression of condition and/or concurrent malignancy

◘ BREAST CANCER

- Definition—a malignant neoplasm of the breast

- Etiology/Incidence
  1. Estimated that one in nine women in the United States will develop breast cancer if they live to be 90 years old
  2. Frequency increases steadily after age 35
  3. Whites have higher incidence than nonwhites in United States
  4. Approximately 182,000 new cases occur annually
  5. Most common cause of cancer in women and second most common cause of cancer death in women
  6. Risk factors include
     a. Increasing age
     b. Postmenopausal long-term estrogen therapy—conflicting data
     c. Nulliparity
     d. Late first pregnancy (over age 30)
     e. Early menarche and late menopause (after age 55)
     f. Cellular atypia
     g. Previous endometrial cancer
     h. Alcohol intake
     i. High-fat diet (polyunsaturated)
     j. Obesity
  7. Patients with higher risk
     a. Positive family history (premenopausal more significant)
     b. Family history suggestive of an inherited predisposition to breast cancer
     c. Confirmation of an inherited mutation ($BRCA_1$ or $BRCA_2$) on a breast cancer susceptibility gene
     d. Prior personal history of breast cancer
     e. Fibrocystic changes associated with cellular atypia

- Signs and Symptoms
  1. Often asymptomatic
  2. Single, firm, nontender, painless mass is usual presenting sign
  3. Later manifestations
     a. Skin erythema, dimpling, ulceration
     b. Breast pain
     c. Nipple retraction, eczema, or ulceration
     d. Nipple discharge

- Differential Diagnosis
  1. Fibrocystic breast changes
  2. Fibroadenoma
  3. Intraductal papilloma
  4. Lipoma
  5. Fat necrosis
  6. Mastitis
  7. Dermatitis (Paget's disease)

- Physical Findings
  1. Most common manifestation is single, firm, nontender, ill-defined lump in breast; associated findings may include
     a. Diffuse nodularity
     b. Skin dimpling
     c. Nipple retraction, discharge (usually bloody)
     d. Lymphadenopathy
     e. Ulcerated/fungating mass (rare)
     f. Palpable supraclavicular and/or axillary lymph nodes
  2. Inflammatory cancer—skin erythema/edema, pain
  3. Paget's disease
     a. Associated with about 5% of mammary carcinomas
     b. Nipple erosion, crusting, bloody discharge
     c. Eczema-like change in skin

- Diagnostic Tests/Findings
  1. Mammography—mass or calcifications indicated; may be negative since 10% of palpable masses are missed on mammogram
  2. Ultrasound—distinguishes cyst vs. solid mass
  3. FNA cytology—fluid vs. solid mass, 10% false negative
  4. Large-needle (core needle) biopsy—histological examination reveals cancer cells (problems with sampling occur)
  5. Excisional biopsy—most reliable diagnostic test where staging of the tumor is done
  6. Determination of hormone receptor tumor cells
  7. Various tests may be conducted if metastasis is suspected including bone and organ scans

- Management/Treatment
  1. Secondary prevention
     a. Clinical breast examination every 3 years to age 40
     b. Clinical breast examination annually over age 40
     c. Mammography annually beginning at age 40 or 10 years before the age of diagnosis in women with first-degree family history
  2. Tertiary prevention
     a. Referral to an oncology team is required
     b. Dependent upon tumor stage, presence of hormone receptors and patient's symptoms/preferences
     c. May include surgery, chemotherapy, radiation therapy, and/or hormonal therapy

3. Discussion of diagnostic and therapeutic plans
4. Encouragement to express concerns and fears
5. Education to patient and family members, especially daughters
6. Encouragement to report new mass or changes
7. Assistance, as appropriate, in meeting physical, psychological, sexual, social, cultural, environmental, and spiritual needs
8. Emphasis on importance of maintaining follow-up with specialists and primary care providers

◻ DYSFUNCTIONAL UTERINE BLEEDING (DUB)

- Definition—excessive, abnormal uterine bleeding, that occurs at irregular intervals, with no demonstrable organic cause

- Etiology/Incidence
  1. Usually results from irregular sloughing of endometrium during anovulatory cycles (90% of cases); but occasionally occurs with poor quality ovulatory cycles
  2. Most frequently due to abnormalities of endocrine function
  3. Estrogen withdrawal or estrogen breakthrough bleeding
  4. Progesterone breakthrough bleeding—continuous low-dose contraceptives
  5. Heaviest bleeding due to high sustained levels of estrogen and seen with
     a. Polycystic ovarian disease
     b. Obesity
     c. Immaturity of the hypothalamic-pituitary-ovarian axis (postmenarchal teenagers)
     d. Late ovulations (perimenopausal women)
     e. Unopposed estrogen replacement therapy
  6. Not related to oral contraceptive use

- Signs and Symptoms
  1. A carefully obtained history and character of bleeding pattern is critical to assist in ruling out other conditions
  2. Bleeding is usually characterized by one or more of the following
     a. Persistent or intermittent uterine bleeding
     b. Episodes of extremely heavy bleeding
     c. Oligomenorrhea
  3. DUB bleeding patterns
     a. Intermenstrual bleeding—variable amounts of bleeding that occur between regular menstrual periods
     b. Menometrorrhagia—prolonged, frequent, excessive uterine bleeding that occurs at irregular intervals
     c. Menorrhagia (hypermenorrhea)—prolonged (> 7 days) and excessive (> 80 mL) uterine bleeding occurring at regular intervals

d. Metrorrhagia—uterine bleeding between normal cycle
e. Polymenorrhea—frequent, irregular bleeding < 18 day intervals
f. Oligomenorrhea—infrequent, irregular uterine bleeding that occurs at intervals > 40 days

- Differential Diagnosis
  1. *Inappropriate* to assume that abnormal uterine bleeding is endocrine in origin; other conditions must be ruled out according to reproductive age
  2. Adolescents
     a. Vaginal trauma secondary to athletics or early sexual exposure
     b. Hypothalamic-pituitary dysfunction secondary to exercise
     c. Pregnancy
     d. Genital infection
     e. Oral contraceptive use/misuse
     f. Blood dyscrasias
  3. Women in reproductive years
     a. Previously noted causes
     b. Endocrine-related anovulatory abnormal uterine bleeding, common with exercise
     c. Organic pathology
        (1) Uterine fibroids
        (2) Endometrial polyps
        (3) Chronic systemic illness, e.g., liver cirrhosis, renal failure
     d. Neoplasia
     e. Secondary to stress
     f. Excessive weight change
  4. Perimenopausal women
     a. Previously listed causes
     b. Follicular dysfunction (predominant cause)
  5. Postmenopausal women
     a. Previously noted causes
     b. Hormone replacement therapy
     c. Cancer

- Physical Findings
  1. A thorough general and pelvic examination should be performed to assist in ruling out conditions included in the differential diagnosis; source of bleeding must be determined
  2. For DUB, the examination may be essentially negative, or an adnexal mass may indicate polycystic ovaries or other pathology

- Diagnostic Tests/Findings
  1. Of secondary importance and usually only substantiates a diagnosis already determined by history and physical examination findings
  2. Three most important initial tests
     a. Pregnancy test (quantitative beta hCG)
     b. Prolactin determination (hyperprolactinemia may initially present as ovulatory dysfunction or anovulation and abnormal

uterine bleeding)—may be elevated after breast examination

c. Thyroid stimulating hormone (TSH)
3. Additional initial tests should include
   a. Follicle stimulating hormone (FSH) and luteinizing hormone (LH)
   b. Complete blood count, blood smear, platelet count
   c. Cervical Pap smear
   d. STD screening tests
4. Additional tests may be done to rule out other conditions as indicated by the history and physical examination, such as
   a. Coagulation profile
   b. Serum iron studies if anemic
   c. Pelvic ultrasound
5. Tests more important in older women
   a. Endometrial biopsy
   b. D&C

- Management/Treatment
  1. Should be considered according to amount of blood loss and with an age-related perspective
  2. Physician consultation may be required
  3. Arrest of heavy, acute, or prolonged bleeding may require intravenous conjugated estrogens followed by combined oral contraceptives or medroxyprogesterone acetate to prevent recurrence
  4. Induction of ovulation is reserved for those desiring pregnancy (use of clomiphene citrate)
  5. Iron supplementation if indicated
  6. Patient should maintain a basal body temperature chart and record symptoms during cycles
  7. Provide instruction regarding basal body temperature monitoring
  8. Discuss therapeutic and diagnostic plans
  9. Review emergency instructions for acute, heavy bleeding
  10. Review nutritional requirements and encourage intake of iron-rich foods
  11. Encourage expression of concerns and fears
  12. Emphasize importance of maintaining follow-up

◘ ENDOMETRIOSIS

- Definition—presence of endometrial glands and stroma outside the endometrial cavity and uterine musculature

- Etiology/Incidence
  1. Etiology is unknown, theories include
     a. Familial tendency, sevenfold increase if first-degree female relative
     b. Alteration in the immune system
     c. Retrograde menstruation
     d. Metaplastic transformation of epithelium to endometrial tissue at extrapelvic sites
     e. Spread of endometrial tissue through lymphatic and vascular channels

2. Estimated to affect 5–20% of all women of reproductive age
3. Median age at diagnosis 29 years

- Signs and Symptoms
  1. Presence and severity of symptoms correlate poorly with degree of disease
  2. Pain (most common complaint)
     a. Cyclic pelvic pain due to blood and menstrual debris in surrounding tissues
     b. Constant pain with secondary dysmenorrhea
     c. Pelvic heaviness
     d. Chronic pelvic pain
  3. Dysmenorrhea, primary or secondary
  4. Dyspareunia from fixed uterine retroversion
  5. Infertility
  6. Menstrual irregularities, especially premenstrual spotting

- Differential Diagnosis
  1. Chronic pelvic inflammatory disease
  2. Pelvic adhesions
  3. Ovarian cyst or tumors

- Physical Findings
  1. Uterosacral ligament nodularity and/or tenderness
  2. Fixed uterine retroversion
  3. Adnexal enlargement and/or tenderness
  4. Endometrioma
  5. Tenderness in vaginal cul de sac or cervical motion tenderness

- Diagnostic Tests
  1. Visualization of disease by laparoscope gold standard "powder burn lesions"
  2. Ultrasound—detection of endometrioma (cannot be used as specific test of endometriosis)
  3. Cancer antigen-125 (CA-125)—chemical marker and noninvasive test; of limited value in following course of disease and response to treatment (Danforth, Scott, & Gibbs, 2008)

- Management/Treatment (since condition is chronic and recurrent, long-term integrative care is required)
  1. Medication
     a. Combined low-estrogen monophasic oral contraceptive pills taken continuously to produce amenorrhea
     b. Nonsteroidal anti-inflammatory medications for pain relief
     c. Medroxyprogesterone acetate (MPA)—30 mg orally daily causes atrophy of endometrial tissue
     d. Depot MPA—100–400 mg intramuscularly monthly causes atrophy of endometrial tissue

e. Danazol—200–400 mg orally twice a day creates anovulation and amenorrhea

f. GnRH agonists—leuprolide acetate 1 mg subcutaneously daily or 3.75 mg (depot) intramuscularly monthly or nafarelin acetate 200 μg intranasally twice a day creates anovulation and amenorrhea

g. Aromatase inhibitors being investigated as a new treatment

2. Surgery
   a. Ablation of endometrial implants via laser or electrocautery
   b. Hysterectomy with salpingo-oophorectomy is curative 90%

3. Optimal treatment depends on goal, pain relief, or fertility

4. Complications—infertility

☐ DYSPLASIA—ABNORMAL PAPANICOLAOU (PAP) SMEAR MANAGEMENT

• Definition—squamous intraepithelial lesions (SIL) refers to precancerous cellular development of the cervix (includes mild, moderate, and severe dysplasia) and carcinoma in situ (CIS) of the cervix

• Etiology/Incidence
  1. Etiology is most likely related to a sexually transmitted factor; the human papillomavirus (HPV) is suspected to be an initiator of malignant transformation
  2. Suspected HPV cofactors include cigarette smoking and folate deficiency
  3. Major risk factors for cervical cancer
     a. Sexual intercourse prior to age 18
     b. More than three sexual partners in a lifetime
     c. Intercourse with a male who has had multiple sexual partners
     d. Smoking or history of smoking
     e. Presence or history of HPV (types 16, 18, 31, 33, 35) more commonly associated with high-grade lesions—see section on Genital Warts (Condylomata acuminata)
     f. Intercourse with man who has HPV
  4. SIL may persist, spontaneously regress, or advance to invasive disease
  5. Globally, carcinoma of the cervix is a leading cause of death; in the United States it ranks as the third most common gynecological malignancy (behind endometrial and ovarian cancer)

• Cervical Cancer Screening
  1. The Papanicolaou (Pap) smear has reduced disease-related mortality in the United States by 50% in the past 40 years
  2. Screening has also increased detection of preinvasive cervical neoplasms including dysplasia and CIS

3. 30% of Pap smears may have false-negative results

4. Risk of invasive cervical cancer significantly increases when screening exceeds 3-year intervals

5. Recommended screening criteria (U.S. Preventive Service Task Force, 2004)
   a. Initiate at age 21 or within 3 years of onset of sexual activity
   b. Up to age 70 Pap smears should be repeated every 3 years depending in patients with normal Pap history and no increased risk factors
   c. After age 70 routine screening may be discontinued if findings are normal on three or more consecutive Pap smears and no abnormal/positive cytology tests occurred within the last 10 years
   d. Routine Pap smear screening in women who have had a total hysterectomy for benign disease is NOT recommended

• Pap smear interpretation—the Bethesda Classification System is most commonly used
  1. Specimen type—indicate conventional smear (Pap smear) vs. liquid-based preparation vs. other
  2. Specimen adequacy
     a. Satisfactory for evaluation—(describe presence or absence of endocervical/transformation zone component and any other quality indicators, e.g., partially obscuring blood, inflammation, etc.)
     b. Unsatisfactory for evaluation (specify reason)
        (1) Specimen rejected/not processed (specify reason)
        (2) Specimen processed and examined, but unsatisfactory for evaluation of epithelial abnormality because of (specify reason)
  3. Interpretation/Result
     a. Negative for intraepithelial lesion or malignancy—(when there is no cellular evidence of neoplasia); the presence of organisms or other non-neoplastic findings should be noted
        (1) Organisms
            (a) *T. vaginalis*
            (b) Fungal organisms morphologically consistent with *Candida* spp
            (c) Shift in flora suggestive of bacterial vaginosis
            (d) Bacteria morphologically consistent with *Actinomyces* spp
            (e) Cellular changes consistent with Herpes simplex virus
        (2) Other non-neoplastic findings (optional to report; list not inclusive)

(a) Reactive cellular changes associated with
  (i) Inflammation (includes typical repair)
  (ii) Radiation
  (iii) Intrauterine contraceptive device (IUD)
(b) Glandular cells status post-hysterectomy
(c) Atrophy

b. Endometrial cells (in a woman ≥ 40 years of age)—specify if negative for squamous intraepithelial lesion
c. Epithelial cell abnormalities
  (1) Squamous cell
    (a) Atypical squamous cells
      (i) Of undetermined significance (ASC-US)
      (ii) Cannot exclude HSIL (ASC-H)
    (b) Low-grade squamous intraepithelial lesion (LSIL) encompassing: HPV/mild dysplasia/CIN 1
    (c) High-grade squamous intraepithelial lesion (HSIL) encompassing: moderate and severe dysplasia, CIS; CIN 2 and CIN 3
      (i) With features suspicious for invasion (if invasion is suspected)
    (d) Squamous cell carcinoma
  (2) Glandular cell
    (a) Atypical
      (i) Endocervical cells, not otherwise specified (NOS) or specify in comments
      (ii) Endometrial cells, NOS or specify in comments
      (iii) Glandular cells, NOS or specify in comments
    (b) Atypical
      (i) Endocervical cells, favor neoplastic
      (ii) Glandular cells, favor neoplastic
    (c) Endocervical adenocarcinoma in situ
    (d) Adenocarcinoma
      (i) Endocervical
      (ii) Endometrial
      (iii) Extrauterine
      (iv) NOS
    (e) Other malignant neoplasms (specify)

4. Ancillary testing
5. Automated review

- Management of Pap smear results
  1. Within normal limits—repeat annually or as indicated according to cervical cancer risk factors and age

2. Infection
   a. Treat based on agent causing inflammation
   b. Repeat Pap smear in 1 year
3. Reactive or reparative changes
   a. Treat if infectious agent present
   b. May be related to contraceptive mechanical devices (IUD), atrophic changes, chemotherapy, and/or radiotherapy, etc.
   c. Repeat Pap in 4–6 months
4. Atypical squamous cells of undetermined significance (ASC-US)
   a. 10–40% risk of SIL and 5–10% of these are HSIL
   b. Repeat Pap smear every 4–6 months, three times
   c. Colposcopy and cervical biopsies with endocervical curettage (ECC) if HSIL develops or HIV positive
   d. If peri- or postmenopausal, treat with vaginal estrogen cream prior to repeat Pap or colposcopy (even if patient is on hormone therapy (HT)
5. Low- and high-grade SIL
   a. Colposcopy and cervical biopsies with ECC
   b. Low-grade lesions may be monitored with Pap smears every 6 months for 2 years if ECC is negative
   c. Common treatments include cryotherapy, large loop excision of transformation zone (LLETZ), laser vaporization
   d. Referral to physician specialist if carcinoma in situ present
6. Squamous cell carcinoma, adenocarcinoma, and other epithelial or nonepithelial malignant neoplasm—refer to physician specialist
7. Hormonal evaluation—treat atrophic changes if present (see Pregnancy, Contraception, and Menopause chapter)
8. Discuss therapeutic and diagnostic plans along with common complications of treatment
9. Emphasize importance of regular screening
10. Review patient's individual risk factors as appropriate
11. Educate regarding recommended management and treatment as appropriate
12. Encourage patient to discuss concerns and/or fears

❑ AMENORRHEA

- Definition
  1. Primary amenorrhea—absence of normal spontaneous menstrual period by age 16
  2. Secondary amenorrhea—cessation of menses after a variable period of normal function, usually 3–6 consecutive cycles

- Etiology—potential underlying conditions
  1. Primary amenorrhea
     a. Hypergonadotropic hypogonadism
     b. Turner syndrome (gonadal dysgenesis)

    c. Severe malnutrition

    d. Pituitary tumors

    e. Head trauma

    f. Encephalitis

    g. Uterine malformations, congenital absence of uterus

    h. Imperforate hymen, cervical stenosis

    i. Androgen insensitivity

    j. Polycystic ovaries

2. Secondary amenorrhea

    a. Pregnancy (most common cause)

    b. Oral contraceptives

    c. Menopause

    d. Emotional stress

    e. Malnutrition

    f. Excessive exercise

    g. Lactation

    h. Hyperprolactinemia (pituitary tumor)

    i. Anorexia/obesity

    j. Drug use

    k. Polycystic ovaries, anovulation

    l. Hypothalamic suppression

    m. Hyper- and hypothyroidism

    n. Addison's disease

    o. Cervical stenosis

- Signs and Symptoms
  1. Primary amenorrhea
     a. Absence of menarche
     b. Failure to develop pubic hair and other secondary sex characteristics may or may not occur
     c. Abnormal growth and development may be present
     d. Normal breast development may or may not occur
     e. Patient symptoms are dependent upon the etiology of the amenorrheic condition
  2. Secondary amenorrhea
     a. Absence of menses at expected time intervals
     b. Previous regular menses

- Differential Diagnosis
  1. First rule out pregnancy
  2. All the potential underlying conditions listed under etiology should be considered in the differential diagnosis
  3. A thorough and complete history/physical examination, with supplemental diagnostic/laboratory testing will assist in ruling out unrelated etiologies

- Physical Findings
  1. A thorough general and pelvic examination should be performed, partially directed by the history

  2. Findings will be related to the underlying etiology
  3. The examination may be essentially negative if the amenorrhea is secondary to such conditions as oral contraceptive use or unreported emotional stress

- Diagnostic Tests/Findings
  1. Primary amenorrhea—refer to endocrinologist if suspected
  2. Secondary amenorrhea
     a. Pregnancy test (quantitative beta hCG)—initial test
     b. Prolactin (if negative pregnancy test), FSH, LH
        (1) Elevated prolactin—rule out micro- and macroadenomas with CT scan of sella turcica
        (2) Physician consult may be required if prolactin, FSH, or LH elevated
     c. Progestin challenge test
     d. TSH
        (1) Elevated TSH—hypothyroid
        (2) Normal TSH—rule out pituitary adenoma
     e. Cervical Pap smear
     f. STD screening tests
     g. Urinalysis
  3. Additional tests may be done to rule out other conditions as indicated by the history and physical examination

- Management/Treatment
  1. Dependent upon underlying etiology
  2. Medical consult is often required
  3. Discuss therapeutic and diagnostic plans
  4. Encourage expression of concerns and fears
  5. Emphasize importance of maintaining follow-up

◘ DYSMENORRHEA

- Definition—crampy pain that occurs prior to or during menses, often with a constellation of other symptoms
  1. Primary—usually begins in women under 20 years; related to menses with no other organic cause
  2. Secondary—usually occurs after age 20 in women with pelvic pathology or IUD use

- Etiology/Incidence
  1. Primary—probably the result of excessive uterine prostaglandin production; usually appears shortly after onset of ovulatory cycles; affects approximately 50% or more of all menstruating females
  2. Secondary—usually occurs in the presence of organic disease, e.g., endometriosis, pelvic

adhesions, adenomyosis, cervical stenosis, uterine fibroids, chronic pelvic infection, or with the use of an IUD

- Signs and Symptoms
  1. Primary
     a. Pain usually crampy in nature, may radiate to back, thighs, and lower abdomen
     b. May also have other symptoms, e.g., nausea, vomiting, diarrhea, headache, fatigue
     c. Usually begins at onset of menstruation or several hours before; duration is usually 48–72 hours
  2. Secondary
     a. Signs and symptoms associated with organic disease listed under Etiology/Incidence
     b. Pain occurs at any point in cycle
     c. Associated symptoms may include dyspareunia, infertility, and abnormal bleeding

- Differential Diagnosis
  1. Differentiation between primary and secondary dysmenorrhea
  2. Rule out secondary pathologic conditions as noted under Etiology/Incidence

- Physical Findings
  1. Primary—usually no significant physical findings; uterine corpus may be tender during menstruation; no pelvic masses or uterine fixation
  2. Secondary—findings associated with organic disease

- Diagnostic Tests/Findings
  1. Primary—usually none, but if diagnosis unclear, CBC, erythrocyte sedimentation rate and genital culture for pathogens
  2. Secondary—tests related to suspected organic pathology; may include pelvic ultrasound, hysterosalpingogram, laparoscopy, hysteroscopy, or dilatation and curettage

- Management/Treatment
  1. Primary
     a. Prostaglandin synthetase inhibitors (PGSI), e.g., naproxen, indomethacin, mefenamic acid, ibuprofen
     b. Oral contraceptives for sexually active individuals
     c. Moderate exercise on a regular basis
     d. Diet high in whole grains, beans, vegetables, fruit
     e. Elimination of or decreased salt, sugar, caffeine
     f. Alternative therapies that have been shown to be more effective than placebo are omega-3 fatty acids, thiamine (B_1), magnesium supplements, and vitamin E
  2. Secondary—treatment related to organic pathology

☐ PREMENSTRUAL SYNDROME (PMS)

- Definition—a group of somatic and affective symptoms occurring during the luteal phase of the menstrual cycle, decreasing shortly after onset of menstruation

- Etiology/Incidence
  1. Exact cause unknown
  2. Postulated etiologic factors include insufficient progesterone, fluid retention, nutritional problems, glucose metabolism disorders, vitamin deficiencies, ovarian infections, altered serotonin, endorphin levels, elevated prolactin levels
  3. Peak prevalence in the thirties with a decline noted in the forties
  4. Incidence ranges from 5–95%; generally agreed about 40% of women are significantly affected at one time or another; only 2–3% of women of childbearing age suffer severe symptoms
  5. Premenstrual dysphoria may be considered a severe subtype of PMS
  6. Most women experience some physical and emotional changes before onset of menstrual flow

- Signs and Symptoms
  1. Bloated feeling, feeling of weight increase
  2. Breast pain or tenderness
  3. Skin disorders
  4. Hot flashes
  5. Headache
  6. Pelvic pain
  7. Change in bowel habits
  8. Irritability, aggression, tension, anxiety, depression, crying, lethargy
  9. Insomnia, fatigue
  10. Change in appetite, thirst
  11. Change in libido
  12. Loss of concentration
  13. Poor coordination, clumsiness, accidents

- Differential Diagnosis
  1. Depression
  2. Anxiety disorders
  3. Marital discord
  4. Substance abuse
  5. Thyroid disease
  6. Impaired glucose tolerance or diabetes
  7. Early menopause
  8. Dysmenorrhea

9. Endometriosis
10. Anemia
11. Polycystic ovaries

- Physical Findings
  1. Because etiology is still unknown, diagnosis is made by history
  2. Complete history and physical examination should be conducted to rule out any medical problems that could be influencing symptomatology

- Diagnostic Tests/Findings
  1. Thyroid profile
  2. Fasting blood sugar, HgbA$_{1c}$
  3. FSH, LH (if early menopause suspected)
  4. CBC with differential
  5. Complete metabolic panel

- Management/Treatment
  1. Exercise 3–4 times per week, especially during luteal phase
  2. Appropriate diet with reasonable amounts of protein (from fish and poultry rather than red meats), vegetables, and fruit
  3. Elimination of tobacco, alcohol, caffeine
  4. Pyridoxine, multiple vitamins
  5. Diuretics, if fluid retention predominates
  6. Progesterone is controversial; in several studies no more effective than placebo
  7. Prostaglandin inhibitors, e.g., mefenamic acid, naproxen sodium
  8. Oral contraceptives
  9. Danazol
  10. Bromocriptine for mastalgia
  11. PMS support group referral
  12. Selective serotonin reuptake inhibitors (SSRIs) for severe cases

◘ QUESTIONS

Select the best answer.

1. Which of the following statements regarding HIV/AIDS is correct?

   a. The greatest increase in cases is in those 15–24 years old
   b. Close to 4 million people in the United States are infected
   c. 21% of cases are undiagnosed
   d. The Western blot is a screening test

2. During the acute phase of HIV infection (first 2–8 weeks), which of the following symptoms may be present?

   a. Rash
   b. Shingles
   c. Oral candida
   d. Pulmonary symptoms

3. Which of the following is not considered in a new HIV treatment program?

   a. NRTIs
   b. Protease inhibitors
   c. Nutritious diet and stress management
   d. Integrase inhibitors

4. Secondary prevention of AIDS includes:

   a. Condom use
   b. Virologic monitoring every 3–6 months
   c. Educating about safe sex practices
   d. ELISA assessment of men who have sex with men

5. Which of the following is a diagnostic test for gonorrhea?

   a. Western blot assay
   b. VDRL
   c. Wet prep with WBC
   d. Culture of endocervix on Thayer-Martin media

6. Which of the following is not a correct statement regarding *Neisseria gonorrhoeae*?

   a. One of the leading causes of infertility among U.S. females
   b. The majority of male patients are asymptomatic
   c. PID is a possible complication
   d. In most cases it is confined to the genitorurinary tract

7. You are evaluating a male patient who is concerned because he has developed a profound purulent penile discharge. He admits to unprotected casual sex. His symptom is most consistent with:

   a. Chlamydia
   b. Epididymitis
   c. Gonorrhea
   d. Prostatitis

8. The most common serious gonococcal complication that occurs in women is:

   a. PID
   b. Cervicitis
   c. Arthritis
   d. Conjunctivitis

9. Patients with gonorrhea should also be treated for:

   a. Chlamydia
   b. Syphilis
   c. Trichomonas
   d. Herpes

10. The causative organism of chlamydia is:

    a. *Chlamydia coli*
    b. *Chlamydia megalovirus*
    c. *Chlamydia trachomatis*
    d. *Chlamydia hominos*

11. A 20-year-old female presents to your clinic with dysuria, dyspareunia, mucopurulent discharge. She reports that her boyfriend was recently treated for nongonococcal urethritis. What STD has she most likely been exposed to?

    a. Gonorrhea
    b. HPV
    c. Chlamydia
    d. Trichomonas

12. Which of the following represents the best description of chlamydia in women?

    a. It is the third most common bacterial STD
    b. It is frequently asymptomatic
    c. It is characterized by "strawberry spots" on the cervix
    d. Coinfection with HPV is common

13. Which of the following is true with respect to syphilis?

    a. It can affect every body system
    b. Over 350,000 cases are diagnosed annually
    c. Treatment with fluoroquinolones is no longer recommended due to resistance
    d. It is frequently asymptomatic in the early stages

14. Which of the following is not a characteristic of secondary syphilis?

    a. Skin rash
    b. Arthralgias
    c. Chancre
    d. Malaise

15. The treatment of choice for a 32-year-old male with early syphilis who is allergic to penicillin is:

    a. Ciprofloxacin
    b. Doxycycline
    c. Erythromycin
    d. Amoxicillin/clavulanate

16. During laboratory assessment, syphilis is characterized by:

    a. A fishy odor with KOH testing
    b. > 20 clue cells/HPF
    c. The presence of multinucleated cells
    d. Treponemes on darkfield microscopy

17. Which of the following is a confirmatory test for syphilis?

    a. VDRL
    b. FTA-Abs
    c. STS
    d. RPR

18. A 24-year-old female seen in your clinic has been diagnosed with urethral strictures. What STD is probably included in her past history?

    a. Chlamydia
    b. Herpes genitalis
    c. Syphilis
    d. HPV

19. Which of the following statements regarding herpes genitalis is not true?

    a. Causative agent is a virus
    b. Genital lesions are painless
    c. Infection during pregnancy can lead to spontaneous abortion
    d. Treatment focuses on relieving symptoms

20. The most common symptomatic viral STD in the United States is:

    a. Gonorrhea
    b. Chlamydia
    c. Genital warts (HPV)
    d. Herpes genitalis

21. Which of the following statements regarding genital warts is incorrect?

    a. More than 40 types of HPV cause genital warts
    b. They increase risk of developing cervical, penile, and vulvar cancer
    c. There is a vaccine available
    d. RPR aids in diagnosing cervical lesions

22. PID is typically characterized by cervical wall motion tenderness, adnexal tenderness, and:

    a. Hypotension
    b. Grouped vesicles on an erythematous base
    c. Solitary papules, macules, or pustules
    d. Lower abdominal discomfort

23. Which of the following is the best treatment regimen for PID?

    a. Ciprofloxacin 500 mg p.o. b.i.d. for 10 days with or without metronidazole
    b. Augmentin 875 mg p.o. b.i.d. for 14 days with azithromycin 1 gm, single dose
    c. TMP/SMX DS tab p.o. b.i.d. for 14 days
    d. Ceftriaxone 250 mg IM with doxycycline 100 mg b.i.d. for 14 days

24. Which of the following is not considered an STD?

    a. Chlamydia
    b. Trichomoniasis
    c. Bacterial vaginitis
    d. Epididymitis

25. A 22-year-old female seen in your clinic has the following signs and symptoms—malodorous, greenish discharge, perineal itching, red macular cervical lesions, and a vaginal pH of 5.0–7.0. What type of vulvovaginitis does she probably have?

    a. Candidiasis
    b. Gardnerella
    c. Bacterial vaginosis
    d. Trichomoniasis

26. Which of the following is not related to bacterial vaginosis?

    a. Multiple bacterial causative agents
    b. "Curdy" white discharge
    c. Positive "whiff test"
    d. Metronidazole is a treatment of choice

27. A classic description of the discharge associated with candida vaginitis is:

    a. "Cottage-cheese"
    b. "Fishy" odor
    c. Green, frothy
    d. Nonpruritic

28. One of the most common causative organisms of UTI in women is:

    a. Klebsiella
    b. Beta-hemolytic streptococci
    c. Chlamydia
    d. *E. coli*

29. Patient education for the patient with urinary tract infection should include all of the following except:

    a. Reminders to empty the bladder frequently
    b. Counseling that the course of antibiotic therapy must be completed
    c. Instruction to increase intake of grapefruit juice
    d. Information about proper perineal wiping

30. Which of the following is not a characteristic sign or symptom associated with a UTI?

    a. Fever
    b. Pyuria
    c. Urgency
    d. Negative CVA tenderness

31. Which of the following activities is contraindicated in a patient with suspected acute bacterial prostatitis?

    a. Ejaculation
    b. Urinary catheterization
    c. Prostate examination
    d. Masturbation

32. The drug of choice for a 40-year-old, monogamous male with prostatitis is:

    a. Metronidazole
    b. Doxycycline
    c. TMP/SMX
    d. Carbenicillin

33. Assessment of BPH may typically include all of the following except:

    a. Symmetrical enlargement
    b. A prostate the consistency of firm rubber
    c. Obliteration of the central sulcus
    d. Fever

34. Which of the following is a true statement about prostate cancer?

    a. It may be present with hard nodules
    b. A PSA of > 10 ng/dL is diagnostic
    c. It is the third leading cause of cancer in men
    d. Men of Western European descent are at greatest risk

35. What is the most common physical finding associated with prostate cancer?

    a. Boggy prostate
    b. Tender prostate
    c. Enlarged, smooth prostate
    d. Hard, nodular prostate

36. When counseling a patient with suspected prostate cancer, the NP should advise the patient that:

    a. He will likely need a needle biopsy of the prostate for diagnosis
    b. Incontinence is a likely consequence of most treatment options
    c. He should refrain from sexual activity until the diagnosis is confirmed
    d. He may need to take alpha-adrenergic antagonists as an adjunct to treatment

37. The type of fibrocystic breast change that has been associated with malignancy is:

    a. Proliferative changes without atypia
    b. Nonproliferative changes
    c. Cellular atypia
    d. Dysplasia

38. Which physical change is not consistent with fibrocystic breast disease?

    a. Strand of pearls to palpation
    b. A tender lump
    c. Enlarged skin pores
    d. Symptoms that are exacerbated during the menstrual cycle

39. A 30-year-old woman is diagnosed with fibrocystic breast changes in your office. All of the following components may be included in the treatment plan except:

    a. Yearly mammograms starting now
    b. Low-salt diet
    c. Limited consumption of caffeine
    d. Oral contraceptives

40. All of the following are risk factors for breast cancer except:

    a. First-degree family history
    b. Late onset of menarche
    c. Increasing age
    d. Obesity

41. Primary prevention of breast cancer includes:

    a. Mammography beginning at age 40
    b. Clinical breast exam every 3 years until age 40
    c. Self-breast exam monthly
    d. Weight loss for obese women

42. Which description is most characteristic of breast cancer?

    a. Single, firm, nontender, ill-defined breast lump
    b. Multiple, firm, nontender, ill-defined breast lumps
    c. Single, firm, tender, circumscribed breast lump
    d. Single, rubbery, nontender, circumscribed breast lump

43. Which of the following is not true with respect to breast cancer?

    a. 10% of palpable masses are missed on mammography
    b. Core needle biopsy is the most reliable diagnostic test
    c. Paget's disease affects the nipple
    d. Inflammatory breast cancer may be painful

44. Dysfunctional uterine bleeding is most often caused by:

    a. Polycystic ovaries
    b. Low estrogen levels
    c. An endocrine abnormality
    d. Low body fat content

45. Menorrhagia refers to:

    a. Uterine bleeding that occurs at regular intervals < 21 days apart
    b. Prolonged and excessive uterine bleeding occurring at regular intervals
    c. Infrequent uterine bleeding that occurs at intervals > 40 days apart
    d. Uterine bleeding that occurs at irregular but frequent intervals

46. Differential diagnosis of dysfunctional uterine bleeding for a perimenopausal woman includes all of the following except:

    a. Neoplasia
    b. Blood dyscrasias
    c. Pregnancy
    d. Vaginal trauma

47. The diagnostic evaluation of primary amenorrhea should include:

    a. Assessment for Turner syndrome
    b. Serum prolactin
    c. Abdominal ultrasound
    d. Endometrial biopsy

48. The most common cause of secondary amenorrhea is:

    a. Oral contraceptives
    b. Polycystic ovaries
    c. Pregnancy
    d. Anovulation

49. What is the first test that should be ordered in a woman who presents with secondary amenorrhea?

    a. Thyroid profile
    b. Prolactin
    c. Pregnancy test
    d. Progestin challenge

50. Who among the following is not a candidate for Gardasil vaccination?

    a. A 14-year-old female who has had HPV diagnosed on Pap screening
    b. A 27-year-old woman who has never been sexually active
    c. An 11-year-old female who has a family history of cervical cancer
    d. A 24-year-old woman who has had a low-grade SIL

51. Medical treatment options for endometriosis include:

    a. DES
    b. Triphasic oral contraceptives
    c. Methyltestosterone
    d. Medroxyprogesterone acetate

52. Endometriosis:

    a. Is the development and deposition of endometrial tissue in the myometrium
    b. Is not a significant factor in infertility
    c. Is common in postmenopausal women
    d. Is a common cause of pelvic pain

Answers

1. **c**	27. **a**
2. **a**	28. **d**
3. **d**	29. **c**
4. **d**	30. **a**
5. **d**	31. **b**
6. **b**	32. **c**
7. **c**	33. **d**
8. **a**	34. **a**
9. **a**	35. **d**
10. **c**	36. **a**
11. **c**	37. **c**
12. **b**	38. **c**
13. **a**	39. **a**
14. **c**	40. **b**
15. **b**	41. **d**
16. **d**	42. **a**
17. **b**	43. **b**
18. **b**	44. **c**
19. **b**	45. **b**
20. **c**	46. **d**
21. **d**	47. **a**
22. **d**	48. **c**
23. **d**	49. **c**
24. **c**	50. **b**
25. **d**	51. **d**
26. **b**	52. **d**

◘ BIBLIOGRAPHY

ACOG. (2006). ACOG Practice Bulletin: Clinical management guidelines for obstetrician-gynecologists, Number 72, May 2006. Vaginitis. *Obstetrics & Gynecology, 107*(5), 1195–1206.

Branson, B. M. (2003). *Rapid HIV testing: 2003 update.* Atlanta, GA: Centers for Disease Control and Prevention.

Centers for Disease Control and Prevention (CDC). (2007). Sexually Transmitted Disease Surveillance. Atlanta, GA.

U.S. Department of Health and Human Services, Centers for Disease Control and Prevention (CDC). (2006). HIV prevalence estimates—United States, 2006. *Morbidity and Morality Weekly Report, 57*(39), 1073–1076.

Centers for Disease Control and Prevention (CDC). (2008). HPV vaccine information for clinicians. Retrieved from http://www.cdc.gov/std/HPV/STDFact-HPV-vaccine-hcp.htm

Cunha, B. A. (2007). *Urinary tract infection: Females.* Retrieved from http://www.emedicine.com/med/TOPIC2835.htm

Danforth, D. N., Scott, J. R., & Gibbs, R. S. (Eds.). (2008). *Danforth's obstetrics and gynecology* (10th ed.). Philadelphia: Lippincott William & Wilkins.

Hall, H. I., Ruiguang, S., Rhodes, P., Prejean, J., Qian, A., Lee, L. M., Janssen, R. S. (2008). Estimation of HIV incidence in the United States. *Journal of the American Medical Association, 300,* 520–529.

Harris, J. R., Lippman, M. E., & Morrow, M. (Eds.). (2004). *Diseases of the breast.* Philadelphia: Lippincott Williams & Wilkins.

McClain, R., & Gray, M. L. (2002). A prostate cancer primer. *The Clinical Advisor, 5*(3), 37–38, 41, 44–47, 49.

McPhee, S. J., Papadakis, M. A., & Rabow, M.W. (Eds.). (2012). *Current medical diagnosis and treatment* (51st ed.). New York: McGraw-Hill.

Murray, M. T., & Pizzorno. J. (1999). *Textbook of Natural Medicine* (2nd ed.). London, England: Churchill Livingstone.

Panel on Antiretroviral Guidelines for Adults and Adolescents. Guidelines for the use of antiretroviral agents in HIV-1-infected adults and adolescents. Department of Health and Human Services. January 10, 2011, 1–166. Retrieved from http://www.aidsinfo.nih.gov/ContentFiles/AdultandAdolescentGL.pdf

Rakel, R. E., & Bope, E. T. (Eds.). (2004). *Conn's current therapy 2004.* Philadelphia: Saunders, The Curtis Center.

Solomon, D., Davey, D., Korman, R. Moriarty, A., O'Connor, D., Prey, M...Young, N. (2002). The 2001 Bethesda System: Terminology for reporting results of cervical cytology. *JAMA, 16*(287), 2114.

U.S. Preventive Services Task Force. (2007). *The guide to clinical preventive services: Recommendations of the United States Preventive Services Task Force.* Retrieved from http://www.ahrq.gov/clinic/pocketgd.htm

Wein, A.J., Kavoussi, L. R., Novick, A. C., Partin, A. W., & Peters, C. A. (Eds.). (2011). *Campbell's urology* (10th ed.). Philadelphia: W. B. Saunders.

11

Pregnancy, Contraception, and Menopause

Beth M. Kelsey

Susan B. Moskosky

◘ PREGNANCY

- Definition—the condition of having a developing embryo or fetus within the female body (usually within the uterus)

- Incidence
  1. Birth rate, or number of live births per 1,000 estimated population, in the United States for 2009 was 13.5
  2. Birth rate for teenagers during 2009 was 41.5 per 1,000 females aged 15–19 years
  3. Fertility rate, or number of live births per 1,000 females of childbearing age (15–44 years), for 2002 was 68.6

- Preconception Care
  1. Goals
     a. Assistance in preventing unintended pregnancies
     b. Identification of risk factors that could affect reproductive outcomes
     c. Identification and management of medical conditions that could be affected by pregnancy or could affect reproductive outcomes, e.g., diabetes
     d. Initiation of education and desired preventive interventions prior to conception
  2. Timing of preconception care—integrate into well-patient visits for all reproductive-age women

  3. Components of preconception care
     a. Assessment—family history, medical/surgical history, infectious disease history, obstetric history, environmental history, cultural health beliefs/practices, psychosocial history including violence, nutrition assessment, paternal health history
     b. Education/counseling and interventions
        (1) Health promotion/disease prevention/risk reduction
           (a) Rubella, varicella, and hepatitis B vaccinations if needed
           (b) Nutrition counseling for weight loss or gain as needed
           (c) Smoking cessation
           (d) Discontinuation of alcohol use
           (e) Treatment for substance abuse/addiction
           (f) Limit environmental/occupational exposures that may be teratogenic
           (g) Folic acid supplementation
           (h) Optimal glucose control for diabetics
           (i) Dietary management for phenylketonuria
           (j) Sexually transmitted disease (STD) testing and treatment as indicated
           (k) HIV counseling and testing as indicated
           (l) Medication changes as needed to avoid teratogens such as oral

hypoglycemics and some antiseizure medications
- (2) Resources/referrals
  - (a) Genetic testing and counseling as indicated—repeated spontaneous abortions, ethnic background that is high risk for autosomal recessive disorder, previous infant with congenital anomaly, age 35 or older
  - (b) Dietary counseling
  - (c) Substance abuse treatment
  - (d) Domestic violence resources

- Early Diagnosis of Pregnancy Is Essential
  1. Begin prenatal care; physical examination; laboratory tests; risk assessment; discontinue use of tobacco, alcohol, street drugs, and/or teratogenic medications; provide educational materials
  2. If pregnancy is unintended, make timely decision regarding pregnancy options (e.g., continuation, termination, adoption)

- Signs and Symptoms of Pregnancy
  1. Presumptive—subjective; frequently reported with pregnancy, but not conclusive for pregnancy
     a. Nausea with or without vomiting
     b. Urinary frequency
     c. Fatigue
     d. Perception of fetal movement by mother (quickening); with pregnancy, usually occurs 16–20 weeks
     e. Amenorrhea
     f. Breast changes
     g. Vaginal mucosa discoloration (Chadwick's sign)
     h. Increased skin pigmentation and abdominal striae
  2. Probable—more objective; often noted on physical examination or with laboratory testing
     a. Enlargement of abdomen and uterus
     b. Uterine changes in size, shape, consistency; softening of lower uterine segment at 6–8 weeks gestation (Hegar's sign)
     c. Softening of cervix at 6–8 weeks gestation (Goodell's sign)
     d. Braxton-Hicks contractions—often present by fourth month
     e. Ballottement—fetus can be pushed against the mother's abdomen and felt to bounce back against an examining finger in the vagina
     f. Outlining of fetus by examiner
     g. Pregnancy tests—detect human chorionic gonadotropin (hCG) in maternal blood or urine

  3. Positive—noted with absolute confirmation of pregnancy
     a. Detection of fetal heartbeat—auscultation with fetoscope at 17–20 weeks gestation; auscultation with doppler by 10–12 weeks gestation
     b. Palpation of fetal movement by examiner
     c. Visualization of fetus by ultrasonography

- Differential Diagnosis
  1. Myomas, hematometra, adenomyosis
  2. Ovarian tumor or extrauterine mass
  3. Amenorrhea/irregular menses of other origin
  4. Gastrointestinal problem
  5. Gestational trophoblastic disease

- Physiologic Changes (Maternal)
  1. Cardiovascular/respiratory
     a. Blood volume increased by 30–50% at term
     b. Increased cardiac output
     c. Heart displaced by uterus upward and to left
     d. Pulse rate increased by 10–15 beats per minute
     e. Dependent edema of feet and hands by third trimester
     f. Exaggerated heart sounds; functional systolic murmurs common
     g. Physiologic anemia common due to unequal expansion of red cell volume (30%) and plasma volume (50%)
     h. Physiological dyspnea may occur during pregnancy due to increased tidal volume that slightly lowers blood P_{CO_2}
  2. Gastrointestinal
     a. Decreased smooth muscle tone and decreased motility due to progesterone resulting in
        (1) Decreased intestinal peristalsis, which may lead to constipation
        (2) Gastric reflux and heartburn
        (3) Increased risk for gallstones
     b. Hemorrhoids are common during pregnancy; caused by constipation and elevated pressure in veins below the level of the enlarged uterus
     c. Hypertrophy and bleeding of gums possibly due to estrogen
  3. Musculoskeletal
     a. Progesterone-induced relaxation of pelvic structures and joints (may cause discomfort)
     b. Center of gravity shifts causing lordosis and posture changes; lower back pain common; waddling gait develops
     c. Diastasis recti possible (separation of rectus abdominis muscles)

4. Integumentary
   a. Cutaneous vascular changes—spider angiomas, palmar erythema
   b. Increased pigmentation of face (chloasma), areolae, abdomen (linea nigra), and genitalia
   c. Striae gravidarum
   d. Increased sebaceous and sweat gland activity
5. Endocrine
   a. Diffuse thyroid gland enlargement
   b. Insulin resistance increases due to action of human placental lactogen (hPL)
6. Breasts
   a. Early tenderness and tingling
   b. Increase in size and nodularity; striae may develop
   c. Veins prominent
   d. Nipples erectile; areolae darken
   e. Montgomery follicles hypertrophy
   f. Colostrum after first few months
7. Genitalia/reproductive
   a. External genitalia
      (1) Increased pigmentation
      (2) Pelvic congestion; swelling of labia majora near term
      (3) Vulvar varicosities possible
   b. Vagina
      (1) Increased vascularity causing bluish/purple color (Chadwick's sign)
      (2) Rugations of vaginal mucosa prominent
      (3) Increased secretions (leukorrhea)
   c. Cervix
      (1) Pronounced softening and cyanosis (early)
      (2) Proliferation of endocervical glands
      (3) Mucus plug blocks endocervical canal
   d. Musculature—broad ligament softening
   e. Uterus
      (1) Increases in size and weight
      (2) Softening of lower uterine segment (Hegar's sign)
      (3) Blood supply increased
   f. Ovaries
      (1) Anovulation secondary to hormonal interruption of feedback loop
      (2) Corpus luteum—continues for first 10–12 weeks of pregnancy; produces progesterone until placenta develops
   g. Urinary
      (1) Dilation of ureters and kidneys (especially on right), decreased bladder tone—increased risk for urinary stasis and infection
      (2) Urinary frequency common early and late in pregnancy
      (3) Incontinence may occur, particularly with multiparity

- Prenatal Care
1. Initial visit
   a. Laboratory confirmation of pregnancy—urine and serum tests available, all test for hCG
      (1) Agglutination inhibition test—urine test, reliable 14–21 days postconception
      (2) Enzyme-linked immunosorbent assay (ELISA); immunometric test (urine or serum) reliable 7–10 days postconception
      (3) Beta subunit radioimmunoassay (RIA)—serum test, reliable 7 days postconception
   b. Expected date of birth (EDB), expected date of delivery (EDD)—Naegele's rule subtract 3 months from last normal menstrual period (LNMP) and add 7 days; duration of human gestation is 266 days
   c. History—emphasize factors that may affect maternal or fetal outcome
      (1) Menstrual history—extremely important for estimating gestational age
      (2) Sexual history
      (3) Contraceptive history
      (4) Maternal history—attention to acute or chronic health problems
      (5) Family history—multiple gestation, congenital anomalies, inherited diseases, maternal family history of diabetes or hypertension
      (6) Medication history—including OTC and herbal supplements
      (7) Immunizations
      (8) Substance use—tobacco, alcohol, recreational, prescription, or herbal drugs
      (9) Exposure to environmental or occupational toxins or hazards
      (10) History of or current domestic violence
      (11) Risk factors for HIV and other STDs, hepatitis B
      (12) Dietary habits
      (13) Ethnic background
      (14) Reproductive/obstetric history
         (a) Each previous pregnancy including outcome—e.g., **T**erm birth, **P**reterm birth, **A**bortion (spontaneous or induced), and number of **L**iving children (T-P-A-L)
         (b) Complications during previous pregnancy/delivery/postpartum—e.g., gestational diabetes, pregnancy induced hypertension (PIH), preterm labor (PTL) and/or preterm birth, postpartum hemorrhage, postpartum depression

(c) Previous pregnancy loss including gestational age and related factors

(d) Method of delivery for previous pregnancies—vaginal or cesarean

d. Physical examination

(1) Vital signs and complete head-to-toe examination—attention to any preexisting medical conditions

(2) Assess uterine size to confirm pregnancy and determine gestational age—most accurately assessed by bimanual examination up to 14 weeks

(a) 8 weeks—approximately 9 cm

(b) 10 weeks—approximately 10 cm

(c) 12 weeks—uterine fundus at symphysis pubis

(d) 16 weeks—fundus midway between symphysis pubis and umbilicus

(e) 20 weeks—fundus at umbilicus

(f) 20 weeks to term—abdominal measurement of fundal height

(i) Measure from top of symphysis pubis to top of uterine fundus

(ii) Between 18 and 32 weeks gestation, good correlation between gestational age in weeks and measurement of fundal height in centimeters

(3) Evaluate pelvic dimensions (pelvimetry)

(4) Obtain Pap smear and cervical cultures

(5) Auscultation of fetal heart by doppler (usually audible by 10–12 weeks with doppler) or fetoscope (usually audible by 17–20 weeks)

e. Laboratory testing (routine)

(1) ABO blood group/Rh factor determination

(2) Complete blood count (CBC)

(3) Antibody screen and titer

(4) Rubella titer—titer of > 1:10 indicates immunity

(5) Syphilis screening—Venereal Disease Research Laboratories test (VDRL), rapid plasma reagin (RPR)

(6) Hepatitis B surface antigen screening

(7) Urinalysis; urine culture if indicated

(8) Chlamydia/gonorrhea screening

(9) Offer human immunodeficiency virus (HIV) antibody testing

(10) Other tests indicated by individual risk status or general patient population, e.g., postprandial 50-g glucose screen, sickle cell screen, tuberculin testing

f. Risk assessment—major categories for increased risk

(1) Preexisting medical illness

(2) Previous pregnancy complications

(3) Evidence of poor maternal nutrition

(4) Exposure to possible teratogens

g. Referral for genetic counseling if indicated

(1) Maternal age of 35 or older by delivery

(2) Family history of genetic anomaly—e.g., Down syndrome, other chromosomal abnormality, hemophilia, muscular dystrophy, cystic fibrosis

(3) History of three or more spontaneous abortions

(4) Previous unexplained pregnancy loss

(5) Parents possible carriers of sickle cell, thalassemia, or Tay-Sachs disease

h. Education

(1) Nutrition

(a) Dietary assessment

(b) Ideal weight gain during pregnancy is 25–35 pounds for woman of normal weight (BMI 18.6–24.9); 15–25 pounds for overweight women (BMI 25–29.9); 11–20 pounds for obese women (BMI > 30); 28–40 pounds for underweight women (BMI < 18.5)

(i) First trimester—1–4.5 pounds

(ii) Second and third trimesters—1–2 pounds per week

(c) Discourage weight loss during pregnancy

(d) Nutritional requirements

(i) Calories—1,800 daily in first trimester, 2,200 calories daily in second trimester, and 2,400 kilocalories per day in third trimester recommended for women who get less than 30 minutes of exercise each week

(ii) Protein—60 g per day

(iii) Calcium—1,000 mg per day for adult; 1,600 mg per day for adolescent

(iv) Iron—30 mg supplement per day

(v) Zinc—11 mg supplement per day

(vi) Folic acid—0.4 mg per day, higher in first trimester if increased risk of neural tube defect

(vii) Other vitamin and mineral needs can usually be met from a balanced diet; encourage fiber and fluids

(2) Encourage good hygiene; douching not recommended

(3) Exercise
  (a) Regular exercise recommended throughout pregnancy
  (b) May continue with prepregnancy exercise routine, but should not begin new strenuous exercise program
  (c) Walking and swimming are ideal during pregnancy
  (d) Avoid excessive fatigue and excessive overheating

(4) Sexual activity
  (a) Coitus not contraindicated during normal pregnancy
  (b) Changes in position may be required as pregnancy progresses
  (c) Sexual intercourse contraindicated during pregnancy with undiagnosed vaginal bleeding, rupture of membranes, preterm labor, threatened abortion

(5) Warning signs—patient should contact provider promptly
  (a) Signs of ectopic pregnancy or threatened abortion
    (i) Abdominal pain
    (ii) Vaginal bleeding
    (iii) Passage of tissue
    (iv) Syncope
  (b) Hyperemesis—severe nausea and vomiting; unable to retain food or fluids
  (c) Signs of pyelonephritis
    (i) Fever above 100.6° F
    (ii) Dysuria, flank pain
  (d) Signs of PIH
    (i) Severe headache, dizziness
    (ii) Scotomata, blurring of vision
    (iii) Swelling of face; severe dependent edema that does not respond to rest/elevation
    (iv) Epigastric pain
  (e) Signs of PTL
    (i) Loss of fluid from vagina
    (ii) Lower back pain or lower abdominal cramping
    (iii) Frequent, palpable uterine contractions with or without pain
    (iv) Heaviness or pressure
    (v) Increased vaginal discharge, especially if blood-tinged, mucoid or watery
  (f) Decreased or absent fetal movement

(6) Signs and symptoms of labor
  (a) True labor
    (i) Contractions—timed from beginning of one contraction to beginning of the next
      a) Occur at regular intervals, which gradually shorten
      b) Initially felt in back, then radiate to lower abdomen
      c) Duration and strength of contractions increase
      d) Intensity of contractions increase with walking
      e) Sedation does not stop contractions
    (ii) Bloody "show"—pink or blood-tinged mucous discharge from cervix may indicate loss of mucus plug
    (iii) Cervix dilates and effaces
    (iv) Presenting part has descended into pelvis
  (b) False labor
    (i) Contractions irregular in timing, duration, and intensity
    (ii) Discomfort is felt mainly in abdomen
    (iii) Intensity of contractions not affected by walking
    (iv) No changes in cervix; no bloody show, dilatation, or effacement
    (v) Fetal head remains free in pelvis
    (vi) Sedation will stop contractions
  (c) Rupture of membranes
    (i) Occurs spontaneously at onset of labor in 50%
    (ii) Premature rupture of membranes associated with increased risk for
      a) PTL if occurs prior to 37 weeks gestation
      b) Ascending intrauterine infection if not delivered within 24 hours
      c) Prolapse of umbilical cord

2. Interval visits
  a. For low risk, routine monthly visits up to 28 weeks, every 2–3 weeks until 36 weeks, then weekly until delivery
  b. Components of routine visits
    (1) Measurement of maternal weight and blood pressure
    (2) Screen urine for protein and glucose; ketones and nitrites if indicated

(3) Obtain interval history, evaluate client complaints and risk-related symptoms, answer questions and provide anticipatory guidance

(4) Assess fetal heart tones by fetoscope or doppler (normal rate is 120–160 beats per minute)

(5) Evaluate fetal growth
  (a) Determine fundal height
  (b) Leopold's maneuvers—abdominal palpation performed using four maneuvers to determine fetal presentation and position (used later in pregnancy—beginning approximately 26 weeks)

(6) Specific needs or screening tests as indicated by gestational age or patient history
  (a) First trimester (LNMP through 13th week)
    (i) Chorionic villus sampling (CVS)—refer when indicated for genetic reasons; generally performed at 10–13 weeks
    (ii) 1 hour postprandial 50-g glucose screen (initial visit or first trimester) for women of high risk for gestational diabetes mellitus (GDM)—prior history of GDM; first-degree relative with type 2 diabetes; prior delivery of macrosomic infant; previous unexplained stillbirth or spontaneous abortions; obesity; glucosuria
    (iii) Assess physical and psychological impact of pregnancy, including support system
    (iv) Discuss warning signs and early complications
  (b) Second trimester (14th–27th week)
    (i) Maternal serum alpha-fetoprotein (MSAFP) and multiple marker (quad) screening—screen at 15–19 weeks (16–18 weeks optimal)
      a) Elevated levels of MSAFP associated with fetal congenital abnormalities—open neural tube defects, congenital nephrosis, abdominal wall defects; also elevated with multiple gestation
      b) Low levels of MSAFP associated with Down syndrome (trisomy 21)

    (ii) Amniocentesis performed at 15–18 weeks if indicated for genetic screening—mother ≥ 35, history of previous child with chromosomal, congenital, or metabolic abnormality
    (iii) 1 hour post 50-g glucose test —between 24–28 weeks
      a) May choose universal screening of all women or selective screening based on risk factors
      b) Selective screening guidelines—perform blood glucose testing if older than 25, ethnic group with high prevalence of diabetes (Hispanic, African-American, Native American, South or East Asian), obese, strong family history of type 2 diabetes, prior gestational diabetes, or for glucosuria or other signs of hyperglycemia
      c) 1 hour post 50-g glucose test of 130–190 mg/dL— follow with 3-hour glucose tolerance test (GTT)
      d) 1 hour post 50-g glucose test > 190 mg/dL—presumptive diagnosis of gestational diabetes
      e) Diagnosis of gestational diabetes with a 3-hour GTT if two or more values are met or exceeded—FBS 105 mg/dL, 1-hour 190 mg/dL, 2-hour 165 mg/dL, 3-hour 145 mg/dL
    (iv) Assess for fetal movements (quickening)—usually between 16–20 weeks
    (v) Discuss warning signs for complications including PTL
  (c) Third trimester (28th week to term —usually 40 weeks)
    (i) Repeat VDRL and hemoglobin (Hgb)
    (ii) Reevaluate antibody screen titer
    (iii) Rh (D) immune globulin (RhoGAM) to unsensitized Rh-negative mother—28 weeks
    (iv) Discuss importance of monitoring fetal movement as indicator of fetal well-being

(v) Review signs and symptoms of labor

(vi) Perform group B strep screen (35–37 weeks)

(vii) Assess fetal lie and presentation (36–40 weeks)

(viii) Perform cervical assessment for position, consistency, length, and dilation near term

3. Tests for assessment of fetal well-being

a. Ultrasound (ultrasonography)

(1) Definition—high-frequency sound waves reflected from tissues of varying densities and converted into images

(a) Level 1 (basic ultrasound)—establishes gestational age, location, and grade of placenta; determines fetal presentation, number of fetuses, stage of fetal growth, cardiac activity; assesses amniotic fluid volume; detects gross fetal anomalies and maternal pelvic masses

(b) Level II (targeted ultrasound)—confirms information obtained in Level I and surveys fetal anatomy for malformations

(2) Indications—determination of gestational age; assess fetal growth pattern; size/date discrepancy; suspected ectopic pregnancy; suspected hydatidiform mole; determine fetal presentation/lie; suspected hydramnios/oligohydramnios; suspected fetal anomaly or fetal demise; determine placental location, integrity, maturity; identify number of fetuses; aid in diagnostic procedures, e.g., amniocentesis, CVS

b. Nonstress test (NST)

(1) Definition—diagnostic test that monitors fetal heart rate acceleration in response to fetal movement (noninvasive); both NST and contraction stress test (CST) were developed to assess any indication of uteroplacental insufficiency and to predict ability of fetus to endure stress of labor

(2) Indications—decreased fetal movement; post-term pregnancy; intrauterine growth restriction; hypertensive disorders

(3) Procedure—fetal heart rate (FHR), fetal movement and uterine contractions are assessed (using external monitoring) over a 20-minute period; may be extended to 40 minutes if no FHR accelerations occur

(4) Interpretation

(a) Reactive NST—two or more accelerations in FHR of 15 or more beats per minute, lasting for 15 seconds or more; fetal well-being assured for 1 week (repeat weekly)

(b) Nonreactive NST—absence of appropriate heart rate accelerations over a 40-minute period; consider additional testing, e.g., contraction stress test (CST) or biophysical profile

c. Contraction stress test (CST)

(1) Definition—diagnostic test performed to evaluate fetal response to uterine contractions; mimics labor

(2) Procedure—baseline tracing obtained for 10–20 minutes; if fewer than three contractions occur in 10-minute period contractions stimulated by intravenous oxytocin infusion or nipple stimulation

(3) Interpretation

(a) Positive CST—late decelerations following 50% or more of contractions; delivery recommended or further tests (test has 30% false-positive rate)

(b) Negative CST—no late or variable decelerations; subsequent testing based on fetal and maternal conditions and institutional protocol

(c) Equivocal CST—late decelerations in fewer than 50% of contractions, or significant variable decelerations; repeat in 24 hours or do biophysical profile

(4) Contraindications—premature rupture of membranes, history of PTL during current pregnancy, incompetent cervix or cerclage, previous vertical uterine incision, third trimester bleeding, polyhydramnios, placenta previa, multiple pregnancy

d. Biophysical profile (BPP)

(1) Definition—use of real-time ultrasound to assess fetal tone, breathing, body movements, and amniotic fluid volume combined with NST to evaluate FHR accelerations (total of five variables)

(2) Indications—high-risk pregnancy, e.g., post-date pregnancy, decreased fetal movement, maternal disease, suspected oligohydramnios, intrauterine growth restriction

(3) Interpretation—each of five variables is scored as 2 (normal) or 0 (abnormal), with total possible score of 10
   (a) 8–10—normal (in absence of oligohydramnios)
   (b) 6—equivocal (repeat according to agency protocol)
   (c) ≤ 4—abnormal (consider delivery)
e. Fetal movement/kick counts
   (1) Definition—fetal movement assessment by mother
   (2) Indications—generally start at 28 weeks if identifiable risks present or 34–36 weeks if low risk for uteroplacental insufficiency
   (3) Interpretation—various methods of counting are used
      (a) Optimal number of movements and ideal duration of counting has not been established
      (b) Cardiff "count to 10" method—start at approximately same time each day and chart how long it takes to count 10 movements; if fewer than 10 movements in 10 hours or amount to reach 10 movements increases consider NST
      (c) More important than a quantitative guideline is the mother's perception of a decrease in fetal activity in relation to a previous level

- Common Complaints in Pregnancy
  1. Nausea and vomiting
     a. Etiology—high levels of hCG in first trimester, changes in carbohydrate metabolism, delayed gastric emptying
     b. Management
        (1) Rule out hyperemesis gravidarum, pyelonephritis
        (2) Small, frequent high-carbohydrate meals; avoid high-fat or spicy meals; avoid empty or overdistended stomach
        (3) Ginger in the form of ginger ale or supplement
  2. Backache
     a. Etiology—softening and relaxation of pelvic structures and joints; increased lordosis of spine caused by shift in center of gravity
     b. Management
        (1) Rule out pyelonephritis, labor, musculoskeletal disease
        (2) Teach pelvic tilt exercise; use proper body mechanics; avoid excessive twisting, bending, and stretching
  3. Varicosities
     a. Etiology—pressure of enlarged uterus causing impaired venous circulation and increased venous pressure in lower extremities; relaxation of vein walls and valves; hereditary factors; weight gain
     b. Management
        (1) Rule out thrombophlebitis
        (2) Support pantyhose; frequent leg elevation; avoid standing for long periods, crossing legs, and knee-high hose
  4. Hemorrhoids
     a. Etiology—pressure of enlarging uterus; constipation; predisposition to varicosities
     b. Management
        (1) Rule out abscessed or thrombosed hemorrhoids
        (2) Topical anesthetics; prevent or treat constipation by increasing fluids and roughage in diet; warm or cool sitz baths; ice packs or cold compresses
  5. Constipation
     a. Etiology—decreased intestinal motility caused by progesterone and compression of bowel by enlarging uterus; oral iron supplements
     b. Management—increase high-fiber foods and fluids; regular exercise; bulk-forming, nonnutritive laxative
  6. Heartburn
     a. Etiology—decreased gastrointestinal peristalsis and relaxation of cardiac sphincter; reflux of gastric contents into lower esophagus; upward displacement and compression of the stomach by uterus
     b. Management
        (1) Rule out cardiac, gallbladder, epigastric, or pancreatic disease, PIH
        (2) Small frequent meals; avoid fatty foods; fluids between but not with meals; after eating do not lie down for at least 1 hour; low-sodium antacids
  7. Pica and food cravings
     a. Etiology—unknown
     b. Management—evaluate diet to determine adequacy; explain need to maintain healthy diet; problems may occur if craved substance is substituting for nutritious food or is harmful to mother or fetus
  8. Ptyalism (increased salivation)
     a. Etiology—unknown
     b. Management—reassurance of resolution following pregnancy; good oral hygiene; avoid excessive starch intake; adequate fluid intake

9. Fatigue—most common in first and third trimesters
   a. Etiology
      (1) Early pregnancy—increased oxygen consumption, increased progesterone level, fetal demands
      (2) Late pregnancy—sleep deprivation from physical discomforts
   b. Management
      (1) Rule out iron deficiency anemia, depression
      (2) Reassurance; encourage adequate sleep and rest periods
10. Headache
    a. Etiology—increased circulatory volume; vasodilation caused by high progesterone levels; vascular congestion; stress; fatigue; hypoglycemia
    b. Management
       (1) Rule out PIH, migraine headache, sinus infection
       (2) Teach symptoms of PIH; encourage adequate rest; stress reduction; massage; moist hot or cold compresses; avoid intake of foods that trigger headaches; acetaminophen
11. Vaginal discharge (leukorrhea)
    a. Etiology—estrogen-induced increase in vascularity and hypertrophy of cervical glands and vaginal cells
    b. Management
       (1) Rule out ruptured membranes, vaginitis, cervicitis, STD
       (2) Reassurance; cotton underwear and loose clothing; avoid douching or tampon use; keep vulva clean and dry
12. Urinary frequency
    a. Etiology—enlargement of uterus compresses bladder; hyperplasia and hyperemia of pelvic organs and increased kidney output
    b. Management
       (1) Rule out urinary tract infection (UTI)
       (2) Void frequently; maintain adequate fluid intake; discontinue fluids 2–3 hours prior to bedtime; avoid caffeine
13. Leg cramps
    a. Etiology—pressure of uterus on pelvic nerves and blood vessels; imbalance in phosphorus/calcium ratio caused by inadequate or excessive calcium intake (postulated)
    b. Management
       (1) Rule out thromboembolic disease, varicosities
       (2) Avoid stretching legs, pointing toes, and lying on back; dorsiflexion of foot to relieve cramp in calf; diet evaluation to correct excessive or inadequate intake of calcium
14. Round ligament pain
    a. Etiology—growth of uterus causes round ligaments to stretch
    b. Management
       (1) Rule out PTL, ectopic pregnancy, ruptured ovarian cyst, appendicitis
       (2) Reassurance of resolution following pregnancy; avoid sudden, twisting movements; heating pad; avoid excessive exercise, standing or walking
15. Dyspnea (breathlessness)
    a. Etiology—increased sensitivity to lower levels of CO_2 (progesterone effect) in early pregnancy; later in pregnancy caused by displacement of diaphragm by enlarging uterus
    b. Management
       (1) Rule out upper respiratory infection, pulmonary or cardiac problem
       (2) Sleep with head elevated; reassure improvement will occur when fetus drops into pelvis; avoid exercise if a precipitating factor
16. Edema
    a. Etiology—increased capillary permeability (hormonal); pressure of uterus impedes venous return; increased fluid in intracellular spaces
    b. Management
       (1) Assess for PIH
       (2) Instruct about symptoms of PIH; rest in left lateral recumbent position for 1–2 hours during day and at night; elevate legs several times during day; avoid constrictive clothing; avoid long periods of sitting or standing

- Immunizations and Medication Use in Pregnancy
  1. Immunizations
     a. Preconception immunization of women to prevent infections harmful to fetus is recommended
     b. Postpartum vaccination for rubella and varicella in susceptible women is encouraged
     c. The use of live attenuated vaccines during pregnancy is contraindicated—e.g., measles, mumps, rubella, varicella
     d. Women should be advised to not become pregnant for at least 4 weeks after receiving a live attenuated vaccine
     e. Influenza vaccine—indicated for women who are pregnant in the second or third trimester during the flu season and for women

at high risk for pulmonary complications regardless of trimester

    f. Hepatitis A and B—indicated preexposure and postexposure for women at risk of infection

    g. Pneumococcus—indications not altered by pregnancy

    h. Tetanus-diphtheria primary series and booster may be given during pregnancy

    i. Immune globulins for hepatitis A and B, rabies, tetanus, and varicella may be used during pregnancy

    j. Refer to CDC at www.cdc.gov/nip for the most up-to-date immunization recommendations

2. Medication use—FDA risk factor categories for prescription drugs in pregnancy

    a. Category A—adequate, well-controlled studies in pregnant women have not shown an increased risk of fetal abnormalities

    b. Category B—animal studies have revealed no evidence of harm to the fetus; however, there are no adequate and well-controlled studies in pregnant women OR animal studies have shown an adverse effect, but adequate and well-controlled studies in pregnant women have failed to demonstrate a risk to the fetus

    c. Category C—animal studies have shown an adverse effect and there are no adequate and well-controlled studies in pregnant women OR no animal studies have been conducted and there are no adequate and well-controlled studies in pregnant women

    d. Category D—studies, adequate and well-controlled or observational studies in pregnant women have demonstrated risk to the fetus; however, the benefits of therapy may outweigh the potential risks

    e. Category X—studies adequate and well-controlled or observational in pregnant women or animals have demonstrated positive evidence of fetal abnormalities, which clearly outweigh any possible benefit to the woman

- Pregnancy Complications
  1. Bleeding disorders
         a. Spontaneous abortion (SAB)
           (1) Definition—naturally occurring termination of pregnancy before 20 weeks gestation
           (2) Etiology—chromosomal abnormalities of fetus; chronic maternal disease, infection, or endocrine imbalance; faulty implantation; immune factors; advanced maternal age

      (3) Signs and symptoms/physical examination findings
        (a) Threatened abortion—occurs in one of four pregnancies
          (i) Vaginal bleeding with or without cramping; may be accompanied by low backache
          (ii) No cervical changes; cervix closed
        (b) Inevitable
          (i) Vaginal bleeding with contractions; possible gush of fluid from vagina
          (ii) Cervical dilatation and rupture of membranes
        (c) Missed abortion—prolonged retention of fetus after fetal death
          (i) Loss of symptoms of pregnancy; may have brownish vaginal discharge
          (ii) Gradual decrease in uterine size; cervix closed and firm
        (d) Incomplete abortion—incomplete expulsion of products of conception (POC), usually placenta retained
          (i) Bleeding (may be profuse); cramping
          (ii) May observe tissue in cervical canal
        (e) Complete abortion—complete expulsion of all POC
          (i) Bleeding; cramping
          (ii) No retained POC; cervix dilated
      (4) Differential diagnosis
        (a) Vaginal/cervical infection
        (b) Cervical polyp
        (c) Ectopic pregnancy
        (d) Molar pregnancy
        (e) Implantation bleeding
      (5) Diagnostic tests/findings
        (a) Ultrasound for evidence of fetal heart action and uterine size
        (b) Serial hCG levels
        (c) Pelvic exam to evaluate cervical dilation, uterine size, and bleeding
      (6) Management/treatment
        (a) Pelvic rest (nothing in vagina); hydration; counsel regarding signs of infection and when to report symptoms
        (b) May require hospitalization, dilatation and curettage (D&C), transfusion, IV fluids
        (c) RhoGAM for unsensitized Rh-negative women
        (d) Emotional support

b. Ectopic pregnancy
  (1) Definition—implantation of fertilized ovum outside the uterine cavity (usually in fallopian tube)
  (2) Etiology—any condition that prevents or slows passage of fertilized ovum into uterus—e.g., tubal damage from previous pelvic infection, tubal surgery, previous ectopic; progestin-only contraceptive use
  (3) Signs and symptoms/physical findings
    (a) Before rupture—early pregnancy symptoms; amenorrhea followed by spotting/bleeding; lower abdominal pain, unilateral or bilateral; uterus normal to slightly enlarged; may have unilateral, tender adnexal mass
    (b) After rupture—sharp, unilateral abdominal pain, may radiate to shoulder; syncope/fainting/shock; spotting/bleeding; adnexal tenderness, possible fullness; cervical motion tenderness; bulging of posterior cul-de-sac
  (4) Differential diagnosis
    (a) Acute appendicitis
    (b) Pelvic inflammatory disease (PID)
    (c) Ruptured corpus luteum cyst
    (d) SAB
  (5) Diagnostic tests/findings
    (a) Ultrasound—no evidence of intrauterine pregnancy; may be gestational sac with no apparent heartbeat
    (b) CBC—may indicate anemia, slight leukocytosis
    (c) Serum beta hCG—positive, but hCG level lower than expected for gestational age
    (d) Serial beta hCG levels—level rises slowly or plateaus; with intrauterine pregnancy, doubles every 2 days
  (6) Management/treatment—hospitalization; surgery for repair or removal of damaged tube; medical management with methotrexate; fluid replacement; transfusion if needed; RhoGAM administration for Rh-negative woman
c. Placenta previa
  (1) Definition—abnormal implantation of placenta in lower uterine segment
  (2) Etiology—unknown; may be associated with multiparity, multiple gestation, previous cesarean, previous uterine surgery, smoking
  (3) Signs and symptoms/physical findings
    (a) Painless bleeding after 20 weeks gestation; usually in third trimester
    (b) Uterus nontender; usually no evidence of fetal distress
  (4) Differential diagnosis
    (a) Abruptio placentae
    (b) Cervical lesion or cervicitis
    (c) Nonvaginal bleeding (rectal or urinary)
  (5) Diagnostic tests/findings
    (a) Ultrasound—indicates low-lying placenta
    (b) *No* pelvic exam
  (6) Management/treatment
    (a) Gestation is less than 36 weeks—expectant management; hospitalization and bedrest; fetal surveillance; monitor mother for increased bleeding
    (b) Gestation 36 weeks or more—anticipate delivery; may need amniocentesis to assess fetal lung maturity
d. Abruptio placentae
  (1) Definition—partial or complete detachment of normally implanted placenta anytime prior to delivery
  (2) Etiology—unknown; contributing factors include maternal hypertension, cocaine use, smoking, advanced maternal age, multiparity, trauma, preterm rupture of membranes, uterine anomalies
  (3) Signs and symptoms/physical findings
    (a) Vaginal bleeding of varying amount with severe, unremitting abdominal pain
    (b) Uterine tenderness, increased uterine tone, contractions, signs of fetal distress, signs of shock
  (4) Differential diagnosis
    (a) Placenta previa
    (b) Appendicitis
    (c) Labor
  (5) Diagnostic tests/findings—ultrasound for placental location
  (6) Management/treatment
    (a) Immediate transport for emergency care
    (b) Immediate delivery if massive bleeding or fetal distress
    (c) Expectant management in emergency facility if fetus immature, no evidence of fetal distress or maternal hypovolemia or anemia

2. Pregnancy induced hypertension (PIH)
   a. Definitions
      (1) Chronic hypertension (HTN)—blood pressure > 140/90 present before pregnancy, diagnosed before 20 weeks of gestation, or that does not resolve in postpartum; preeclampsia may be superimposed on chronic hypertension
      (2) Preeclampsia—pregnancy specific syndrome of reduced organ perfusion secondary to vasospasm and activation of a coagulation cascade
         (a) Usually occurs after 20 weeks gestation
         (b) Elevated blood pressure (> 140/90) accompanied by proteinuria and edema
         (c) Clinical spectrum ranges from mild to severe forms
      (3) HELLP syndrome—seen with severe preeclampsia, multi-organ system failure; **H**emolytic anemia, **E**levated **L**iver enzymes, **L**ow **P**latelets
      (4) Eclampsia—occurrence of seizures in woman with preeclampsia that cannot be attributed to other causes
   b. Etiology
      (1) Cause is unknown
      (2) Predisposing factors—primigravidas, age < 19 or > 35, family history of preeclampsia, multiple gestation, antiphospholipid antibody syndrome, thromboembolic disorders, diabetes mellitus, or other chronic diseases
   c. Signs and symptoms/physical findings
      (1) Mild preeclampsia—HTN with BP < 160/110, proteinuria, edema, no maternal symptoms
      (2) Severe preeclampsia—BP ≥ 160/100, proteinuria, generalized edema, oliguria, cerebral disturbances (severe headaches, disorientation), visual disturbances (scotoma, blurred vision), hyperreflexia, epigastric or right upper quadrant pain, enlarged liver, pulmonary edema, fetal growth restriction
   d. Differential diagnosis
      (1) Chronic hypertension
      (2) Gestational trophoblastic disease
      (3) Renal disease
      (4) Liver disease
      (5) Brain tumor
   e. Diagnostic tests/findings
      (1) Findings dependent on severity of PIH (laboratory tests other than proteinuria normal with mild preeclampsia)
      (2) Proteinuria—> 300 mg/24 hours or persistent > 30 mg/dL (1+ dipstick) in random urine samples
      (3) Serum creatinine, ALT/AST, uric acid elevated
      (4) Platelet count—< 100,000 cells/mm^3
      (5) Hemoglobin/hematocrit elevated (hemoconcentration)
      (6) Increased LDH—microangiopathic hemolysis
      (7) Ultrasound—may indicate fetal growth restriction
   f. Management/treatment—goal is prevention of seizures, hematologic, renal, and hepatic complications in mother and birth of uncompromised newborn as close to term as possible
      (1) Antepartum
         (a) Intermittent bed rest in left lateral position throughout day
         (b) Adequate nutrition and hydration
         (c) Careful monitoring of mother—BP, proteinuria, edema, weight, intake and output, deep tendon reflexes (DTR), subjective symptoms, laboratory tests
         (d) Careful monitoring of fetus—NST, BPP, fetal movement counts, serial ultrasounds, fetal maturity tests
         (e) Educate mother to report headaches, visual disturbances, disorientation, epigastric/abdominal pain, decreased urinary output
         (f) Hospitalization and early delivery may be necessary
      (2) Intrapartum
         (a) Goal is to prevent seizures and deliver newborn
         (b) Magnesium sulfate—used as an anticonvulsant
            (i) Drug action—interferes with the release of acetylcholine at the synapses decreasing neuromuscular and CNS irritability
            (ii) Side effects/adverse reactions—drowsiness, hypotension, bradycardia, diarrhea, flushing, sweating, respiratory depression, muscular paralysis
            (iii) Monitor for signs of toxicity—vital signs, DTR, magnesium levels, urinary output (decreased output increases chance for toxicity)
            (iv) Overdose antidote is calcium gluconate

(c) Hydralazine—most commonly used antihypertensive for severe HTN

(d) Diuretics should not be used as may further compromise placental perfusion

3. Preterm labor (PTL)

   a. Definition—documented persistent uterine contractions (at least four in 20 minutes or eight in 60 minutes) and at least one of the following (documented cervical change or cervix > 1 cm dilated and/or 80% effaced when gestational age is 20 weeks or greater and less than 37 weeks

   b. Etiology

     (1) Not always known—often multifactorial

     (2) Predisposing factors—maternal chronic disease, PIH, uterine anomalies, trauma to abdomen, genitourinary infection, chorioamnionitis, systemic infections, previous history of PTL, incompetent cervix, multiple gestation, hydramnios, placenta previa or abruption, premature rupture of membranes, lower socioeconomic status

   c. Signs and symptoms/physical findings

     (1) Menstrual-like cramps, pelvic pressure, constant or intermittent low backache, change in vaginal discharge (increased, watery, pink-tinged)

     (2) Contractions documented by fetal monitoring or palpation, cervical dilation and/or effacement, ruptured membranes

   d. Differential diagnosis

     (1) Braxton-Hicks contractions

     (2) Urinary tract infection/pyelonephritis

     (3) Vaginal infection

   e. Diagnostic tests and findings

     (1) Urinalysis—negative for infection

     (2) Positive ferning and nitrazine tests if rupture of membranes

   f. Management/treatment

     (1) Conservative measures if cervical changes not advanced—hydration (no evidence to support but often advised), modified bed rest (up to bathroom, meals, and shower)—prolonged bed rest may increase risk for thromboembolic complications, avoid bladder distention, avoid sexual intercourse and orgasm, avoid breast stimulation, continue to monitor fetal status and status of contractions

     (2) Tocolytics—useful in postponing birth to allow time for administration of corticosteroids to enhance fetal lung maturity

       (a) Use if 20–34 weeks, membranes intact, cervical dilation < 4 cm and effacement < 80% and fetus not in distress

       (b) Contraindications—chorioamnionitis, severe preeclampsia, placenta previa, fetal distress, lethal fetal anomalies, maternal hemodynamic instability, cardiac disease, or cardiac rhythm disturbance

       (c) Beta adrenergic agonists (ritodrine, terbutaline)

         (i) Drug action—interferes with smooth muscle contractility

         (ii) Side effects/adverse reactions—tachycardia, tremors, anxiety, hyperglycemia, hypokalemia, pulmonary edema, fetal tachycardia

       (d) Magnesium sulfate

         (i) Drug action—acts on vascular smooth muscle causing vasodilatation

         (ii) Side effects/adverse reactions—drowsiness, hypotension, bradycardia, diarrhea, flushing sweating, respiratory depression, muscular paralysis

         (iii) Monitor for signs of toxicity—vital signs, DTR, magnesium levels, urinary output (decreased output increases chance for toxicity)

         (iv) Overdose antidote is calcium gluconate

     (3) Corticosteroids (betamethasone, dexamethasone)—stimulates fetal surfactant production and reduces risk for neonatal respiratory distress syndrome

       (a) May be given between 24 and 34 weeks unless there is an indication for immediate delivery

       (b) Optimal benefits begin 24 hours after starting therapy

◘ FERTILITY CONTROL

- Combination Oral Contraceptives (COC)

  1. Description—pill taken daily for contraception or for specific noncontraceptive benefits; combination of estrogen and progestin

   a. Monophasic pills—deliver constant amount of estrogen/progestin throughout cycle

b. Multiphasic pills—vary amount of estrogen and/or progestin delivered throughout cycle; concept is to mimic natural menstrual cycle more closely

2. Mechanism of action
   a. Estrogen—inhibits ovulation through suppression of FSH, alters cellular structure of the endometrium, stabilizes endometrium, potentiates progestin
      (1) Ethinyl estradiol (E_2)—most prevalent synthetic estrogen in COC
      (2) Mestranol—weaker estrogen; utilized in older COC formulations
   b. Progestin—inhibits ovulation through suppression of LH; produces atrophic endometrium; thickens cervical mucus; decreases ovum transport through fallopian tube; may inhibit capacitation of sperm
      (1) Norethindrone
      (2) Norethindrone acetate
      (3) Norgestrel
      (4) Levonorgestrel
      (5) Ethynodiol diacetate
      (6) Norgestimate
      (7) Desogestrel
      (8) Gestodene (not available in United States)
      (9) Drospirenone

3. Effectiveness/first-year failure rate
   a. Perfect use—0.1%
   b. Typical use—5%

4. Advantages
   a. Ease of use
   b. Reversible
   c. Effective
   d. May reduce incidence of/afford protection against
      (1) Acne
      (2) Dysmenorrhea
      (3) Pelvic inflammatory disease
      (4) Ectopic pregnancy
      (5) Endometriosis
      (6) Anemia
      (7) Osteoporosis
      (8) Benign breast disease
      (9) Functional ovarian cysts
      (10) Ovarian cancer; endometrial cancer
      (11) Atherogenesis
      (12) Rheumatoid arthritis
      (13) Migraine headaches
      (14) Premenstrual syndrome
      (15) May be used as emergency contraception

5. Disadvantages/side effects
   a. Does not prevent transmission of STD/HIV
   b. Requires user compliance/daily dosing schedule
   c. Side effects may include
      (1) Estrogenic effects
         (a) Nausea
         (b) Increased breast size
         (c) Cyclic weight gain
         (d) Leukorrhea
         (e) Cervical eversion/ectopy
         (f) Hypertension
         (g) Increased cholesterol concentration in gallbladder bile
         (h) Growth of leiomyomata
         (i) Telangiectasia
         (j) Chloasma
         (k) Hepatocellular adenomas/cancer (rare)
         (l) Cerebrovascular accidents
         (m) Thromboembolic complications including pulmonary emboli
         (n) Stimulation of breast neoplasia
      (2) Progestogenic side effects (alone or in combination with estrogen)
         (a) Breast tenderness
         (b) Headaches
         (c) Hypertension
         (d) Decreased libido
      (3) Androgenic effects
         (a) Increased appetite/weight gain
         (b) Depression, fatigue
         (c) Acne, oily skin
         (d) Increased breast tenderness/size
         (e) Increased LDL cholesterol
         (f) Decreased HDL cholesterol
         (g) Decreased carbohydrate tolerance/increased insulin resistance
         (h) Pruritus

6. Contraindications (World Health Organization [WHO] category 4 use represents unacceptable risk)
   a. Refrain from providing if any of the following conditions exist
      (1) Venous thromboembolism
      (2) Cerebrovascular accident, coronary artery/ischemic heart disease
      (3) Structural heart disease
      (4) Pregnancy
      (5) Breast cancer
      (6) Lactation (less than 6 weeks postpartum)
      (7) Benign hepatic adenoma, liver cancer, or history thereof; active viral hepatitis; severe cirrhosis
      (8) Headaches (migraine) with focal neurologic symptoms
      (9) Major surgery with prolonged immobilization, any surgery on legs
      (10) Age 35 years or older smoking 15 or more cigarettes daily

(11) Hypertension systolic ≥ 160 or diastolic ≥ 100

(12) Vascular disease

(13) Known thrombotic mutations

b. Exercise caution WHO category 3 risks outweigh benefit

(1) Postpartum less than 21 days

(2) Lactation (6 weeks–6 months)

(3) Undiagnosed, abnormal vaginal/uterine bleeding

(4) Age 35 years or older smoking less than 15 cigarettes daily

(5) Past history breast cancer with no recurrence for 5 years

(6) Adequately controlled hypertension or BP of systolic 140–159 or diastolic 90–99

(7) Untreated stage 1 hypertension

(8) Bariatric bypass procedures (only combined oral options)

(9) Age 35 years or older with migraine headache but no focal neurological symptoms

(10) Use of drugs that alter liver enzymes—rifampin, phenytoin, griseofulvin, carbamazepine, barbiturates, topiramate, primidone

(11) Gall bladder disease/history of COC-related cholestasis

(12) DM type 1 or 2 of > 20 years duration and/or comorbid vascular disease

7. Management

a. Health assessment prior to initiation of method

(1) Elicit information from thorough history concerning any contraindications/risk to use of COCs

(2) Blood pressure

(3) Pelvic examination/Pap smear not required but recommended if patient sexually active, now or in past

(4) Clinical breast examination not required but recommended if age ≥ 20

(5) Mammogram not required but recommended if age ≥ 40

b. Health assessment at follow-up visits

(1) Patients may be assessed yearly if no risk factors

(2) Patients with risk factors may be seen at 3–6 month intervals

c. Special considerations

(1) Drug interactions—drugs which may decrease the effectiveness of COC

(a) Rifampin

(b) Griseofulvin

(c) Phenobarbital

(d) Phenytoin

(e) Topiramate

(f) Carbamazepine

(g) Primidone

(h) Saint John's Wort

(2) Drug interactions—COC may potentiate effect of some drugs

(a) Benzodiazepines

(b) Anti-inflammatory corticosteroids

(c) Bronchodilators

(3) Management of breakthrough bleeding/spotting

(a) Common side effect first 3 months of use

(b) Reinforce to take pills daily at the same time

(c) Change to 30–35 mcg estrogen if on 20 mcg COC and bleeding is during first half of cycle

(d) Change to COC with different progestin

(e) If problem persists consider another cause for bleeding, e.g., infection, polyps

(4) Management of absence of withdrawal bleeding

(a) Occurs in about 5% of women after several years of COC use

(b) Rule out pregnancy

(c) No intervention required if woman is okay with no menses

(d) Change to 30–35 mcg estrogen if on 20 mcg COC

(e) Add supplemental estrogen to regimen for first 3 weeks of one cycle

8. Instructions for use

a. General instructions

(1) Backup method used (e.g., condoms) for first 7 days of first pack

(a) Necessary only if patient is on Sunday start pack or begins pills after day 5 of menstrual cycle

(b) Initiation on first day of cycle ensures protection

(2) Pill taken at approximately same time each day

(3) If nausea occurs, pill taken with meals or at bedtime

(4) Backup method (condoms) used if efficacy/absorbency compromised by severe vomiting/diarrhea

(5) Condom use considered for prevention of STD/HIV

b. Missed pills

(1) If 1 pill missed, take as soon as remembered and next pill taken at normal time, use backup method for 7 days if pill missed in week 1

(2) If 2 pills missed in weeks 1 or 2, 2 pills taken on day remembered and 2 pills the next day, pack finished as usual, backup method used for 7 days

(3) If 2 pills missed in week 3

    (a) Sunday start—1 pill taken each day until Sunday; remainder of pack discarded; new pack started; backup method used for 7 days

    (b) First day menses start—remainder of pack discarded and new pack started immediately; backup method used for 7 days

(4) Emergency contraception considered if unprotected intercourse occurred during days when backup method should have been used

  c. Warning signs (ACHES)

    (1) **A**bdominal pain (severe)

    (2) **C**hest pain (sharp, severe, shortness of breath)

    (3) **H**eadache (severe, dizziness, unilateral)

    (4) **E**ye problems (scotoma, blurred vision, blind spots)

    (5) **S**evere leg pain (calf or thigh)

- Progestin-Only Pills (POP)
  1. Description—pill taken daily for purposes of contraception; comprised of synthetic progestins in lower doses than those used in combination oral contraceptive pills
  2. Mechanism of action
     a. Inhibits ovulation through suppression of FSH and LH
     b. Produces atrophic endometrium
     c. Thickens cervical mucus
     d. Slows ovum transport through fallopian tube
     e. May inhibit sperm capacitation
  3. Effectiveness/first-year failure rate
     a. Perfect use—0.5%
     b. Typical use—5%
  4. Advantages
     a. Ease of use
     b. Reversible
     c. Effective
     d. Contains no estrogen for women in whom it is contraindicated or who cannot tolerate estrogenic side effects
     e. Can be used during lactation
  5. Disadvantages and side effects
     a. Effectiveness may be compromised by drug interactions due to low-dose formulation
        (1) Rifampin
        (2) Phenobarbital
        (3) Phenytoin
        (4) Primidone

(5) Carbamazepine

(6) Griseofulvin

  b. Decreased availability/increased expense compared to COC

  c. Strict daily dosing schedule

  d. Possible side effects include

    (1) Increased incidence of functional follicular cysts

    (2) Menstrual cycle irregularities

    (3) Mastalgia

    (4) Depression

  e. No protection against STD/HIV

6. Contraindications (WHO recommendations)
   a. Refrain from providing if any of the following conditions exist
      (1) Pregnancy
      (2) Breast cancer
   b. Exercise caution if any of the following conditions exist
      (1) Use of drugs that alter liver enzymes (same as with COC)
      (2) Lactation (less than 6 weeks postpartum)
      (3) History of breast cancer with 5-year disease-free interval
      (4) Current deep vein thrombosis or pulmonary emboli
      (5) Liver conditions such as cirrhosis, adenoma, cancer, active viral hepatitis
      (6) Current/history of ischemic heart disease or cerebrovascular accident
      (7) Development of migraine headaches with focal neurological symptoms while using the method

7. Management
   a. Health assessment prior to initiation of method—refer to COC section
   b. Health assessment at follow-up visits—refer to COC section
   c. Special considerations—ectopic pregnancy more likely if pregnancy occurs

8. Instructions for using the method
   a. General instruction
      (1) Pills started on cycle day 1 (first day of menses)
      (2) Pill taken at same time each day every day; no placebo/off week
         (a) If more than 3 hours late taking pill, backup method should be used for 48 hours
         (b) If more than 1 pill is missed, 2 pills should be taken for 2 days, backup method should be used for rest of cycle, clinician should be notified if no bleeding occurs in 4–6 weeks

b. Warning signs
    (1) Severe low abdominal pain
    (2) No bleeding after series of regular cycles
    (3) Severe headache

- Transdermal Contraceptive System
  1. Description—patch applied to skin; delivers continuous daily systemic dose of progestin (norelgestromin) and estrogen (ethinyl estradiol), new patch applied each week for 3 weeks followed by 1 week without patch to induce withdrawal bleeding
  2. Mechanism of action—same as COC
  3. Effectiveness/first-year failure rate
     a. Perfect use—0.99%
     b. Typical use—1.24%
  4. Advantages
     a. Ease of use—no daily dosing regimen
     b. Reversible
     c. Effective
     d. Good menstrual cycle control
  5. Disadvantages and side effects
     a. Does not prevent transmission of STD/HIV
     b. Skin irritation at application site
     c. Other side effects similar to those of COC
  6. Contraindications (WHO recommendations)
     a. Refrain from providing if any of the following conditions exist—same as with COC
     b. Exercise caution if any of the following conditions exist—same as with COC
  7. Management
     a. Health assessment prior to initiation—same as with COC
     b. Health assessment at follow-up visits—same as with COC
     c. Special considerations
        (1) May be less effective in women who weigh ≥ 90 kg (198 pounds)
        (2) Probably same drug interactions as with COC
  8. Instructions for using the method
     a. First patch applied on first Sunday after menstrual period starts; backup method used for first 7 days
     b. Patch applied first day of menses; no backup method needed
     c. Patch applied to buttocks, abdomen, upper torso front or back (excluding breasts), upper outer arm
     d. New patch applied on same day each week for total of 3 weeks
     e. Patch not worn on week 4; withdrawal bleeding will occur
     f. Use of condoms considered for STD/HIV prevention
     g. New patch applied if current patch partially or completely pulls away from skin

h. Healthcare provider contacted if warning signs occur—same as COC warning signs

- Contraceptive Vaginal Ring (NuvaRing)
  1. Description—soft, malleable, clear plastic ring; delivers continuous, systemic dose of estrogen (ethinyl estradiol) and progestin (etonogestrel); worn in vagina for 3 weeks followed by 1 week without ring to induce withdrawal bleeding
  2. Mechanism of action—same as COC
  3. Effectiveness/first-year failure rate
     a. Perfect use—data not available
     b. Typical use—2%
  4. Advantages
     a. Ease of use—no daily dosing regimen
     b. Reversible
     c. Effective
     d. Good menstrual cycle control
  5. Disadvantages and side effects
     a. Does not prevent transmission of STD/HIV
     b. Side effects similar to those of COC
     c. Vaginal discharge/vaginal irritation
  6. Contraindications (WHO recommendations)
     a. Refrain from providing if any of the following conditions exist—same as with COC
     b. Exercise caution if any of the following conditions exist—same as with COC
  7. Management
     a. Health assessment prior to initiation—same as with COC
     b. Health assessment at follow-up visits—same as with COC
     c. Special considerations—probably same drug interactions as with COC
  8. Instructions for using the method
     a. First vaginal ring inserted within 5 days of start of menstrual period
     b. Hands washed before inserting
     c. Ring folded and gently inserted into vagina
     d. Exact position of ring in vagina is not important
     e. Ring left in vagina for 3 weeks then removed
     f. New ring inserted in 7 days
     g. If ring is expelled or removed for 3 hours or more, backup method used for next 7 days after ring is reinserted in vagina
     h. If ring is left in vagina for more than 3 weeks but less than 4 weeks it should be removed; new ring inserted after 1-week ring-free period
     i. If ring is left in vagina more than 4 weeks it may not protect from pregnancy; backup method used until new ring in vagina for 7 days
     j. Use of condoms considered for STD/HIV prevention

k.　Healthcare provider contacted if warning signs occur—same as COC warning signs

- Progestin-Only Injectable Contraception (Depo-Provera [DMPA])
  1. Description—intramuscular, injectable progestin administered in 3-month intervals for contraception
  2. Mechanism of action
     a. Inhibits ovulation through suppression of FSH and LH
     b. Produces atrophic endometrium
     c. Thickens cervical mucus
     d. Slows ovum transport through fallopian tube
     e. May inhibit sperm capacitation
  3. Effectiveness/first-year failure rate
     a. Perfect use—0.3%
     b. Typical use—0.3%
  4. Advantages
     a. Ease of use
     b. Effective
     c. Long-term contraceptive option
     d. Does not require compliance with daily/event regimen
     e. Does not have drug interaction profile
     f. Results in absence of menstrual bleeding in up to 50% of women by end of first year of use (4 injections); by end of second year 70% are amenorrheic
     g. Contains no estrogen for women in whom it is contraindicated or who cannot tolerate estrogenic side effects
     h. Can be used during lactation
     i. May decrease the following
        (1) Intravascular sickling in patients with sickle cell disease
        (2) Incidence of seizures in affected individuals
  5. Disadvantages/side effects
     a. Menstrual cycle irregularities
     b. Mastalgia
     c. Depression
     d. No protection against STD/HIV
     e. Not immediately reversible—requires 3 months to be eliminated
     f. Requires routine 3-month injection schedule
     g. Weight gain
        (1) Average 5.4 pounds first year
        (2) 13.8 pounds after 4 years
     h. 6- to 12-month delay in return to fertility in some women
     i. Decreased bone density in long-term (greater than 5 years) user—returned to normal following discontinuance
     j. May decrease HDL cholesterol

  6. Contraindications (WHO recommendations)
     a. Refrain from providing if any of the following conditions exist
        (1) Pregnancy
        (2) Breast cancer
     b. Exercise caution if any of the following conditions exist
        (1) Lactation (less than 6 weeks postpartum)
        (2) History of breast cancer with 5-year disease-free interval
        (3) Current deep vein thrombosis or pulmonary emboli
        (4) Liver conditions such as cirrhosis, adenoma, cancer, or active viral hepatitis
        (5) Current/history of ischemic heart disease or cerebrovascular disease
        (6) Hypertension systolic > 160 or diastolic > 100 or vascular disease
        (7) Multiple risk factors for arterial cardiovascular disease
        (8) Unexplained vaginal bleeding before evaluation
        (9) Development of migraine headaches with neurological symptoms while using the method
  7. Management
     a. Health assessment prior to initiation of method
        (1) Refer to COC section
        (2) Include relevant health history
        (3) Baseline weight assessment
     b. Health assessment at follow-up visits
        (1) Return every 3 months for injection
        (2) Determine bleeding pattern—hematocrit/hemoglobin if excessive
        (3) Assess for side effects/problems
        (4) Weight
     c. Special considerations
        (1) Consider DMPA as contraceptive of choice for women with
           (a) Seizure disorder
           (b) Sickle cell disease
        (2) DMPA may be administered within 7 days postpartum with no adverse effects on breastfeeding
  8. Instructions for using the method
     a. Explain importance of adherence to 3-month injection schedule—contraceptive efficacy maintained for 14 weeks after injection
     b. Administer first injection within first 5 days of menstrual period
     c. Rule out pregnancy prior to first injection if administered other than within first 5 days of menstrual period
     d. Counsel patients regarding possibility of irregular bleeding; use of backup

contraception if more than 3 months between injections; use of condoms for STD/HIV prevention

   e. Procedure for injection

     (1) Deep intramuscular injection in deltoid or gluteal muscle

     (2) Do not massage injection site (alters absorption/efficacy)

     (3) Observe patient for 20 minutes following first injection to rule out allergic reaction

   f. Warning signs

     (1) Frequent intense headache

     (2) Heavy, irregular bleeding

     (3) Depression

     (4) Abdominal pain (severe)

     (5) Signs of infection at injection site (prolonged redness, bleeding, pain, discharge)

- Progestin-Only Implants
  1. Description—long-term contraceptive system of rod-shaped implant placed subdermally that provides low-dose sustained release of progestin; Implanon is the only one currently available in the United States
     a. One rod containing etonogestrel
     b. Effective for 3 years
  2. Mechanism of action
     a. Suppresses LH—ovulation inhibited—more consistent with Implanon
     b. Produces atrophic endometrium
     c. Thickens cervical mucus
     d. Decreases ovum transport through fallopian tubes
     e. May inhibit sperm capacitation
  3. Effectiveness/first-year failure rate
     a. Perfect use—0.05%
     b. Typical use—0.05%
  4. Advantages
     a. Ease of use
     b. Effective
     c. Reversible—fertility returns immediately upon removal
     d. Contains no estrogen for women with contradictions to estrogen or who cannot tolerate estrogenic side effects
     e. Can be used during lactation
     f. Affords long-term contraception
     g. High continuation rate
  5. Disadvantages and side effects
     a. Requires surgical procedure for insertion and removal; insertion/removal fees expensive
     b. Efficacy compromised when taking anti-seizure medications (except valproic acid) and rifampin—more likely with Norplant

   c. Pain, bruising, infection (potential) at insertion site

   d. Irregular bleeding

   e. No protection against STD/HIV

   f. Implants may be visible

   g. Possible side effects include

     (1) Increased incidence of functional ovarian cysts—more likely with Norplant

     (2) Mastalgia

     (3) Depression

     (4) Acne

6. Contraindications (WHO recommendations)
   a. Refrain from providing if any of the following conditions exist
      (1) Pregnancy
      (2) Breast cancer
   b. Exercise caution if any of the following conditions exist
      (1) Use of drugs that alter liver enzymes (same as with COC)
      (2) Lactation (less than 6 weeks postpartum)
      (3) History of breast cancer with 5-year disease-free interval
      (4) Current deep vein thrombosis or pulmonary emboli
      (5) Liver conditions such as cirrhosis, adenoma, cancer, active viral hepatitis
      (6) Current/history of ischemic heart disease or cerebrovascular accident
      (7) Development of migraine headaches with focal neurological symptoms while using method
      (8) Unexplained vaginal bleeding before evaluation
7. Management
   a. Health assessment prior to initiation of method
      (1) Refer to COC section
      (2) Include relevant health history
   b. Health assessment at follow-up visits
      (1) Return 1 month after insertion to assess site
      (2) Routine annual visits
   c. Special considerations
      (1) Drug interaction—same as with COC
      (2) Good option for diabetic women—no impact on carbohydrate metabolism
8. Instructions for using the method
   a. Use backup contraception for 3–7 days following insertion
   b. Insert within 7 days of start of menstrual period
   c. Rule out pregnancy, if inserted other than within 7 days of start of menstrual period
   d. Inform patient of replacement date for implants

e. Discuss efficacy decline after replacement date
f. Discuss use of condoms for STD prevention
g. Discuss possible bleeding changes
h. Warning signs
  (1) Abdominal pain (severe)
  (2) Arm pain
  (3) Increased/heavy vaginal bleeding
  (4) Bleeding/drainage from insertion area
  (5) Missed menses after period of regularity
  (6) Onset of severe headaches

- Emergency Contraception
  1. Definition—method used to prevent conception after unprotected coitus; involves use of either progestin-only pills (POP) or a copper-containing IUD
  2. Mechanism of action
    a. POP
      (1) Inhibits ovulation (refer to POP mechanism of action section)
      (2) Alters sperm/ova transport
      (3) Will not disrupt an established pregnancy—minimal endometrial effect
    b. Copper-containing IUD
      (1) Prevents fertilization (regular use)
      (2) Interferes with implantation
  3. Effectiveness
    a. POP
      (1) Depends on preexisting fertility
      (2) Reduces risk of pregnancy by at least 75%
      (3) Effective up to 5 days after unprotected intercourse; the sooner taken, the greater the efficacy
    b. IUD—reduces risk of pregnancy by more than 99%
  4. Advantages
    a. Provides means of emergency contraception in event of
      (1) Unplanned intercourse
      (2) Method failure—condom breaks/leaks; IUD expelled; cap/diaphragm dislodged/improperly placed
      (3) Missed COC pills at beginning of pack
      (4) Late for contraceptive injection
      (5) POP may be provided with instructions for use for women using any contraceptive method
    b. Can provide continuous contraception (IUD)
  5. Disadvantages and side effects
    a. POP
      (1) Nausea/vomiting—23% and 6% respectively
      (2) Change in next menses

    b. Copper-containing IUD
      (1) Irregular, heavy bleeding
      (2) Uterine cramping/abdominal pain
      (3) Refer to section on IUD
  6. Precautions and risks
    a. POP
      (1) Contraindication—pregnancy
      (2) Consider actual risk of pregnancy vs. theoretical risk
    b. Copper-containing IUD
      (1) Contraindications
        (a) Pregnancy
        (b) Pelvic inflammatory disease
      (2) See IUD section for details
  7. Management
    a. Health assessment prior to initiation of method
      (1) Urine hCG as needed to determine preexisting pregnancy
      (2) If using IUD
        (a) Speculum examination; wet prep/cervical cultures to assess for STD
        (b) Bimanual examination; determine size/position/consistency of uterus
      (3) Discuss/provide ongoing contraception
    b. Health assessment at follow-up visits
      (1) Follow-up visit if no menses within 1 month or if pregnancy symptoms
      (2) Check placement of IUD (visible string) after first menses
      (3) Perform pregnancy test as needed to determine efficacy
      (4) Discuss/provide ongoing contraception
      (5) Discourage use of emergency contraception as contraceptive method
  8. Instructions for using the method
    a. Progestin-only pills
      (1) Begin first dose within 120 hours after coitus (most effective if initiated within 72 hours)
      (2) Two-dose and single-dose options available
    b. IUD—can be inserted up to 5 days after intercourse

☐ INTRAUTERINE DEVICES/SYSTEMS

1. Description—device placed in uterus for purpose of long-acting contraception
   a. Copper T 380A
     (1) "T" shaped plastic device with copper wrapped around both vertical stem and horizontal arms
     (2) Effective for 10 years

b. Progesterone T
   (1) "T" shaped plastic device with steroid reservoir in vertical stem that contains progesterone
   (2) 65 mcg of progesterone released daily into uterine cavity
   (3) Effective for 1 year
c. Levonorgestrel intrauterine system (LNG IUS)
   (1) "T" shaped plastic frame with steroid reservoir in vertical stem that contains levonorgestrel
   (2) 20 mcg of levonorgestrel released daily into uterine cavity
   (3) Effective for 5 years

2. Mechanism of action
   a. Copper T 380A
      (1) Copper may inhibit sperm capacitation
      (2) Alters tubal/uterine transport of ovum
      (3) Enzymatic influence on endometrium
   b. Progesterone T and LNG IUS—progestin influence
      (1) Thickens cervical mucus
      (2) Produces atrophic endometrium
      (3) Slows ovum transport through tube
      (4) Inhibits sperm motility and function

3. Effectiveness/first-year failure rate
   a. Perfect use
      (1) Copper T—0.6%
      (2) Progesterone T—1.5%
      (3) LNG IUS—0.71%
   b. Typical use
      (1) Copper T—0.8%
      (2) Progesterone T—2.0%
      (3) LNG IUS—0.71%

4. Advantages
   a. Ease of use
   b. Not coitally dependent
   c. Effective
   d. Reversible
   e. No systemic side effects
   f. Cost effective (if used longer than 1 year)
   g. Progestin IUD/IUS can decrease blood loss during menses
   h. Effective choice for women who cannot use other hormonal methods
   i. Can be used during lactation

5. Disadvantages and side effects
   a. Altered menstrual bleeding patterns
      (1) Increased amount and length of menstrual bleeding—Copper T; first few months of LNG IUS
      (2) Increased dysmenorrhea—Copper T
      (3) Absence of bleeding—LNG IUS
   b. Risk of PID
      (1) Increased risk first few weeks following insertion

   (2) Poor choice for women exposed to STD
      (a) Recent history of STD
      (b) Multiple sexual partners
   c. Risk of spontaneous expulsion
      (1) May go undetected by the woman
      (2) More likely at time of menses

6. Contraindications (WHO category 4)
   a. Refrain from providing if any of the following conditions exist
      (1) Known/suspected pregnancy
      (2) PID current or within past 3 months
      (3) Severely distorted uterine cavity
         (a) Leiomyomata
         (b) Endometrial polyps
         (c) Cervical stenosis
         (d) Bicornuate uterus
         (e) Small uterus
      (4) Unexplained vaginal bleeding before evaluation
      (5) Cervical cancer awaiting treatment
      (6) Breast cancer
      (7) Endometrial cancer
   b. Exercise caution WHO category 3 theoretical risks outweigh benefit
      (1) Increased risk for STD—multiple partners, partner with multiple partners
      (2) AIDS-defining illness
      (3) Active hepatitis, severe cirrhosis, benign/malignant liver tumor—LNG IUS only

7. Management
   a. Health assessment prior to initiation of method
      (1) History to include
         (a) STD/PID—current, history of, or symptoms
         (b) Risk factors for STD
         (c) Vaginitis symptoms
         (d) Contraceptive history (e.g., condom use)
         (e) HIV status/exposure
         (f) Pap smear—abnormal results
         (g) Heavy menses/anemia
         (h) Menstrual history
      (2) Physical examination to include
         (a) Speculum examination with wet prep to assess for possible vaginal/cervical infection
            (i) Cervicitis/cervical discharge
            (ii) Suspect infection if numerous WBC
         (b) Pap smear (if none within past year)
         (c) Cervical cultures (if history/physical examination indicates)

(d) Bimanual examination—contour; size; consistency; mobility; position of uterus

(e) Hgb/Hct if history of anemia

b. Health assessment at follow-up visits

(1) Speculum examination at first menses after insertion—check for IUD strings

(2) Assessment for any signs/symptoms of pelvic infection

(3) Hgb/Hct if increased bleeding

c. Special considerations

(1) Prophylactic antibiotics at time of insertion

(a) No consensus regarding risk reduction for postinsertion infection

(b) May use doxycycline 1-time dose at time of insertion

(2) Timing of insertion

(a) Not necessary to wait for menses if evidence patient is not pregnant

(b) May be inserted at any time if patient not pregnant

(i) May be inserted immediately after childbirth

(ii) May be inserted when breast feeding

(iii) May be inserted immediately after spontaneous or induced abortion

(3) Menstrual abnormalities (spotting, bleeding)

(a) Hgb/Hct

(i) Ferrous sulfate for 2 months if Hgb less than 11.5 g—repeat Hgb/Hct 3 months

(ii) Remove IUD if Hgb less than 9 g—repeat Hgb/Hct 1 month

(b) Assess for endometritis/PID if associated with pain

(i) Cervical cultures

(ii) Uterine tenderness

(iii) Treat with antibiotics if suspicious

(c) If more than 40 years old and prolonged heavy bleeding, remove IUD

(4) Cramping and pain

(a) If severe—rule out perforation

(b) If mild—NSAID/other analgesic or remove IUD

(c) May indicate infection, pregnancy

(5) Expulsion

(a) Symptoms—cramping, spotting, dyspareunia, lengthening of string

(b) Partial expulsion

(i) Remove IUD

(ii) Rule out pregnancy/infection

(iii) Replace IUD if patient desires

(iv) Doxycycline for 5–7 days

(c) Complete expulsion

(i) Pregnancy test

(ii) Replace IUD if patient desires

(6) Pregnancy

(a) SAB

(i) Remove IUD

(ii) Doxycycline/ampicillin for 7 days

(iii) Ferrous sulfate if anemic/heavy bleeding

(b) Patient requests abortion—refer

(c) Patient wants to continue pregnancy—visible strings

(i) Advise concerning risk for spontaneous abortion—decreased risk with IUD removal early in pregnancy

(ii) Gently remove IUD

(iii) Warning about possible ectopic

(d) Patient wants to continue pregnancy—no visible strings

(i) Advise concerning risk for spontaneous abortion

(ii) Ultrasound to determine if IUD present

(iii) Monitor for intrauterine infection throughout pregnancy and retrieve IUD at delivery

(iv) If intrauterine infection occurs refer for evacuation of uterus

(7) Perforation, embedding

(a) Perforation occurs 1 in 1,000 insertions

(i) Ultrasound to determine location—refer for treatment

(ii) If protrusion through cervix, can be removed in office with local anesthetic

(iii) May/may not be associated with severe pain

(b) Embedding

(i) Can remove IUD from uterus with forceps if visualized

(ii) May need to be removed with D&C

(8) PID

(a) Most IUD-related PID occurs within the first 20 days after insertion

(b) If symptomatic PID occurs, antibiotic therapy should be initiated and the IUD removed

(9) Actinomycosis on Pap smear
    (a) Asymptomatic
        (i) Repeat Pap smear in 1 year
        (ii) If actinomycosis present on repeat Pap smear
           a) Remove IUD; replace after one menstrual cycle
           b) Keep IUD and treat with doxycycline for 14 days; repeat Pap smear
           c) Keep IUD and do not treat; advise to notify healthcare provider if PID symptoms develop
    (b) Symptoms of PID
        (i) Preload with antibiotic
        (ii) Remove IUD
        (iii) Treat PID

8. Instructions for using the method
    a. Check IUD strings
      (1) After each menses
      (2) If increased cramping
      (3) If absent—use backup birth control and notify healthcare provider
      (4) If longer
        (a) May be in process of expulsion
        (b) Use backup birth control and notify healthcare provider
    b. Signs of infection—notify healthcare provider if
      (1) Pelvic pain
      (2) Vaginal discharge
      (3) Unexplained vaginal bleeding
    c. Monitor menses—notify provider if
      (1) Heavy, irregular bleeding
      (2) Missed menses
      (3) Increased cramping
    d. Warning signs (PAINS)
      (1) **P**eriod late/missed; abnormal spotting or bleeding
      (2) **A**bdominal pain
      (3) **I**nfection—vaginal discharge
      (4) **N**ot feeling well—fever, aches, chills
      (5) **S**tring missing, shorter or longer

- Vaginal Spermicides
  1. Description—cream, foam, suppository, tablet, film, gel, or other preparation that destroys sperm when placed in vagina
  2. Mechanism of action
     a. Nonoxynol-9 or octoxynol-9 is active ingredient
     b. Destroys sperm cell membrane
  3. Effectiveness/first-year failure rate
     a. Perfect use—6%
     b. Typical use—21–28%
  4. Advantages
     a. Accessible
     b. Inexpensive
     c. Readily available backup method
     d. No systemic effects
  5. Disadvantages and side effects
     a. Coitally dependent
     b. Does not protect against STD/HIV
     c. Potential for allergy/sensitivity/irritation
     d. Must follow instructions for effective use
  6. Precautions and risks
     a. Individuals with skin sensitivities may want to test/avoid use
     b. Individual must be capable of following instructions for use
     c. Vaginal abnormalities (septa, prolapse) may preclude use
  7. Management
     a. No health assessment needed prior to initiation of method
     b. Special considerations—encourage use of spermicide with condom for increased effectiveness
  8. Instructions for using method
     a. Spermicide used with each act of intercourse
     b. All instructions read carefully
     c. Spermicide left in place (no douching) for 6 hours following last intercourse
     d. Instructions should be followed regarding how long prior to intercourse the spermicide may be inserted—if too much time has lapsed, pregnancy may occur
     e. Spermicide placed deep within vagina
     f. Adequate time should be allowed for spermicide to dissolve (if film, tablets, or suppositories)
     g. With foam use—canister should be shaken well, as directed, prior to filling applicator

- Male Condoms
  1. Description—latex/polyurethane/natural membranous sleeve placed over erect penis prior to intercourse to prevent transmission of semen/sperm into vaginal vault
  2. Mechanism of action—barrier; prevents transmission of semen/sperm into vagina
  3. Effectiveness/first-year failure rate
     a. Perfect use—3%
     b. Typical use—14%
  4. Advantages
     a. Accessible
     b. Cost effective
     c. Prevents transmission of STD (except membrane condoms)

    d. Active involvement of male partner

    e. Prevents allergic reaction to semen

    f. Arrests development of antisperm antibodies in infertility patients

    g. May help prevent premature ejaculation

    h. Does not require visit to healthcare provider

5. Disadvantages and side effects
    a. Decreased penile sensitivity
    b. Interrupts act of love making
    c. Not appropriate for men with erectile dysfunction
    d. Requires active involvement of male partner
    e. Possibility of condom rupture

6. Contraindications
    a. Latex allergy (male or female partner)—use polyurethane
    b. Spermicide allergy (if condoms lubricated with spermicide)

7. Management
    a. No health assessment needed prior to initiation of method
    b. Special considerations
      (1) Membrane condoms may not protect against STD/HIV
      (2) Petroleum/oil-based lubricants may decrease effectiveness of latex condoms (okay for polyurethane condom)

8. Instructions for using method
    a. New condom used with each act of intercourse
    b. Use only water soluble lubricants—K-Y jelly, Astroglide, Replens, Lubrin
    c. Condom unrolled over penis completely (to the base)
    d. Penis withdrawn from vagina soon after ejaculation—condom secured at base of penis to prevent spillage
    e. If condom slips/breaks
      (1) Before ejaculation—apply new condom
      (2) After ejaculation—consider emergency contraception

- Female Condom
1. Description—polyurethane sheath placed in the vagina that acts as a barrier to prevent direct contact with seminal fluid during intercourse
2. Mechanism of action—barrier, protects vagina/vulva from direct contact with penis/seminal fluid
3. Effectiveness/first-year failure rate
    a. Perfect use—5%
    b. Typical use—21%
4. Advantages
    a. Prevents transmission of STD
      (1) Decreases risk of cervical dysplasia/neoplasia related to HPV

      (2) Decreases risk of PID and sequelae due to decreased transmission of gonococcal (GC) and chlamydia
    b. Does not require use of spermicide
    c. Accessible
    d. Controlled by the woman
    e. Does not require visit to healthcare provider

5. Disadvantages and side effects
    a. Coitally dependent
    b. Noisy
    c. May be aesthetically unappealing
    d. Expensive

6. Precautions and risks
    a. Must be properly inserted/positioned
    b. Polyurethane allergy

7. Management
    a. No health assessment needed prior to initiation of method
    b. Special considerations—women with vaginal abnormalities should not use this method

8. Instructions for using the method
    a. Pouch held with open end down—inner ring should be at bottom of pouch
    b. Inner ring squeezed together and inner ring and pouch inserted into vagina
    c. Inner ring pushed deep into vagina
    d. Outer ring should rest outside vulva
    e. Condom removed immediately after intercourse
    f. Outer ring squeezed together and twisted to prevent spillage
    g. Discard
    h. New condom used with each act of intercourse
    i. Male condom should not be used when using female condom—may adhere together causing dislodgement

- Diaphragm
1. Description—reusable latex dome that covers anterior vaginal wall, including cervix; spermicide placed in dome covers cervix affording increased contraceptive protection; types include
    a. Flat spring
      (1) Good for women with firm vaginal tone
      (2) Gentle spring strength
    b. Coil spring
      (1) Good for women with average vaginal tone
      (2) Firm spring strength
    c. Arcing spring
      (1) Good for women with lax vaginal tone
      (2) Firm spring strength

d. Wide seal
 (1) Good for women with average/lax vaginal tone
 (2) Available as arcing or coil spring

2. Mechanism of action
 a. Barrier—prevents direct cervical contact with seminal fluid
 b. Spermicide—nonoxynol-9/octoxynol-9 destroys sperm cell membrane

3. Effectiveness/first-year failure rate
 a. Perfect use—6%
 b. Typical use—20%

4. Advantages
 a. Cost effective—may be used for 1–2 years
 b. Affords some protection against STD—possible decreased incidence of PID
 c. No systemic effects

5. Disadvantages and side effects
 a. Requires sizing by trained clinician and instructions in use
 b. May have sensitivity to latex/spermicide
 c. Increased risk of bacterial vaginosis and UTI
  (1) Due to increased colonization with *E. coli*
  (2) Related to use of spermicide
  (3) Mechanical irritation/compression against urethra
 d. Does not afford absolute protection from STD/HIV
 e. Risk of toxic shock—2–3/100,000 per year
 f. Inability to learn correct insertion technique

6. Contraindications
 a. Known allergy to latex or spermicide
 b. Inability to follow directions for insertion
 c. Significant vaginal relaxation—prolapse/cystocele/rectocele
 d. Frequent/recurrent UTI
 e. History of toxic shock

7. Management
 a. Health assessment prior to initiation of method
  (1) Routine annual Pap smear
  (2) Proper fit by trained professional—determine appropriate size and type for woman's anatomy
 b. Health assessment at follow-up visits—recheck fit following childbirth or if patient gains/loses 15 pounds or more

8. Instructions for using the method
 a. General instructions (patient)
  (1) Insert just prior to intercourse or up to 6 hours before
  (2) Coat inner dome with 1 tablespoon of spermicide

  (3) Pinch sides of diaphragm and insert fully into vagina
   (a) Tuck anterior rim behind symphysis
   (b) Be certain that dome covers cervix
  (4) If repeated intercourse, insert another application of spermicide in vagina; do not remove diaphragm
  (5) Leave diaphragm in place for at least 6 hours following last intercourse
  (6) Do not leave in place for more than 24 hours
  (7) After each use wash and store diaphragm in clean, cool, dark environment
  (8) Do not use with oil-based lubricants or vaginal medications
  (9) Replace diaphragm yearly
  (10) Assess for holes/tears periodically by filling with water and inspecting for leaks
 b. Warning signs (toxic shock)
  (1) High fever
  (2) Nausea, vomiting, diarrhea
  (3) Syncope, weakness
  (4) Joint/muscle aches
  (5) Rash resembling sunburn

- Cervical Cap
1. Description—reusable rubber cap, fits over cervix providing barrier contraception; spermicide placed in dome affords additional contraceptive efficacy
2. Mechanism of action
 a. Barrier—prevents direct cervical contact with seminal fluid
 b. Spermicide—nonoxynol-9/octoxynol-9 destroys sperm cell membrane
3. Effectiveness/first-year failure rate
 a. Perfect use
  (1) Parous women—26%
  (2) Nulliparous women—9%
 b. Typical use
  (1) Parous women—40%
  (2) Nulliparous women—20%
4. Advantages
 a. Cost effective—may be used for 1 year
 b. Affords some protection against STD
 c. Possible decreased incidence of PID
 d. Possible decreased incidence of cervical dysplasia/neoplasia
 e. No systemic effects
 f. May be left in place for 48 hours
 g. Does not require insertion of more spermicide with repeat intercourse
 h. Does not increase incidence of bladder infection

5. Disadvantages and side effects
   a. Requires trained clinician for sizing
   b. Sensitivity to latex/spermicide
   c. Does not afford absolute protection against STD/HIV
   d. Not every woman can be fitted appropriately
   e. May become dislodged during intercourse
6. Contraindications
   a. Known allergy to latex or spermicide
   b. Inability to insert properly
   c. History of toxic shock
   d. Full-term vaginal delivery within past 6 weeks; recent abortion/vaginal bleeding
   e. Known/suspected cervical/uterine cancer
   f. Current abnormal Pap smear
7. Management
   a. Health assessment prior to initiation of method
      (1) Pap smear within past year
      (2) Visualization of cervix to rule out abnormalities
         (a) Extensive lacerations
         (b) Cervicitis
         (c) Asymmetry
      (3) Palpation of cervix
         (a) Length
         (b) Position
         (c) Circumference
   b. Health assessment at follow-up visits—re-evaluate cap fit especially if patient complains of dislodgement during intercourse
   c. Special considerations
      (1) Not all women can achieve a good cervical cap fit
         (a) Cervix too short
         (b) Cap sizes not appropriate
      (2) Efficacy significantly decreased in parous women
      (3) Using cap without spermicide is common but not recommended
8. Instructions for using method
   a. Insert cap at least 30 minutes prior to intercourse to create suction
   b. Fill one-third of cap with spermicide
   c. Compress rim prior to insertion
   d. Advance into vagina so rim can slide over cervix
   e. Check that cap covers cervix
   f. Not necessary to reinsert spermicide with repeated intercourse
   g. FDA recommends removal within 48 hours
   h. Cap should be refit and replaced yearly
   i. Warning signs (toxic shock)
   j. Refer to diaphragm section for warning signs of toxic shock

- Fertility Awareness Methods
  1. Description—method of contraception using abstinence during estimated fertile period based on all or some of the following methods
     a. Menstrual cycle pattern (calendar method)
     b. Basal body temperature (BBT)—determines ovulation
     c. Evaluation of cervical mucus (ovulation/Billings method)—determines ovulation
     d. Sympto-thermal method—combines BBT with evaluation of cervical mucus and cervical position/consistency
  2. Mechanism of action—intercourse is avoided during fertile period
     a. Ovum remains fertile for 24 hours
     b. Sperm viability approximately 72 hours
     c. Most pregnancies occur when intercourse occurs before ovulation
  3. Effectiveness/first-year failure rate
     a. Perfect use
        (1) Calendar method—9%
        (2) BBT—2%
        (3) Ovulation method—3%
        (4) Sympto-thermal—2%
     b. Typical use for all methods—25%
  4. Advantages
     a. Minimal cost
     b. Natural
        (1) No systemic effects
        (2) No localized side effects, e.g., latex allergy
     c. Can be utilized for contraception and conception planning
  5. Disadvantages and side effects
     a. Requires motivation from both partners
     b. Requires periodic abstinence
     c. No protection against STD/HIV
  6. Precautions and risks
     a. Not reliable for women
        (1) With irregular menses (consider sympto-thermal and ovulation methods)
        (2) Who are perimenopausal
        (3) Who are recently postpartum
        (4) Who have had recent menarche
     b. Not a suitable method for
        (1) Women who cannot accurately evaluate their fertile period
           (a) Inability to use/read thermometer
           (b) Inability to understand cervical mucus/changes
           (c) Inability to time intercourse based on calendar evaluation
        (2) Couples unwilling to abstain during fertile time period
        (3) If nonconsensual coitus is likely to occur

7. Management
   a. Health assessment prior to initiation of method
      (1) History to reflect pattern of menses
      (2) Evaluation of client's willingness/ability to check cervical mucus/consistency/position
   b. Health assessment at follow-up visits—BBT/sympto-thermal chart evaluation
   c. Special considerations—combination of fertility awareness methods more effective than single method
8. Instructions for using the method
   a. Calendar method
      (1) Keep record of menstrual cycle intervals for several months
      (2) From the shortest cycle length, subtract 18 days—this determines first fertile day
      (3) From the longest cycle length, subtract 11 days—this determines last fertile day
      (4) Use these numbers to determine days of abstinence for every cycle
   b. BBT method
      (1) Take temperature each morning before rising
         (a) BBT thermometer
         (b) Temperature can be oral, vaginal, or rectal (maintain same route)
      (2) Record on BBT chart
      (3) Temperature increase of 0.4° F or higher at ovulation—remains elevated for at least 3 days
      (4) Abstain from intercourse until 3-day temperature increase occurs
   c. Ovulation method
      (1) Inspect cervical mucus/secretions on underwear, toilet tissue with fingers, beginning day after menses
      (2) Determine consistency—elastic, slippery, wet by touch indicates pre-ovulatory
         (a) Amount increases; becomes thinner and more elastic around time of ovulation
         (b) After ovulation, mucus becomes thick, tacky, and cloudy
      (3) Abstain from intercourse during "wet days" at onset of increased, slippery, thin mucus discharge until 4 days past the peak day (last day of clear, stretchy, slippery secretions)
      (4) Abstain from intercourse during menses due to inability to assess mucus

   d. Sympto-thermal method—combines ovulation, BBT, and assessment of consistency/position of cervix in vagina
      (1) Uses cervical assessment method and BBT
      (2) Ovulatory pain "mittelschmerz" may be indicator
      (3) Abstain until latter of two methods indicates "safe" time

- Lactational Amenorrhea Method
   1. Description—method of contraception for women who are breastfeeding without supplementation or with minimal supplementation and have not had a postpartum menstrual cycle
   2. Mechanism of action—high prolactin
      a. FSH normal; LH decreased—no ovarian follicular development
      b. Inhibits pulsatile GnRH
      c. Results in anovulation
   3. Effectiveness/first-year failure rate
      a. Perfect use—0.5–1.5% (if amenorrheic)
      b. Typical use—data not available
   4. Advantages
      a. Temporary
      b. No cost
      c. Highly effective until infant nutritional requirements mandate supplementation (approximately 6 months)
      d. Not coitally dependent
      e. Advantageous for infant
         (1) Nutritional
         (2) Bonding
      f. Requires no devices
      g. Minimal systemic effects
   5. Disadvantages and side effects
      a. Woman must breastfeed completely or with minimal supplementation—may lead to exhaustion
      b. Decreased estrogen due to absence of follicular development
         (1) Atrophic vaginitis
         (2) Decreased vaginal lubrication
         (3) Dyspareunia
      c. Affords no protection against STD/HIV
   6. Precautions and risks
      a. Efficacy decreases with resumption of menses
      b. Must breastfeed completely or with minimal supplementation
   7. Management
      a. No health assessment needed prior to initiation of method

b. Special considerations—should not use vaginal estrogen cream to treat atrophic vaginitis
  (1) Absorption can inhibit milk production
  (2) Recommend use of vaginal lubricants
8. Instructions for using method
  a. Minimal or no supplementation should be used
  b. Alternative contraceptive method should be considered when any of the following occur
    (1) Menses
    (2) Regular supplementation is being used
    (3) Long periods without breastfeeding
    (4) Baby is 6 months old
  c. Ovulation may occur before onset of menses

- Coitus Interruptus (Withdrawal)
1. Description—contraceptive method whereby male withdraws penis from vagina prior to ejaculation
2. Mechanism of action—no contact between sperm and ovum
3. Effectiveness/first-year failure rate
  a. Perfect use—4%
  b. Typical use—19%
4. Advantages
  a. Requires no devices
  b. No systemic effects
  c. No expense
  d. May result in decreased transmission of HIV (man to woman)
5. Disadvantages and side effects
  a. Requires self-control on part of male partner
  b. Requires ability to predict time of ejaculation
  c. Does not afford protection from STD
6. Precautions and risks—should not be used by men with premature ejaculatory disorder
7. Management
  a. No health assessment needed prior to initiation of method
  b. Special considerations
    (1) In itself, preejaculatory fluid contains no sperm
    (2) If multiple acts of coitus occur, efficacy is decreased as subsequent preejaculatory fluid may have "carry over" sperm from previous ejaculation
8. Instructions for using the method
  a. Male partner should void prior to intercourse
  b. Penis is withdrawn prior to ejaculation—ejaculation occurs away from vaginal area
  c. Repeated orgasms may result in presence of sperm in preejaculatory fluid

- Abstinence
1. Description—contraception based on abstaining from penile-vaginal or penile-rectal contact
2. Mechanism of action—no possibility of conception as genital contact does not occur
3. Effectiveness/first-year failure rate
  a. Perfect use—100%
  b. Typical use—data not available
4. Advantages
  a. No cost
  b. No side effects
  c. Protection against sexually transmitted diseases
5. Disadvantages—requires motivation and acceptance by both partners
6. Precautions and risks—couples should refrain from alcohol/drug use to "stay in control"
7. Management—no health assessment needed prior to initiation of method
8. Instructions for using the method
  a. Avoid any penile-vaginal/rectal contact
  b. Consider alternative means of intimacy/sexual expression, e.g., mutual masturbation
  c. Avoid alcohol or drug use, may affect commitment to method

- Female Sterilization
1. Description—permanent contraception for woman achieved through surgical means; commonly performed on outpatient basis or postpartum prior to discharge using laparoscopy
2. Mechanism of action
  a. Fallopian tubes are obstructed to prevent union of sperm and ovum
    (1) Surgical ligation—Pomeroy procedure
    (2) Surgical ligation and attachment to uterine body—Irving procedure
    (3) Electrocauterization
    (4) Section of tube excised—Pritchard procedure, fimbriectomy
    (5) Occluded—compressed with falope ring
    (6) Transcervical method—micro insert device inserted into fallopian tubes with catheter; expands and occludes tubes
3. Effectiveness/first-year failure rate
  a. Perfect use—0.5%
  b. Typical use—0.5%
4. Advantages
  a. Affords permanent contraception
  b. Highly effective
  c. Cost effective over long term
  d. Not coitally dependent

5. Disadvantages and side effects
   a. Invasive surgical procedure requiring anesthesia
   b. Reversal is difficult, expensive, and often unsuccessful
   c. No protection against STD/HIV
   d. Initially expensive
6. Precautions and risks
   a. Surgical procedure
      (1) Operative complications—bladder/uterine/intestinal injury may occur
      (2) Anesthetic complications—death (rare)
   b. Wound infection
   c. If pregnancy occurs following procedure, increased risk of ectopic
7. Management
   a. Health assessment prior to initiation of method
      (1) Is patient candidate for surgery
      (2) Assess psychological readiness for permanent contraceptive method
   b. Health assessment at follow-up visits—assess for signs/symptoms of infection
      (1) Fever
      (2) Wound tenderness
      (3) Wound drainage
      (4) Abdominal pain
   c. Special considerations
      (1) Consent form signed in advance
      (2) Patient should be advised procedure is irreversible
8. Instructions for using the method
   a. Nothing by mouth at least 8 hours prior to procedure
   b. Need transportation assistance from hospital/clinic to home
   c. Rest for at least 24 hours recommended following procedure
   d. Light lifting only for 1 week
   e. No coitus for 1 week
   f. Warning signs (notify healthcare provider)
      (1) Fever greater than 100° F
      (2) Severe pain
      (3) Drainage from incision
      (4) Dizziness/fainting/vertigo

- Male Sterilization
  1. Description—permanent contraception involving occlusion of vas deferens, preventing transmission of sperm through semen
     a. Surgical resection—surgical incision made in scrotum; vas deferens is resected
     b. Occlusion—surgical incision made in scrotum; vas deferens is divided and fulgurated/tied/cauterized
     c. No scalpel—ring forceps secures vas deferens; dissecting forceps punctures skin of scrotum; vas deferens lifted out and occluded
  2. Mechanism of action—sperm not present in ejaculate
  3. Effectiveness/first-year failure rate
     a. Perfect use—0.10%
     b. Typical use—0.15%
  4. Advantages
     a. Cost effective
     b. Highly effective
     c. Affords permanent contraception
     d. Not coitally dependent
     e. No systemic effects/artificial devices
  5. Disadvantages and side effects
     a. Initial expense
     b. Should be considered irreversible
     c. Invasive surgical procedure
     d. No protection against STD/HIV
  6. Precautions and risks
     a. Surgical procedure
     b. Wound infection
  7. Management
     a. Health assessment prior to initiation of procedure—assess psychological readiness for permanent contraceptive method
     b. Health assessment at follow-up visits—assess for signs/symptoms infection
        (1) Fever
        (2) Wound tenderness
        (3) Wound drainage
        (4) Swelling
     c. Special considerations
        (1) Relationship between vasectomy and prostate cancer unclear
           (a) Study data conflicting
           (b) Prostate screening post-vasectomy is same as for men in general population
        (2) Procedure does not confer immediate sterility—up to 20 ejaculations will contain sperm
  8. Instructions for using the method
     a. Rest recommended for approximately 48 hours following procedure
     b. Apply ice pack to scrotum for minimum of 4 hours after procedure
     c. Avoid lifting/exercise for minimum of 1 week
     d. Keep area dry for 48 hours
     e. Abstain from intercourse for 48 hours
     f. Continue using other contraception until minimum of 20 ejaculations; obtain semen analysis to confirm azoospermia
     g. Warning signs
        (1) Fever greater than 100° F
        (2) Increasing pain
        (3) Increasing swelling/tension on stitches
        (4) Bleeding/drainage from incision

- Abortion
  1. Medical methods
     a. Mifepristone plus misoprostol
        (1) Most effective at 7 weeks gestation or earlier
           (a) 95% effective at 7 weeks LMP or earlier
           (b) 80% effective in the 9th week LMP
        (2) Mifepristone
           (a) 19-nor steroid
           (b) Progesterone antagonist
        (3) Misoprostol—prostaglandin analogue
        (4) Avoid use of nonsteroidal anti-inflammatory medications during procedure; may inhibit action of misoprostol
        (5) Method requires three clinic visits
           (a) Mifepristone orally at initial visit
           (b) Misoprostol 48 hours later if expulsion not complete—observe for 4 hours
           (c) 1–2-week follow-up appointment to assess for complete abortion
     b. Methotrexate plus misoprostol
        (1) 95% effective in early pregnancy
        (2) Methotrexate
           (a) Destroys trophoblastic tissue
           (b) Blocks folic acid preventing cell division
        (3) Two clinic visits
           (a) Methotrexate IM at initial visit
           (b) Misoprostol vaginally 3–7 days later
        (4) Avoid use of folic acid during procedure; may inhibit action of methotrexate
     c. Hypertonic saline (2nd trimester)—instilled intra-amniotically
     d. Hypertonic urea (2nd trimester)—instilled intra-amniotically
     e. Misoprostol (2nd trimester)
     f. Dinoprostone—prostaglandin vaginal suppository
  2. Surgical methods
     a. Vacuum aspiration (1st trimester)
        (1) Suction curettage
        (2) Local anesthetic
     b. Dilation and evacuation (D&E)—can be performed up to 20 weeks gestation
  3. Pre-abortion health assessment and counseling
     a. History
        (1) LMP and menstrual history
        (2) Surgical history including gynecological surgeries
        (3) Contraceptive history
        (4) Medical history
        (5) Current medications/history of allergic responses
     b. Physical examination
        (1) Size of uterus
        (2) Note uterine/cervical position
        (3) Presence of uterine/cervical/adnexal abnormalities
           (a) Fibroids
           (b) Adnexal masses (rule out ectopic)
        (4) Laboratory tests
           (a) Pregnancy test—urine/serum
           (b) Hgb/Hct
           (c) Blood type and Rh
           (d) STD evaluation if warranted, e.g., sexual assault/patient concern
     c. Counseling
        (1) Discuss all pregnancy options
        (2) Discuss options for termination—medical, surgical
  4. Postabortion health assessment and counseling
     a. Contraceptive counseling
     b. Rh immunization if patient Rh negative
     c. Prophylactic antibiotics may be given to surgical patients
     d. Tissue examined to rule out molar pregnancy
  5. Potential postabortion complications
     a. Infection
     b. Retained products of conception
     c. Trauma to uterus/cervix
     d. Excessive bleeding
     e. Warning signs
        (1) Fever
        (2) Persistent/increasing lower abdominal pain
        (3) Prolonged/excessive vaginal bleeding
        (4) Purulent vaginal discharge
        (5) No return of menses within 6 weeks

◘ MENOPAUSE

  1. Definitions
     a. Menopause—cessation of menses; average age in United States is 51 years; genetically predetermined; confirmed after 12 consecutive months without a period
     b. Climacteric—term used to describe the physiologic changes associated with the change from reproductive to nonreproductive status; 2–8 years before menopause until 1 year after last period
     c. Perimenopause—another term for climacteric
     d. Postmenopause—phase of life following menopause
     e. Premature menopause (premature ovarian failure)—cessation of menses before age 40

2. Physiology
   a. As climacteric begins the rhythmic ovarian and endometrial responses of the menstrual cycle decline and eventually stop
   b. Number of responsive follicles decreases with resultant decreased production of estradiol throughout climacteric
   c. With decreasing estradiol, FSH levels increase
   d. At the end of the climacteric, ovary contains no follicles and endometrium atrophies so that reproductive capability is terminated
   e. After menopause, estrone becomes principal estrogen
   f. Estrone produced through aromatization of androstenedione; androstenedione is an androgen produced by adrenal cortex and ovarian stroma; converted to estrone in peripheral fat cells
   g. After menopause, both FSH and LH levels are elevated
   h. Generally rely on cessation of menses, hypoestrogenic symptoms, age, and consistently elevated FSH for diagnosis of menopause
3. Laboratory findings
   a. FSH—> 40 mIU/mL
   b. LH—threefold elevation after menopause (20–100 mIU/mL)
   c. Estradiol—< 20 pg/mL
4. Possible menstrual changes in climacteric
   a. No change
   b. Oligomenorrhea/olymenorrhea—cycles shorter or longer than usual
   c. Hypomenorrhea/hypermenorrhea—bleeding lighter/shorter or heavier/longer than usual
   d. Metrorrhagia—irregular intervals, amount variable
5. Physical changes
   a. Reproductive organs
      (1) Labia—decrease in subcutaneous fat and tissue elasticity
      (2) Vagina
         (a) Thinning of epithelium; decreased rugae, increase in pH (>5.0)
         (b) May have pruritus, leukorrhea, friability, increased susceptibility to infection
         (c) May have dyspareunia
      (3) Cervix—decrease in size, or may become flush with vaginal walls, may become stenotic
      (4) Uterus and ovaries—decrease in size and weight; ovaries usually not palpable
   b. Urinary tract
      (1) Decreased muscle tone—urethra and trigone area of bladder
      (2) Atrophic changes in urethra and periurethral tissue—stress incontinence may occur
      (3) Hypoestrogenic effects in trigone area; lowered sensory threshold to void—sensory urge incontinence may occur
      (4) Urinary urgency, frequency, and dysuria due to atrophic changes in urethra and periurethral tissue
   c. Breasts—reduction in size and flattened appearance; decrease in glandular tissue
   d. Skin
      (1) Thinning/decreased activity of sebaceous and sweat glands
      (2) Hyperpigmentation/hypopigmentation
      (3) Scalp, pubic, and axillary hair becomes thinner and drier
   e. Bone integrity
      (1) Increased bone loss associated with decrease in estrogen
      (2) See section on Osteoporosis in Musculoskeletal Disorders chapter for more information
6. Vasomotor symptoms—hot flashes
   a. Observed in 75% of women during climacteric
   b. Mechanism responsible not known; gonadotropin-related effect on the central thermoregulatory function of the hypothalamus (measurable increase in body surface heat and decrease in core temperature)
   c. Sudden feeling of warmth followed by visible redness of upper body and face
   d. May be associated with profuse sweating and palpitations
   e. May awaken during the night leading to insomnia, sleep disturbance, cognitive (memory) and affective (anxiety) disorders with loss of REM sleep
   f. Generally cease within 2–3 years after menopause
7. Cardiovascular system effects
   a. Lipid levels—increase in low-density lipoproteins (LDL), very-low-density lipoproteins (VLDL), and triglycerides; possible decrease in high-density lipoproteins (HDL)
   b. Regulation of clotting processes—increase in certain fibrinolytic and procoagulation factors
   c. Vasoactive substances—increase in endothelin and decrease in angiotensin-converting enzyme (vasoconstrictors),

increase in nitric oxide, and decrease in prostacyclin (vasodilators)

d. Extent of impact of decreased estrogen levels on cardiovascular disease not definitively established

8. Alterations in mood
    a. Majority of women do not have psychological problems attributable to menopause
    b. Depression in menopause often related to history of previous depression
    c. Depression/irritability may be related to sleep disturbances caused by hot flashes
    d. Perceived health shown to be a major factor related to depression in perimenopausal women; individual characteristics and self-perception appear to be important determinants of each woman's experience of the climacteric
    e. More research is needed to establish hormonal influences on mood changes that occur during the perimenopause

9. Cognitive function
    a. Memory impairment may be indirectly related to decreased estrogen secondary to hot flashes and sleep disturbance
    b. Women's Health Initiative Memory Study (2002)—use of estrogen plus progestin does not prevent dementia or mild cognitive impairment

10. Sexuality
    a. Diminished genital sensation, less vaginal expansion, and decreased vasocongestion may cause some changes in orgasm experience—increased time to reach orgasm, shorter duration of orgasm, decreased strength of orgasmic contractions
    b. Freedom from fear of pregnancy, freedom from contraceptives, and increased privacy as children leave home may increase sexual enjoyment
    c. Dyspareunia, loss of partner, medications, and chronic illness may affect sexual desire and activity

11. Health assessment/health promotion
    a. Health history
        (1) Family and personal history—focus on risks for cancer, heart disease, osteoporosis
        (2) High-risk behavior evaluation—smoking, alcohol, drugs, STD/HIV risks
        (3) Menstrual history—focus on irregular bleeding problems
        (4) Nutrition and exercise assessment
        (5) Psychosocial assessment—sexuality, stressors, support system, domestic violence

b. Physical assessment
    (1) Blood pressure
    (2) Height and weight
    (3) Complete physical examination

c. Screening tests
    (1) Pap smear every 3 years to age 70
    (2) Colorectal cancer screening beginning age 50—fecal occult blood test annually; colonoscopy every 10 years, or double contrast barium enema every 5 years
    (3) Mammography every year starting at age 40
    (4) Cholesterol with HDL every 5 years beginning at age 20, more frequent and additional lipid tests as needed (National Cholesterol Education Program [NCEP] of the National Heart, Lung, and Blood Institute)
    (5) Plasma glucose every 3 years age 45 years or older and for younger women with risk factors
    (6) Bone mass density screening—age 65 and older, earlier in postmenopausal women with risk factors (National Osteoporosis Foundation)
    (7) Screening for visual acuity and glaucoma by ophthalmologist every 2–4 years from age 40–64 and every 1–2 years beginning at age 65, earlier and more frequent screening if risk factors are present (American Academy of Ophthalmology)
    (8) Other as determined by risk factors

d. Immunizations—see section on immunizations in Health Promotion and Evaluation chapter

e. Counseling and education
    (1) High-risk behaviors
    (2) Nutrition
        (a) Food guide pyramid
        (b) Calcium
            (i) National Institutes of Health recommendations (National Institutes of Health, 2000)—for older adults, calcium intake should be maintained at 1,000–1,500 mg/day
            (ii) Calcium—National Osteoporosis Foundation (2003)
                a) All adults—at least 1,000 mg/day of elemental calcium
                b) Vitamin D 400–800 IU per day if risk for deficiency
            (iii) Dietary sources of calcium—dairy products, canned sardines

and salmon with bones, some dark green leafy vegetables, tofu, calcium-fortified foods
   (iv) Average dietary intake of calcium—450–650 mg/day
   (v) Calcium supplements—calcium carbonate most common preparation; provides most elemental calcium (40%)
   (vi) Take in two divided doses with meals if more than 600 mg/day needed
   (vii) Avoid taking with very-high-fiber foods
   (viii) Do not use aluminum-containing antacids for calcium; aluminum binds with phosphorus in GI tract and interferes with calcium absorption
   (ix) Calcium citrate better absorbed by elderly with less stomach acid
   (x) Factors interfering with calcium absorption
      a) Phosphorus in canned and processed meats, soft drinks, some packaged foods
      b) Caffeine
      c) High-protein diet
      d) Tobacco
      e) Heavy alcohol use
   (xi) Calcium interferes with iron absorption
   (xii) Vitamin D supplement (400–800 IU/day) may be necessary if ≥ 65 years old or if minimal sun exposure
   (c) Fat intake—total fat < 30% of total calories; saturated fat < 10% of total calories; cholesterol < 300 mg/day
   (d) May need decrease in calories with decrease in basal metabolic rate and physical activity
(3) Self-examination—breasts, skin, vulva
(4) Physical activity
   (a) 30 minutes or more of moderate exercise most days of the week
   (b) Weight bearing exercise—walking, stair climbing, jogging, dancing, cross country skiing
   (c) Exercises for flexibility, muscle strength, relaxation
(5) Kegel exercises

(6) Injury prevention—seat belts, safety helmets for bike riding, smoke detectors, fall prevention
(7) Sexuality
(8) Management of menopausal symptoms
(9) Benefits and risks of hormone therapy (HT)
(10) Health maintenance checkup schedule
f. Contraception for women over 40
   (1) Continue contraception until FSH level indicates no longer fertile or no menses for 1 year
   (2) Nonsmokers with no CVD risk factors may continue combination hormonal methods until age 53–55, then assume menopause and discontinue contraception
   (3) A single elevated FSH during hormone-free week is not a reliable indicator of menopause
   (4) Options
      (a) Low-dose combination oral contraception (COC)—Noncontraceptive benefits of COC may be especially attractive to the perimenopausal woman
         (i) Decreased incidence of endometrial and ovarian cancer
         (ii) Relief of vasomotor symptoms
         (iii) Increased menstrual regularity and decreased dysmenorrhea
         (iv) Possible increased bone density
      (b) Other hormonal contraception methods are also options if there are no contraindications
      (c) IUD/IUS
         (i) Long-lasting, effective contraceptive option
         (ii) Levonorgestrel IUS (LNG IUS) may also be therapeutic for perimenopausal women with heavy bleeding
      (d) Barrier methods are acceptable options
      (e) Sterilization—most prevalent contraceptive method among married women in the United States
      (f) Fertility awareness methods less effective during perimenopause with irregular menstrual cycles
12. Hormone therapy (HT)
   a. Indications
      (1) Relief of moderate to severe menopausal symptoms related to estrogen

deficiency—vasomotor instability, vulvar/vaginal atrophy

 (2) Prevention of osteoporosis—consider nonestrogen medications if not also treating for vasomotor and/or vulvo-vaginal symptoms

b. Other potential benefits—reduction in risk for colon cancer

c. Contraindications

 (1) Active or recent arterial thromboembolic disease (MI, angina)

 (2) Untreated hypertension

 (3) Venous thromboembolic disorders or thrombophlebitis

 (4) Known or suspected breast cancer

 (5) Endometrial hyperplasia

 (6) Estrogen-dependent cancer

 (7) Liver dysfunction or disease

 (8) Undiagnosed abnormal uterine bleeding

 (9) Known or suspected pregnancy

 (10) Porphyria cutanea tarda

d. Potential risks

 (1) Endometrial hyperplasia/cancer

 (2) Breast cancer

  (a) Relationship with HT inconclusive

  (b) Possible small but significant increase of breast cancer with long-term HT

 (3) Gallbladder disease

 (4) Thromboembolic disorders

e. Assessment prior to initiation of HT

 (1) Health history with attention to specific contraindications and precautions

 (2) General physical examination, gynecological examination with Pap smear, breast examination, mammogram

 (3) Base decisions concerning HT use on woman's symptoms, treatment goals, benefit-risk analysis

f. Routine follow-up after HT initiation

 (1) Reevaluate in 3 months—assess therapeutic effectiveness and any problems

 (2) Annual follow-up thereafter if no problems

  (a) Evaluate continuing need for HT—limit use to shortest duration consistent with treatment goals and risks for individual woman

  (b) Consider nonhormonal drugs for osteoporosis prevention if long-term therapy needed

g. Regimen options

 (1) Consider use of lowest dose of estrogen needed for symptom relief—0.3–0.625 mg conjugated estrogen or equivalent

 (2) 10–14 days each month of 5–10 mg of medroxyprogesterone acetate (MPA) or equivalent or daily doses of 1.5–5.0 mg recommended for prevention of endometrial hyperplasia

 (3) Continuous-combined regimen

  (a) Estrogen and progestin every day

  (b) Lower cumulative dose of progestin than with cyclic regimens

  (c) May have unpredictable bleeding

  (d) After several months endometrium atrophies and amenorrhea usually results

  (e) No estrogen-free period during which vasomotor symptoms can occur

 (4) Continuous-cyclic regimen

  (a) Estrogen every day

  (b) Progestin added 10–14 days each month

  (c) No estrogen-free period during which vasomotor symptoms can occur

  (d) Withdrawal bleeding when progestin withdrawn each month

 (5) Cyclic regimen

  (a) Estrogen days 1–25

  (b) Progestin added last 10–14 days

  (c) Followed by 3–6 days of no therapy

  (d) Withdrawal bleeding when progestin withdrawn each month

 (6) Continuous unopposed estrogen—for woman without uterus

h. Types of estrogen—estradiol, conjugated estrogen, esterified estrogen, estropipate (estrone), estriol (plant based)

i. Types of progesterone/progestin—medroxyprogesterone acetate, norethindrone, norethindrone acetate, micronized progesterone (plant based)

j. Routes of administration

 (1) Oral

  (a) Estrogen, progestin, or combination

  (b) First-pass metabolism determines bioavailability

  (c) Increased HDL

  (d) Increased triglycerides

 (2) Transdermal patches/gel

  (a) Estrogen and progestin or estrogen only

  (b) Can use with continuous-cyclic regimen or continuous-combined regimen

  (c) No significant impact on HDL or triglycerides

(3) Vaginal estrogen creams
  (a) Treatment of vulvar and vaginal symptoms
  (b) May use initially with oral estrogen to get more immediate relief
  (c) Will not provide relief from vasomotor symptoms
  (d) Some systemic absorption possible
  (e) Need cyclic progestin with intact uterus

(4) Estrogen vaginal rings
  (a) Low dose (0.0075 mg/day estradiol ring—indicated for treatment of vulvar and vaginal symptoms)
  (b) 0.05–1.0 mg estradiol acetate ring indicated for both vasomotor and vulvovaginal symptoms
  (c) 90 days duration
  (d) Do not need cyclic progestin with low-dose ring but do need with other ring

k. Progestin only may be used if estrogen is contraindicated
  (1) Effective in relieving vasomotor symptoms; may have a positive impact on calcium balance
  (2) Not effective in relief of vulvovaginal symptoms; may have adverse effect on lipid metabolism

l. Testosterone may be added if extreme vasomotor symptoms not relieved by estrogen alone; oral, transdermal, injections, subcutaneous implants
  (1) May be especially useful after surgical menopause
  (2) May increase energy level, feeling of well-being, libido
  (3) Side effects—acne, hirsutism, clitoromegaly
  (4) Long-term effects of low-dose testosterone treatment in women are not known

m. Side effects of HT
  (1) Breast tenderness—estrogen or progestin (usually subsides after first few weeks)
  (2) Nausea—estrogen (relieved if taken at mealtime or at bedtime)
  (3) Skin irritation with transdermal patches
  (4) Fluid retention and bloating—estrogen or progestin
  (5) Alterations in mood—estrogen or progestin

n. Management of side effects may include
  (1) Lowering dose
  (2) Altering route of administration
  (3) Changing to different formulation

o. Management of bleeding during HT
  (1) Continuous-cyclic regimen—usually experience some uterine bleeding; starts last few days of progestin administration or during hormone-free days; earlier bleeding, heavy or persistent bleeding may indicate endometrial hyperplasia and warrants endometrial evaluation
  (2) Continuous-combined regimen—erratic spotting and light bleeding of 1–5 days duration in first year; endometrial biopsy if bleeding heavier or longer than usual

13. Nonhormonal management of vasomotor symptoms
  a. Drugs FDA approved for other indications that have shown some effectiveness in relieving hot flashes—clonidine, gabapentin, SSRIs
  b. Avoiding caffeine, alcohol, cigarettes, spicy foods, and big meals
  c. Regular, moderate exercise—may also help alleviate insomnia
  d. Wearing layers and natural fibers
  e. Sleeping in a cool room
  f. Keeping a thermos of ice water available
  g. Stress management and relaxation techniques
  h. Vitamin E—anecdotal reports of relief, placebo controlled studies not supportive
  i. Soy foods and isoflavone supplements

14. Nonhormonal management of vulvovaginal symptoms
  a. Water-soluble lubricants
  b. Regular sexual activity
  c. Noncoital methods of sexual expression—massage, mutual masturbation if penetration is painful

Note: This chapter was written by Susan Moskosky in her private capacity. No official support or endorsement by the Department of Health and Human Services or any component thereof is intended or should be inferred.

◘ QUESTIONS

Select the best answer.

1. Which of the following is a positive sign of pregnancy?

   a. Goodell's sign
   b. Urinary frequency/urgency
   c. Braxton-Hicks contractions
   d. Fetal movement felt by examiner

2. Which of the following statements is correct regarding maternal physiologic changes in pregnancy?

    a. Pulse rate decreases
    b. Insulin requirements decrease
    c. Increased sweat gland activity
    d. Increased intestinal peristalsis

3. Examination of the breasts in pregnancy may normally show:

    a. Increased nodularity
    b. Linea nigra
    c. Retractions in skin
    d. Loss of nipple pigmentation

4. Examination of a woman in the 30th week of pregnancy would normally reveal:

    a. Cervical dilation of 2 cm
    b. Diastolic heart murmur
    c. Fundal height of 29 cm
    d. Thyroid nodularity

5. Examination of a woman in her 14th week of pregnancy would normally reveal:

    a. Fundal height of 14 cm
    b. Fetal heart tones audible with fetoscope
    c. Milk expressed from breasts
    d. Cyanosis of the cervix

6. Chadwick's sign is described as:

    a. Softening of the uterine isthmus
    b. A bluish discoloration of the cervix
    c. Palpable uterine softening to palpation
    d. Manipulation of the uterus displaces fetus to examiner's finger in the vagina

7. Which of the following complications is most likely to occur in the first trimester?

    a. Pregnancy induced hypertension
    b. Bleeding
    c. Placenta previa
    d. Gestational diabetes

8. What is the recommended weight gain in pregnancy for a woman beginning pregnancy with a BMI of 27?

    a. Less than 20 pounds
    b. 20 pounds
    c. 25 pounds
    d. Over 30 pounds

9. How is the EDD determined using Naegele's rule?

    a. Subtract 3 months from LNMP and add 7 days
    b. Subtract 7 days and add 9 months from the start of the LNMP
    c. Add 9 months from start of the LNMP
    d. Subtract 7 from last day of LNMP and count back 3 months

10. During pregnancy, sexual intercourse is contraindicated when:

    a. Increased whitish vaginal discharge is present
    b. 36 weeks gestation has been reached
    c. Rupture of membranes is suspected
    d. Weight gain is inadequate

11. Which of the following statements is true regarding diagnostic testing during pregnancy?

    a. Chorionic villus sampling is performed between weeks 14 and 24 when indicated for genetic reasons
    b. Alpha-fetoprotein in maternal blood is assessed between weeks 16 and 18
    c. Gestational diabetes screening is performed between weeks 15 and 18
    d. Amniocentesis between weeks 22 and 26 when indicated for advanced maternal age

12. Laboratory testing ordered in the first trimester of pregnancy should include all of the following except:

    a. HbsAg screening
    b. VDRL screening
    c. HIV test
    d. Quad screening

13. True labor is characterized by:

    a. Contractions initially felt in back and radiate to lower abdomen
    b. Decrease of intensity of contractions with walking
    c. Discomfort of contractions felt mainly in abdomen
    d. Contractions relieved with sedation

14. A predisposing factor for preterm labor is:

    a. Hypothyroidism
    b. Gestational diabetes
    c. Pyelonephritis
    d. Oligohydramnios

15. Which of the following is a risk factor for the development of gestational diabetes?

    a. Multiple gestation
    b. Prior macrosomic infant
    c. Oligohydramnios in prior pregnancy
    d. Maternal age under 19

16. A 19-year-old female patient reports that she has not had a normal period in 6 weeks, but she has had bleeding for several days and bilateral lower abdominal/groin pain. A urine hCG is positive. Further evaluation must include:

    a. A serum hCG
    b. A pelvic examination
    c. A transvaginal ultrasound
    d. Serial quantitative hCGs

17. Which of the following increases a woman's chances of having an ectopic pregnancy?

    a. Use of combined oral contraceptives
    b. Uterine myoma
    c. Maternal age over 30
    d. Previous ectopic pregnancy

18. Inevitable abortion refers to:

    a. Death of embryo or fetus without expulsion
    b. Gross rupture of membranes in the presence of cervical dilatation
    c. Expulsion of products of conception without medical intervention
    d. Presence of bleeding and uterine cramping without cervical dilation

19. Which of the following is a sign of increasingly severe preeclampsia?

    a. Hemoconcentration with decreased platelets
    b. Increased urinary output
    c. Patellar hyporeflexia
    d. Elevated serum glucose

20. Presentation with placenta previa is differentiated from abruptio placentae by:

    a. Abruptio placentae occurs earlier in gestation
    b. Amount of bleeding is more with placenta previa
    c. Severe abdominal pain with abruptio placentae
    d. PIH usually accompanies placenta previa

21. Which of the following patterns in laboratory values would be expected in menopause?

    a. Decreased FSH, increased LH, decreased estradiol
    b. Decreased LH, increased FSH, increased estradiol
    c. Increased FSH, increased LH, decreased estradiol
    d. Increased LH, decreased FSH, increased estradiol

22. All of the following are contraindications to hormone therapy (HT) in menopause except:

    a. A history of angina chest pain currently managed with beta adrenergic blockade
    b. Hypothyroidism currently managed with 100 mcg/day of synthetic thyroxine
    c. Endometrial hyperplasia
    d. Breast cancer treated 6 years ago

23. What is the most prevalent contraceptive method among married women in the United States?

    a. Combination oral contraceptives
    b. Condoms
    c. Sterilization
    d. Withdrawal

24. A 54-year-old female with vaginal dryness causing irritation and dyspareunia has no problem with hot flashes. Bone densiometry reveals a T score of 1.0. What is the best treatment?

    a. Continuous combined regimen HT
    b. Cyclic HT with added testosterone
    c. Estrogen vaginal ring
    d. Progestin-only therapy

25. Which of the following women should have an endometrial biopsy/evaluation?

    a. Woman on continuous-cyclic HT regimen with amenorrhea
    b. Woman on continuous-cyclic HT regimen with bleeding starting last few days of progestin administration each month
    c. Woman on continuous-combined HT regimen with irregular bleeding in the first year of use
    d. Woman on continuous-combined HT regimen with spotting that occurs after several months of amenorrhea

26. A 53-year-old female who had a hysterectomy 10 years ago for dysfunctional uterine bleeding presents with complaints of severe hot flashes and night sweats for the past few months. Her lipid profile is significant for cholesterol of 220 mg/dL and triglycerides of 350 mg/dL. What is the most appropriate therapy for her vasomotor symptoms at this time?

    a. Continuous-combined oral HT
    b. Selective estrogen receptor modulator (raloxifene)
    c. Transdermal estrogen patch
    d. Vaginal estrogen cream

27. A 24-year-old female presents to your office with a request for combination oral contraceptives. Her current medications include a bronchodilator for asthma. Management for this client should include advising her that:

    a. Combination oral contraceptives are not recommended for women with asthma
    b. Combination oral contraceptives may potentiate the action of her bronchodilator
    c. She should use a backup method if using the bronchodilator several days in a row
    d. Use of progestin-only contraceptive injections may reduce her asthma attacks

28. Which of the following contraceptive methods would be best for a woman with a seizure disorder who is taking phenytoin?

    a. Combination oral contraceptives
    b. Combination contraceptive injections
    c. Progestin-only oral contraceptives
    d. Progestin-only contraceptive injections

29. A 22-year-old female calls the clinic on Monday morning stating that the condom broke when she and her partner had sex on Saturday night at about 11:00 P.M. She is interested in emergency contraception. In discussing options with this client it is important to explain that the latest she should wait before initiating emergency contraception is:

    a. Monday at 11:00 A.M.
    b. Monday at 11:00 P.M.
    c. Tuesday at 11:00 A.M.
    d. Thursday at 11:00 P.M.

30. The second dose of emergency contraceptive pills should be taken _____ hours after the first dose.

    a. 4
    b. 6
    c. 12
    d. 24

31. A 28-year-old female who has had a copper T 380 IUD for 2 years has a Pap smear showing actinomycosis. She has no symptoms of infection. Appropriate management would include:

    a. Removing the IUD and repeating the Pap smear in 6 months
    b. Removing the IUD, treating with doxycycline and repeating the Pap smear in 1 year
    c. Keeping the IUD and repeating the Pap smear in 1 year
    d. Keeping the IUD, treating with doxycycline and repeating the Pap smear in 3 months

32. When counseling a woman about the use of POP emergency contraception, it is appropriate to tell her:

    a. There is an increased risk of birth defect if pregnancy does occur
    b. It is not safe to use if she has a history of arterial or venous thromboembolic disease
    c. There is a 25% chance she will experience nausea as a side effect
    d. The same contraindications apply to any hormonal contraception

33. What is an advantage of progestin-only hormonal contraception?

    a. It is significantly less expensive than combined forms
    b. It has a lesser side effect profile
    c. It provides an option for women who have contraindications to estrogen
    d. It can be taken within 4 weeks of giving birth

34. Following a vasectomy, another method of contraception should be used until the man has had a minimum of _____ ejaculations.

    a. 5
    b. 10
    c. 15
    d. 20

35. A woman who is undergoing a medically induced abortion using mifepristone and misoprostol should be advised to avoid which of the following during the procedure?

    a. Acetaminophen
    b. Folic acid supplements
    c. Nonsteroidal anti-inflammatory drugs
    d. Vitamin B$_6$ supplements

36. Which of the following abortion methods may be used in the second trimester?

    a. Hypertonic saline instillation
    b. Methotrexate and misoprostol
    c. Mifepristone and misoprostol
    d. Vacuum aspiration

37. According to National Osteoporosis Foundation recommendations a 50-year-old woman not on estrogen therapy who obtains at least 600 mg of calcium each day in her diet should take a daily calcium supplement of:

    a. 400 mg
    b. 600 mg
    c. 900 mg
    d. 1,200 mg

38. Although not an approved indication, studies have indicated that HT may have the benefit of decreasing the risk for:

    a. Colon cancer
    b. Rheumatoid arthritis
    c. Osteoarthritis
    d. Cognitive dysfunction

39. A woman who is requesting contraception and who also wants to get pregnant in 1 year should avoid using:

    a. Combination oral contraceptives
    b. Fertility awareness methods
    c. Progestin-only oral contraceptives
    d. Progestin-only contraceptive injections

40. A woman plans to use the calendar method for contraception. She has charted her menstrual cycles for several months and has noted her longest cycle to be 30 days and her shortest cycle to be 27 days. She should abstain from sexual intercourse each cycle from day _____ through day _____.

    a. 9; 19
    b. 10; 15
    c. 11; 18
    d. 12; 16

41. Which of the following statements by a client indicates she needs additional information about use of the contraceptive vaginal ring?

    a. I should insert a new ring every 7 days
    b. I should expect to have regular periods while using the ring
    c. My partner can use a male condom while I am wearing the ring
    d. The exact position of the ring in the vagina is not important

42. Your patient is on combined oral contraceptives and calls to tell you that she has missed her pills for 2 days in a row. It is the second week of her cycle. You advise her to:

    a. Double her pills for the next 2 days; no backup is required
    b. Take 1 pill daily until Sunday; discard the pack and start a new one at that time
    c. Take 2 pills a day for the next 2 days, using backup contraception for 7 days
    d. Begin a new pack immediately; use a backup method for 7 days

43. A 3-week postpartum woman who is breastfeeding presents in your office to discuss her contraceptive options. Currently she is breastfeeding on demand and is not providing any supplements. She plans to continue breastfeeding for at least 6 months. She wants to know if she should restart her birth control pills or if she is protected from getting pregnant as long as she is breastfeeding. Information for this woman concerning the lactational amenorrhea method of contraception should include:

    a. The expected failure rate for this method of contraception is about 20%
    b. This method is considered effective for only 3 months postpartum
    c. The woman can rely on this method as long as she is not having periods
    d. Another method of contraception should be considered when the infant begins sleeping through the night

44. The woman in the preceding question asks if she can restart birth control pills now as she wants to be sure that she does not become pregnant. The best response would be:

    a. Combination oral contraceptives are contraindicated during the duration of breastfeeding
    b. All hormonal methods of contraception should be avoided while she is breastfeeding
    c. She should wait until she is having regular periods before restarting her birth control pills
    d. Progestin-only pills may be a better option for her to start at 6 weeks postpartum

45. A woman using a diaphragm for contraception has sexual intercourse at 8:00 A.M. on Friday, at 2:00 A.M. on Saturday, and again at 8:00 A.M. on Saturday. When can she safely remove her diaphragm for effective contraception while minimizing problems related to leaving the diaphragm in for extended periods of time?

    a. 10:00 A.M. on Saturday
    b. 2:00 P.M. on Saturday
    c. 10:00 P.M. on Saturday
    d. 8:00 A.M. on Sunday

46. When counseling patients about emergency contraception, in the interest of full disclosure it is important to advise that:

    a. Depending upon the timing in the cycle, it may interrupt an established pregnancy
    b. There is a possibility of teratogenicity if a pregnancy does occur
    c. An increased risk of embolic disease occurs due to the relatively large dose
    d. While it may be taken up to 5 days later, it is most effective when used earliest

47. Which of the following is an advantage of the female condom?

    a. It can be used with a male condom for added protection
    b. It can be used for repeated acts of intercourse
    c. It may be used by individuals with latex allergy
    d. It has a lower failure rate than the male condom

48. Noncontraceptive benefits of combination oral contraceptives include all of the following *except*:

    a. Decrease in risk for benign breast disease
    b. Decrease in risk for cervical cancer
    c. Decrease in risk for endometrial cancer
    d. Decrease in risk for ovarian cancer

49. For which of the contraceptive methods is there the least difference between the perfect use and typical use failure rates?

    a. Combination oral contraceptives
    b. Diaphragm
    c. Intrauterine device
    d. Male condom

50. A woman who weighs 200 pounds or greater may have decreased effectiveness with which of the following contraceptive methods?

    a. Combination injectable contraception
    b. Contraceptive vaginal ring
    c. Levonorgestrel intrauterine system
    d. Transdermal contraceptive system

51. When performing a routine assessment of a woman who is 18 weeks gestation, what would you expect her to report?

    a. Worsening nausea and heartburn
    b. Round ligament discomfort
    c. Having just recently felt fetal movement
    d. Increased leukorrhea

52. A 20-year-old female who is 30% overweight presents for her first Depo Provera injection. Concerns in administering Depo-Provera to this woman include:

    a. She may need a larger dose than the usual 150 mg
    b. She should return for repeat injections every 2 months
    c. You should massage the injection site well to assure absorption
    d. You should choose a site that assures deep IM injection

53. Instructions for progestin-only oral contraceptive users should include:

    a. If you are more than 3 hours late taking a pill use a backup method for 48 hours
    b. If 2 pills are missed in the third week of the pack, throw away the pack and start a new one
    c. If you miss pills in the fourth week of the pack you do not have to use a backup method
    d. If you miss 2 pills in the first week of the pack, make them up and use a backup method for 7 days

54. The menopausal woman may experience some changes in sensation or the orgasmic experience during sexual activity related to:

    a. Decreased vasocongestion and decreased vaginal expansion
    b. Decreased vasocongestion and increased vaginal expansion
    c. Increased vasocongestion and decreased vaginal expansion
    d. Increased vasocongestion and increased vaginal expansion

55. Which of the following contraceptive choices should not be recommended for the perimenopausal woman who is having irregular menses?

    a. Combination oral contraceptives
    b. Diaphragm
    c. Fertility awareness methods
    d. LNG intrauterine system

56. A 26-year-old female is planning to use basal body temperatures for contraception. Which of the following statements would indicate that she needs further instruction on this method?

    a. I will take my temperature the same time each day before getting out of bed
    b. I know that I am about to ovulate when my temperature rises at least 0.4 degrees
    c. I will need to use a special thermometer to take my basal body temperature
    d. After a rise of 0.4 degrees above my baseline for 3 days it is safe to have sex

57. The mechanism of action of mifepristone in inducing abortion is:

    a. Antiprogesterone effect on the endometrium
    b. Cervical dilatation effect
    c. Stimulatory effect on the myometrium
    d. Toxic effect on the fertilized egg

58. When a patient on combined oral contraceptives has persistent breakthrough bleeding during the first half of the cycle, the appropriate intervention is to:

    a. Advise that this may occur for up to 1 year
    b. Consider progestin-only options
    c. Counsel regarding the need to switch to non-hormonal methods
    d. Increase the estrogen component of the method

59. What is considered to be the main mechanism of action of oral contraceptives when used for emergency contraception?

    a. Disruption of implanted fertilized ovum
    b. Inhibition of ovulation
    c. Prevention of implantation of fertilized ovum
    d. Toxic effect on the fertilized ovum

60. According to WHO recommendations which of the following is considered to be a condition that represents an unacceptable health risk (refrain from providing) for the use of the indicated contraceptive method?

    a. Initiation of progestin-only oral contraceptives by a woman with a history of deep vein thrombosis
    b. Initiation of progestin-only injectable contraception for a woman with hypertension
    c. Initiation of combination injectable contraception in a lactating woman who is less than 6 weeks postpartum
    d. Insertion of an IUD in a woman who is at risk for HIV infection

61. Which of the following statements concerning coitus interruptus is not correct?

 a. It has a lower perfect use failure rate than the cervical cap

 b. It may result in a decreased risk for HIV transmission to female partner

 c. Men are typically not able to predict the timing of ejaculation

 d. There is a decreased chance for the presence of preejaculatory sperm with repeat acts of intercourse

Answers

1. **d**	32. **c**
2. **c**	33. **c**
3. **a**	34. **d**
4. **c**	35. **c**
5. **d**	36. **a**
6. **b**	37. **b**
7. **b**	38. **a**
8. **c**	39. **d**
9. **a**	40. **a**
10. **c**	41. **a**
11. **b**	42. **c**
12. **d**	43. **d**
13. **a**	44. **d**
14. **c**	45. **b**
15. **b**	46. **d**
16. **c**	47. **c**
17. **d**	48. **b**
18. **b**	49. **c**
19. **a**	50. **d**
20. **c**	51. **b**
21. **c**	52. **d**
22. **b**	53. **a**
23. **c**	54. **a**
24. **c**	55. **c**
25. **d**	56. **b**
26. **c**	57. **a**
27. **b**	58. **d**
28. **d**	59. **b**
29. **d**	60. **c**
30. **c**	61. **d**
31. **c**	

◘ BIBLIOGRAPHY

American Association of Clinical Endocrinologists' (AACE) Menopause Guidelines Revision Task Force. (2006). Endocrinologists' guidelines for the diagnosis and treatment of menopause. *Endocrine Practice, 12*(3), 315–337.

American College of Obstetricians and Gynecologists (ACOG). (2007). *Guidelines for women's health care* (3rd ed.). Washington, DC: Author.

American College of Obstetricians and Gynecologists (ACOG) and American Academy of Pediatrics (AAP). (2007). *Guidelines for perinatal care* (6th ed.). Washington, DC: Author.

Centers for Disease Control and Prevention (CDC). (2009). National Vital Statistics System; birth data. Retrieved from http://www.cdc.gov/nchs/births.htm

Freeman, S. (2004). Lower-dose hormone therapy for postmenopausal women. *American Journal for Nurse Practitioners, 8*(3), 9–20.

Hatcher, R., Trussell, J., Nelson, A. L., & Cates, W. (2008). *Contraceptive technology* (19th ed.). New York: Thomas Reuters Publishing.

Khan, M. I., & Klachko, D. M. (2006). *Polycystic ovarian syndrome.* Retrieved from http://www.emedicine.com/med/TOPIC2173.htm

Leveno, K., Cunningham, F., Alexander, J., Bloom, S., Bloom, S. L., Casey, B. . . . Roberts, S. (2007). *Williams manual of obstetrics: Pregnancy complications* (22nd ed.). New York: McGraw-Hill.

National Institutes of Health. (2000). *NIH Consensus Statement: Osteoporosis prevention, diagnosis, and therapy.* Washington, DC: Author.

National Institutes of Health. (2000). *Working group report on high blood pressure in pregnancy.* Washington, DC: Author.

National Osteoporosis Foundation. (2003). *Physician's guide to prevention and treatment of osteoporosis.* Washington, DC: Author.

North American Menopause Society. (2002). *Menopause core curriculum study guide* (2nd ed.). Cleveland, OH: Author.

North American Menopause Society (NAMS). (2004). Treatment of menopause associated vasomotor symptoms: Position statement of the North American menopause society. *Menopause: The Journal of NAMS, 11*(1), 11–33.

The American Cancer Society. (2011). *Breast cancer: Early detection.* Retrieved from http://www.cancer.org/acs/groups/cid/documents/webcontent/003165-pdf.pdf

Wright Jr., T. C., Massad, L., Dunton, C. J., Spitzer, M., Wilkinson, E. J., & Solomon, D. (2006). 2006 consensus guidelines for the management of women with cervical intraepithelial neoplasia or carcinoma in situ. *American Journal of Obstetrics and Gynecology, 197*(4), 223–239.

Writing Group for the Women's Health Initiative Investigators. (2002). Risks and benefits of estrogen plus progestin in healthy postmenopausal women: Principal results from the Women's Health Initiative randomized controlled trial. *Journal of the American Medical Association, 288,* 321–333.

Youngkin, E., & Davis, M. (2003). *Women's health: A primary care clinical guide* (3rd ed.). Stamford, CT: Appleton & Lange.

Musculoskeletal Disorders

Madeline Turkeltaub

12

◘ OSTEOARTHRITIS (OA)

- Definition—a noninflammatory, degenerative disorder of movable joints characterized by an imbalance between synthesis and degradation of articular cartilage, leading to classic cartilaginous and joint destruction. Subsequent formation of osteophytes, bony cysts, and hypertrophy may occur.

- Etiology/Incidence
  1. Idiopathic
     a. Occurs without obvious cause
     b. Familial tendency
     c. Obesity—exacerbates stress on weight-bearing joints
  2. Secondary osteoarthritis—results from underlying abnormality
     a. Trauma
     b. Congenital
     c. Metabolic/endocrine/neuropathic
     d. Other underlying medical causes
  3. Overall affects 26.9 million adults
  4. Higher incidence in females, especially after age 50

- Signs and Symptoms
  1. Pain
     a. Worsens throughout the day; patient feels best upon awakening and discomfort progresses
     b. Aggravated by activity and relieved with rest; may become persistent as disease progresses
  2. Joints affected become edematous but not hot or red
  3. Limitation of movement in affected joint
  4. Joints most frequently involved
     a. Weight bearing—hips, knees, lower back
     b. Distal interphalangeal joints (DIP), proximal interphalangeal joints (PIP)
     c. Neck, metatarsophalangeal (MTP)

- Differential Diagnosis
  1. Rheumatic disease
  2. Pseudogout
  3. Reiter's syndrome
  4. Arthritis of chronic ulcerative colitis
  5. Fibromyalgia
  6. Multiple myeloma

- Physical Findings
  1. Hands
     a. Heberden's nodes—enlargement of DIP joints
     b. Bouchard's nodes—enlargement of PIP joints
  2. Joints
     a. Localized tenderness
     b. Crepitus on movement
     c. Bony consistency to enlargement
     d. Decreased range of motion (ROM)
     e. No gross deformity
  3. Neurologic—pain due to pressure on nerves by affected joints
  4. Knee—instability
  5. Hips—reduced internal rotation, pain may be referred to knee

- Diagnostic Tests/Findings
  1. Radiograph—cardinal radiologic features
     a. Unequal loss of joint space
     b. Osteophytes
     c. Juxta-articular sclerosis
     d. Subchondral bone
     e. Sharpened articular bone
  2. Synovial fluid aspirate is usually normal
  3. Serologic markers of inflammation within normal limits

- Management/Treatment
  1. Preserving function and decreasing pain are goals of treatment
  2. Treating biomechanical factors
     a. Weight loss in obese patients
     b. Correct uneven leg length with heel wedge
     c. Use canes on opposite side or crutches to decrease weight bearing on affected joint
     d. Quadriceps setting for knee involvement
     e. Cervical collar for cervical spine pain
     f. Isometric exercises for abdominal muscles decreases lumbosacral spine pain
     g. Orthotic shoe modification
  3. Local measures
     a. Ice to improve range of motion ROM and exercise performance
     b. Moist heat to decrease muscle spasm and relieve morning stiffness
     c. Temporary rest such as removable splint to decrease motion
  4. Medications
     a. Acetaminophen 500 mg to 1 g t.i.d. or q.i.d.
        (1) Caution with high doses over extended periods
        (2) May cause significant GI upset and liver toxicity
     b. Nonsteroidal anti-inflammatory drugs (NSAID), e.g., ibuprofen 400–800 mg t.i.d.; indomethacin 50–200 mg/day up to 1 g q.i.d.
        (1) COX-2 inhibitors for selected patients with history of or high risk for GI bleeding, e.g., Celebrex 100–200 mg/d
        (2) Consider risk of GI toxicity and cardiovascular events with all COX inhibitors
        (3) Consider H_2 blocker or PPI when using NSAID
        (4) Instruction on side effects of NSAID including
           (a) Gastrointestinal intolerance
           (b) Fluid retention
           (c) Platelet abnormalities
           (d) Hepatic and renal dysfunction
     c. NSAIDs may be added to acetaminophen when acetaminophen alone is inadequate
        d. Topical therapies such as lidocaine patches and capsaicin may contribute to pain control
        e. Adjuvant medications such as antiepileptics and antidepressants for neuropathic component
        f. Opioids when other measures are inadequate
        g. Intra-articular injections of hyaluronic acid, e.g., Hyalgan, Synvisc
        h. Intra-articular steroid injection 2–3 times yearly as alternate option
  5. Surgery—refer to orthopedics for procedures, such as fusion or joint replacement when other options fail
  6. Educate regarding body mechanics, muscle strengthening, rang-of-motion exercises, and weight-reduction strategies

◘ RHEUMATOID ARTHRITIS (RA)

- Definition—chronic multisystem disease resulting in symmetrical joint inflammation, loss of synovial joint and bone, increased risk for a variety of systemic diseases, and shortened life expectancy

- Etiology/Incidence
  1. Cause unknown—may have autoimmune component
  2. Other diseases of joints, such as gout and OA may predispose to RA
  3. Affects approximately 1% of the adult population
  4. 30% of patients have mild disease with remissions and little deformity
  5. 10% have a single period of active disease with only occasional exacerbations
  6. About one-half of patients have progressive disease
  7. Two to three times more common in women
  8. Peak age of onset 40–60 years

- Signs and Symptoms
  1. Morning stiffness lasting several hours
  2. Pain—joint pain and/or stiffness develops insidiously over several weeks to months in three or more joints symmetrically
  3. Fatigue, malaise, weakness, low-grade fever
  4. Proximal interphalangeal (PIP) and metacarpophalangeal (MCP) joints are the most commonly affected; distal interphalangeal (DIP) joints not affected in RA
  5. The first ROM loss is full extension
  6. Patient may report decrease in ability to perform specific functions such as
     a. Turn on faucets
     b. Hold a hairbrush or toothbrush

c. Open jars

d. Hold cups or drinking glasses

- Differential Diagnosis
  1. Ankylosing spondylitis
  2. Rheumatic fever
  3. Systemic lupus erythematosus
  4. Arthritis of inflammatory intestinal disease
  5. Psoriatic arthritis
  6. Reiter's syndrome
  7. Lyme disease

- Physical Findings
  1. Soft-tissue swelling
     a. Most frequently in MCP joints, wrists, and PIP joints
     b. Usually symmetrical
     c. Positive squeeze test precedes radiographic or laboratory evidence of disease—vigorous squeeze of metacarpals produces significant pain
  2. Tenderness and pain on passive motion
  3. Warmth at site of inflamed joint
  4. Limited ROM at joint
  5. Permanent deformity in chronic disease
     a. Flexion contractures
     b. Subluxation
     c. Ulnar deviation of fingers at MCP joints or deformities of fingers (swan neck, boutonniere)
  6. Synovial cysts can be visualized and palpated; Baker's cysts (synovial cysts of popliteal space) are common
  7. Extra-articular manifestations
     a. Ocular manifestations
     b. Skin and/or muscle atrophy
     c. Splenomegaly
     d. Lymph node enlargement

- Diagnostic Tests/Findings
  1. Anti-cyclic citrullinated peptide antibodies (anti-CCP)
     a. Higher specificity for RA than rheumatoid factor
     b. Similar or higher sensitivity than rheumatoid factor; present in 40% of people with negative rheumatoid factor
     c. Higher predictive value than rheumatoid factor
     d. Not all patients anti-CCP positive
  2. Rheumatoid factor can be isolated in 70–80% of patients at some course in disease
     a. Less than 50% patients positive in first 6 months of disease
     b. Not specific to RA

c. High titer early suggests poor prognosis

d. Titers not useful to follow—once positive, no need to check again

3. Erythrocyte sedimentation rate may be elevated; not particularly helpful or useful in diagnosis or prognosis
4. Antinuclear antibodies are present in 20% of patients
5. Radiograph findings
   a. Early changes are often limited to periarticular osteoporosis and soft-tissue swelling, joint effusion; radiograph not helpful in diagnosing early disease
   b. Primary value is to assess degree of joint destruction
6. Joint fluid shows inflammatory changes
7. CBC—mild to moderate anemia

- Management/Treatment
  1. The goals of treatment are
     a. To arrest or delay disease progression with disease modifying antirheumatic drugs (DMARDs)
     b. To relieve pain
     c. To relieve inflammation
     d. To maintain optimal function
     e. To prevent deformity
     f. To lower rates of complications
     g. To decrease rates of extra-articular manifestations; patients with RA have
        (1) Cardiovascular disease risk 10 years earlier
        (2) Increased incidence of pulmonary disease
        (3) Increased GI bleeding
        (4) Twice the risk for certain cancers
        (5) Six to nine times higher incidence of serious infection
     h. To educate the patient
  2. Conservative management includes
     a. Education
     b. Rest
     c. Physical therapy
     d. Nonsteroidal anti-inflammatory agents
     e. Cold and heat therapies
  3. If patient is unresponsive, additional medications from the following categories may be added
     a. Disease-modifying antirheumatic drugs (DMARDs)—methotrexate preferred, supplemented with folate 1 mg daily or 7 mg once weekly
     b. Tumor necrosis factor (TNF) inhibitors
        (1) Etanercept, infliximab, adalimumab
        (2) Very effective in modifying/treating RA

(3) Concern over serious risk of infections

(4) Patients must be well screened and monitored closely for infection

c. Antimalarials, e.g., hydroxychloroquine sulfate

d. Gold salts—intramuscular or orally

e. Corticosteroids (not more than 10 mg of prednisone or equivalent per day) on short-term basis to relieve disabling symptoms; may be used at start of therapy as a bridge to DMARDs

f. Intra-articular corticosteroids if medications do not relieve symptoms

4. Education

a. Explanation of autoimmune disease

b. Stress management and relaxation techniques

c. Abstinence from alcohol while taking methotrexate

d. Methotrexate is contraindicated in pregnancy (category X) and in those with impaired renal function

5. Multidisciplinary management

a. Physical therapy

b. Occupational therapy

6. Management plan for daily living

◘ GOUT

- Definition—gout is a metabolic disease associated with abnormal accumulation of urates in the body and characterized by recurring acute arthritis; classic gouty attack is podagra, involving the big toe

- Etiology/Incidence
  1. Due to deposition of crystals of monosodium urate (MSU)
  2. Related to either excess production or decreased excretion of uric acid
  3. Decreased uric acid excretion is present in 90% of patients
  4. 90% of patients with primary gout are men over 30 years of age
  5. The onset in women is usually at menopause plus 20–30 years
  6. Rapid fluctuation of serum urate levels may be precipitated by alcohol and food excess; surgery, infection, diuretics, or uricosuric drugs
  7. Gout is the most common cause of monoarticular joint inflammation

- Signs and Symptoms
  1. Acute onset, frequently monoarticular, affecting the first metatarsophalangeal joint, called podagra
  2. Tophi due to accumulation of urate crystals may be found in ears, hands, feet

3. Remissions and exacerbations; exacerbations may occur years apart

4. Involved joint is swollen, tender, warm, red; pain may wake patient from sleep and interfere with ADLs

5. Temperature elevation to 39° C

6. May become chronic with progressive loss and disability

- Differential Diagnosis
  1. Diagnosis may be confirmed based on dramatic response to NSAID or colchicine
  2. Acute stage may be confused with cellulitis or septic joint, e.g., gonorrhea, staphylococcal infection
  3. Pseudogout presents with similar symptoms but normal serum uric acid
  4. Chronic gout may mimic rheumatoid arthritis
  5. Chronic lead intoxication may result in attacks of gout
  6. See rheumatoid arthritis

- Physical Findings
  1. Limited, painful ROM in affected joint
  2. Elevated temperature during acute attack
  3. Palpation of tophi in areas indicated above
  4. Affected area hot to touch

- Diagnostic Tests/Findings
  1. Synovial fluid aspirate contains monosodium urate crystals
  2. In later stages of disease, radiograph may show punched-out areas in bone
  3. Erythrocyte sedimentation rate elevated
  4. White cell count elevated
  5. Uric acid elevated
  6. Hyperuricemia—serum urate > 7.5 mg/dL

- Management/Treatment
  1. Acute attack should be treated first, hyperuricemia later
  2. NSAID—indomethacin, 50 mg every 8 hours, continued until symptoms resolve
  3. Colchicine
     a. Most effective during first 24–48 hours
     b. Dose—0.5–0.6 mg orally, every hour, until pain relieved or GI symptoms occur or maximum dose of 6 mg
  4. Corticosteroids—used for patients who cannot tolerate NSAID
  5. Analgesics—codeine or meperidine may be indicated; ASA is *contraindicated*
  6. Bed rest—for 24 hours after acute attack subsides
  7. Discontinue thiazide diuretics if in use
  8. Diet to maintain daily output of 2,000 cc of urine; avoid obesity and prevent dehydration; low purine diet has little effect on blood levels

9. Support is needed during remissions for patient to maintain medical regimen, including
   a. Diet instruction
   b. Prophylactic medication
      (1) Xanthine oxidase inhibitors—begin 40 mg daily, may increase to 80 mg daily if no effect within 2 weeks; liver function abnormalities most common adverse effect
      (2) Allopurinol—100 mg/day for 1 week initially, then 200–300 mg daily; observe for rash associated with hypersensitivity
10. Comfort may be obtained with cold or hot compresses and elevation of affected area during acute attack

◘ OSTEOPOROSIS

- Definition—demineralization of bone, resulting in decrease in bone mass with an otherwise normal structural matrix

- Etiology/Incidence
  1. Most common metabolic bone disease in the United States
  2. Clinically evident in middle years and beyond
  3. Type I—affects women more frequently than men, especially postmenopausal women
  4. Type II—in men and women older than 75
  5. Caucasians have highest incidence, then Asians, then African-Americans
  6. Most frequently associated with
     a. Lack of estrogen (postmenopausal or post-oophorectomy)
     b. Lack of activity (immobilization)
     c. Malabsorption (post-gastrectomy, lactase deficiency)
     d. Vitamin D deficiency
     e. Low calcium intake
  7. Family history of osteoporosis
  8. Sedentary lifestyle
  9. Smoking (greater than one pack per day)
  10. Excessive alcohol intake
  11. Small body frame
  12. Secondary causes—drug related, endocrine, gastrointestinal, neoplastic, renal, rheumatologic disorders
  13. Affects 25 million women and over 5 million men in the United States

- Signs and Symptoms
  1. Loss of height
  2. Kyphosis
  3. Backache
  4. Spontaneous fracture or collapse of vertebrae

- Differential Diagnosis
  1. Adrenal cortical excess
  2. Hyperthyroidism
  3. Metabolic bone disease, such as hyperparathyroidism and osteomalacia
  4. Multiple myeloma
  5. Metastatic bone disease

- Physical Findings
  1. There may be no specific physical findings, unless a fracture is present; FRACTURE IS THE CARDINAL FINDING OF OSTEOPOROSIS
  2. Loss of height is most common
  3. Kyphosis ("dowager's hump") is evident with vertebral compression fractures

- Diagnostic Tests/Findings
  1. Serum calcium, phosphorus, and alkaline phosphatase are within normal limits
  2. Standard radiography is not a reliable indicator since more than 25–30% of bone loss must occur for detection with this method
  3. Lateral radiograph of spine might show
     a. Anterior wedging of thoracic vertebral bodies
     b. Widening intervertebral bodies
     c. New or old fractures of vertebrae
  4. Dual-energy x-ray absorptiometry (DEXA)—more sensitive to bone loss
     a. Results reported as standard deviation in the general population (T-score)
     b. T-score above –1 is normal
     c. T-score between –2.5 and –1 is osteopenia
     d. T-score below –2.5 is osteoporosis
  5. Additional laboratory tests may be ordered for older patients, including
     a. Albumin (to allow interpretation of serum calcium)
     b. Serum and urine protein electrophoresis (differentiate multiple myeloma)
     c. BUN and creatinine (to rule out chronic renal disease)
  6. Record accurate serial height measurements

- Management/Treatment—treatment of established osteoporosis must take into consideration severity of disease, age, and coexisting medical problems; prevention is key factor
  1. Prevention and treatment of osteoporosis includes
     a. Balanced diet—protein not to exceed 20% of total calories; diet counseling to include dietary sources high in calcium and low in fat
     b. Exercise
        (1) Prevention
            (a) Weight-bearing, at least 30 minutes 3–4 times per week

(b) Encourage lifestyle changes related to importance of exercise

(c) Strength training, e.g., lifting weights, swimming

(2) Moderate walking for those with diagnosed osteoporosis, depending upon severity

(3) Active or passive ROM exercises for bedridden patients

c. Estrogen therapy in postmenopausal women or postoophorectomy—decreases rate of bone resorption

(1) Indicated for prevention

(2) Consider other medications unless also using estrogen to treat vasomotor symptoms or vulva/vaginal atrophy

(3) Use short term—5 years

(4) Progestin required for women with intact uterus

d. Bisphosphonates—inhibit osteoclast mediated bone resorption

(1) Indicated for treatment of osteopenia and osteoporosis

(2) A variety of weekly, monthly, and annual oral and infusion options available

(3) Oral forms taken with 8 ounces of water at least one-half hour prior to eating

e. Salmon calcitonin—decreases bone resorption

(1) Indicated for treatment only

(2) Alleviates bone pain

f. Selective estrogen receptor modulators (SERMs)—agonist and antagonist effects on estrogen receptors

(1) Indicated for prevention and treatment

(2) Raloxifene

(3) Estrogen-like effect on bone

(4) Estrogen-like effect on lipid levels

(5) Estrogen antagonist effect on breast and endometrial tissue

g. Adequate calcium intake

(1) Ages 13–18—1,300 mg/day (adolescents)

(2) Ages 19–50—1,000 mg/day (adults and pregnant women)

(3) Ages 51–70 years

   (a) Men 1,000 mg/day

   (b) Women 1,200 mg/day

(4) Adults 71+ years—1,200 mg/day

h. Calcium may be obtained through dietary sources or through calcium supplements; calcium carbonate—least expensive; calcium citrate—absorbed easily; calcium phosphate—decreased chance of constipation

i. 400–600 IU vitamin D daily

2. Elderly patients must be protected from falls—educate family regarding safe environment

3. Alcohol and smoking should be avoided

4. Judicious use of glucocorticoids

5. Regular follow-up with mammogram and pelvic examination for women on hormone therapy (HT)

6. Educate teens and young women regarding adequate calcium intake and dangers of excessive exercise

7. Treatment for acute back pain includes

a. Rest

b. Analgesia

c. External support

d. Heat

e. Stool softeners

◘ LOW BACK PAIN (LBP)

- Definition—acute, chronic, or recurrent pain occurring in the lumbosacral spine region and associated musculoskeletal areas; in the absence of contributory history and physical exam findings, most LBP is a consequence of lumbosacral strain or radiculopathy

- Etiology/Incidence

1. Most acute back pain is caused by muscle strain and spasm of the paraspinal muscle groups

2. Low back pain from trauma or mechanical causes is most common between 30 and 40 years of age

3. 80% of the population will experience low back pain (LBP) sometime during their lifetime

4. LBP is a self-limited condition

a. 40% remit in 1 week

b. 60–80% in 3 weeks

c. 90% in 2 months

5. Risk factors include

a. Obesity

b. Poor body mechanics

c. Physical deconditioning

- Signs and Symptoms

1. Lumbarsacral strain

a. Discomfort confined to the lower back region; may radiate to the anterior superior iliac crest but no farther

b. Symptoms exacerbated by activity/movement

c. Tenderness reproducible with palpation of paraspinal muscles

2. Lumbar radiculopathy

a. Pain radiates beyond the back and hip dependent upon the nerve path affected

b. Discomfort described as electric, burning, numbness, and other manifestations of neuropathic involvement

c. Symptoms exacerbated by maneuvers that increase intra-abdominal pressure, e.g., straining for a bowel movement, Valsalva maneuver

- Differential Diagnosis
  1. Congenital disorders, e.g., asymmetry
  2. Tumors involving nerve roots or meninges
  3. Trauma
     a. Lumbar strain
     b. Compression fracture
  4. Spondylosis and spondylolisthesis
  5. Metabolic disorders, e.g., osteoporosis
  6. Arthritis of the spine
  7. Degenerative diseases
  8. Herniated nucleus pulposus
  9. Infections
  10. Mechanical causes, e.g., weak abdominal muscles, pelvic tumors, prostate disease
  11. Cauda equina syndrome
  12. Psychogenic

- Physical Findings
  1. Lumbosacral strain
     a. Physical findings typically normal
     b. Possible decreased ROM to lumbosacral spine as a function of pain
     c. No neurological findings
     d. Normal straight leg raise
  2. Lumbar radiculopathy
     a. Abnormal straight leg raise
     b. Other neurological abnormalities depending upon area affected
        (1) Altered deep tendon reflexes
        (2) Great toe dorsiflexion
        (3) Sensory impairment
        (4) Foot eversion
        (5) Atrophy of calf muscle
        (6) Flexing thigh on pelvis (femoral stretch test)—associated with L_3 problems
        (7) L_{3-4} disc
           (a) Pain in lower back, hip, anterior leg to great toe
           (b) Numbness in anteromedial thigh and knee
           (c) Weakness in quadriceps leading to atrophy
           (d) Diminished patellar reflex
        (8) L_{4-5} disc
           (a) Pain over sacroiliac joint, hip, lateral thigh
           (b) Numbness of lateral leg, web of great toe
           (c) Weakness on dorsiflexion, difficulty walking on heels
           (d) Reflexes usually unchanged
        (9) L_5-S_1 disc
           (a) Pain over sacroiliac joint, hip, back of thigh, and leg to heel
           (b) Numbness in back of calf and lateral foot to small toe
           (c) Difficulty walking on toes
           (d) Atrophy of gastrocnemius
           (e) Diminished or absent Achilles tendon reflex
  3. Complete physical examination to rule out nonmusculoskeletal etiology—urgent findings that require immediate referral
     a. Bilateral leg weakness
     b. Saddle anesthesia
     c. Pain unrelieved by rest
     d. Pain worsens at night

- Diagnostic Tests/Findings
  1. None indicated in the presence of an otherwise normal history and physical examination; conservative management of a clinical diagnosis is indicated
  2. If conservative management is not effective in 4–6 weeks or referral to specialty service is being considered, an MRI is indicated
  3. Standard radiography—anterior-posterior (AP), lateral and oblique only if bony structure abnormalities, fracture, metastasis, or other abnormal conditions need to be ruled out

- Management/Treatment—key elements include
  1. Bed rest not indicated—limit select activities that increase pain
  2. Analgesia
     a. Salicylates or acetaminophen
     b. Nonsteroidal anti-inflammatory drugs
     c. Occasionally, opiates may be required
  3. Muscle relaxants
     a. Limit use to 1–2 weeks
     b. Avoid in older patients
  4. With radiculopathy
     a. 5-day steroid dose pack at first visit if pain severe
     b. Schedule second visit 1 week after first visit, if no improvement consider referral to specialist for epidural steroid injection (ESI)
  5. Patient education
     a. Good body mechanics
     b. Diet—weight loss if indicated
     c. Appropriate exercise
     d. Sleeping posture
  6. Traction

7. Back and abdominal exercises for prevention and recurrences; contraindicated during acute episode; walking better than jogging
8. Back massage
9. Many times there is a psychosocial overlay—a psychosocial assessment should be conducted for
   a. Stress
   b. Depression
   c. Domestic violence
   d. Inadequate coping ability
   e. Marriage/family problems
10. Early return to work with limited activity
11. Stress management

□ BURSITIS

- Definition—inflammation of the synovial membrane lining of a bursal sac; more than 150 bursae throughout the body

- Etiology/Incidence
  1. Infection in a joint space
  2. Inflammation as part of a systemic process, such as RA or gout
  3. Occurs most commonly in middle and old age, following trauma or unaccustomed repetitive use of the part
  4. Most common locations
     a. Subdeltoid
     b. Olecranon
     c. Ischial
     d. Prepatellar

- Signs and Symptoms
  1. Abrupt onset of pain that increases on motion (superficial)
  2. Local tenderness
  3. Fluctuant edema
  4. Erythema may be present
  5. Regional tenderness and limited motion (deep bursitis)

- Differential Diagnosis
  1. RA
  2. Gout or pseudogout
  3. Septic arthritis

- Physical Findings
  1. Restriction of movement
  2. Tenderness over rotator cuff
  3. Swelling and redness (prepatellar/olecranon)

- Diagnostic Tests/Findings
  1. None indicated in chronic, stable, painless disease

2. Aspirate fluid with 18-gauge needle and request laboratory analysis
   a. Culture
   b. WBC count—elevation is associated with bacterial infection
   c. RBC count—associated with trauma
   d. Glucose—decreased with bacterial infection
   e. Crystals—associated with microcrystalline bursitis
   f. Mucin clot—poor clot associated with bacterial infection

- Management/Treatment
  1. If bursitis is traumatic
     a. Splint part
     b. Apply heat 30 minutes t.i.d. or q.i.d.
     c. ASA or NSAID—naproxen 250 mg b.i.d. or t.i.d.
  2. If symptoms recur and fluid reaccumulates inject long-acting corticosteroids into bursa
  3. If septic bursitis
     a. Incision and drainage
     b. Parenteral antibiotics
  4. Education regarding care of injured part
     a. Ice for first 24 hours
     b. After swelling is stabilized, warm, moist heat several times daily

□ EPICONDYLITIS (TENNIS ELBOW)

- Definition—an overuse syndrome resulting in inflammation in the region of the lateral epicondyle of the humerus at the origin of the common extensor muscles

- Etiology/Incidence
  1. Repetitive stress on the tendons
  2. Specific pathogenesis of tennis elbow is not known
  3. Occurs most frequently in the dominant extremity during midlife (may be athletic or work related)

- Signs and Symptoms
  1. Pain exacerbated by constant motion of the forearm and twisting motions, aggravated by hand and wrist movements
  2. Gradual onset of dull pain along lateral aspect of elbow
  3. Point tenderness over the epicondyle
  4. Limited motion

- Differential Diagnosis
  1. RA
  2. Localized intra-articular pathology
  3. Radial tunnel syndrome

4. Trauma
5. Septic joint

- Physical Findings
  1. Burning or aching pain with grasping or lifting
  2. Point tenderness present at or just distal to lateral epicondyle

- Diagnostic Tests/Findings—radiographs usually normal or show small calcium deposits

- Management/Treatment
  1. Pain relief
     a. Mild analgesics
     b. Rest
     c. Ice to tendon
  2. Counterforce brace; wrist splint
  3. Peri-tendon cortisone injection
  4. For continued pain
     a. Immobilize for 6–8 weeks in a long arm cast with 90° elbow flexion
     b. Physical therapy to restore strength and motion when cast is removed
  5. Reinforce an exercise program to condition muscle groups in the forearm and wrist
  6. If associated with a sport, evaluate whether improper technique was responsible for injury
  7. If nonoperative management fails, surgical intervention recommended

◻ CARPAL TUNNEL SYNDROME

- Definition—median nerve compression of wrist beneath transverse carpal ligament

- Etiology/Incidence
  1. Related to repeated forceful wrist flexion
  2. More common in women
  3. Frequently involves dominant hand
  4. May be associated with
     a. Pregnancy (likely to resolve within 6 weeks after delivery)
     b. Endoneural edema in diabetes mellitus
     c. Thyroid disease
     d. Occupational activities

- Signs and Symptoms
  1. Burning, tingling, numbness sensation along distribution of median nerve
  2. Pain exacerbated with dorsiflexion of wrist
  3. Night pain that interferes with sleep
  4. Clumsiness in performing fine hand movements
  5. May be unilateral or bilateral

- Differential Diagnosis
  1. Compression syndromes of median nerve
  2. Mononeuritis multiplex

3. Cervical radiculopathy
4. Tendonitis

- Physical Findings
  1. Decreased two-point discrimination on affected side
  2. Positive Tinel's sign—sensation of electric shock on percussion of volar aspect of wrist
  3. Positive Phalen's sign—pain and/or paresthesia when hands are held in forced flexion for 30–60 seconds
  4. Decreased sensation and muscle atrophy of thenar eminence

- Diagnostic Tests/Findings
  1. Electromyography—assists in documenting motor involvement
  2. Segmental sensory and motor conduction testing
  3. Abnormal monofilament test—used to determine sensation
  4. Radiography not routinely indicated but appropriate when there is history of trauma

- Management/Treatment
  1. Elevate extremity
  2. Splint hand and forearm
  3. Injection of corticosteroids into carpal tunnel if bursitis is involved
  4. Refer to surgeon for surgical intervention
  5. Notification of healthcare provider if symptoms increase
     a. Numbness and tingling persists
     b. Sensation in fingers decreases
  6. Take NSAID with food and report any gastric distress
  7. Consideration of occupational changes if appropriate

◻ KNEE PAIN

- Definition—knee pain is due to mechanical, inflammatory, and/or degenerative problems

- Etiology/Incidence
  1. Trauma
  2. Most frequently an exercise-related condition
  3. Tears of medial meniscus 10 times more common than lateral meniscus
  4. Increasingly overweight population has resulted in an increased prevalence of osteoarthritis of the knee

- Signs and Symptoms
  1. Locking—most frequently indicative of meniscal tear or loose bodies

2. "Giving way" or "buckling"—related to patella dislocation or ligamentous instability or anterior cruciate tear
3. Effusions around knee—associated with hemarthrosis and anterior cruciate ligament; fluid under patella noted on ballottement
4. Crepitus

- Differential Diagnosis
  1. Single painful knee with minimal edema
     a. Dislocated patella
     b. Degenerative joint disease (DJD)
     c. Prepatellar bursitis
  2. Single edematous knee
     a. Baker's cyst
     b. Torn ligaments
     c. Loose bodies
     d. Meniscal tears

- Physical Findings—the physical examination is confirmatory, following a careful history
  1. McMurray's test—a palpable or audible click when knee is raised slowly with foot externally rotated; examiner's hand rests on joint line; positive = medial meniscal injuries
  2. Anterior drawer test—positive = anterior cruciate ligament (ACL) tear; posterior drawer test—positive = posterior cruciate ligament (PCL) tear
  3. Lachman test—(anterior drawer test for ACL tear) most sensitive and easy to perform test on a swollen, painful knee; place knee in 20–30° flexion, grasp leg with one hand with anterior force to proximal tibia (to stress ACL) while opposite hand stabilizes thigh; graded 1+ to 3+ grade of displacement
  4. Pain on resisted knee extension
  5. Apley's grind test—flex knee to 90° with patient prone; put pressure on heel with one hand while rotating the lower leg internally and externally; pain or click = positive = medial or lateral collateral ligament damage

- Diagnostic Tests/Findings
  1. Radiographs of knees—AP and lateral to rule out fracture, arthritis
  2. MRI to assess tendon and ligament disease if unresponsive to conservative therapies or physical examination inconsistent with symptoms

- Management/Treatment
  1. Rest, cold pack, immobilization for acute sprain/strain, fractures
  2. NSAID for pain management
  3. ROM of knee, if possible, to prevent stiffness
  4. Hinged knee brace for grades I, II, III collateral ligament sprains

5. Cruceate ligament sprains may require surgical repair, physical therapy
6. Meniscal tears require arthroscopic repair
7. Review ROM and muscle-strengthening exercises

◘ ANKLE SPRAIN

- Definition—stretched, partially torn, or completely ruptured ligaments; usually a consequence of forced inversion or eversion—ankle sprain is most common sports-related injury

- Etiology/Incidence
  1. Lateral ankle sprains most frequent sports-related injury
  2. Between 5 and 10 million ankle sprains occur annually
  3. Most commonly involved structures include the anterior talofibular and fibulocalcaneal ligaments
  4. 10% of ankle sprains are injuries to the medial ligament as a result of pronation and eversion of the ankle

- Signs and Symptoms
  1. Sprains are classified on a grading system of 1–3; signs and symptoms are associated with each grade as follows
     a. Grade 1—related to a stretched ligament; mild or minimal sprain
        (1) Mild localized tenderness
        (2) Normal ROM
        (3) No functional disability
     b. Grade 2—characterized by incomplete or partial rupture of ligament fibers
        (1) Moderate to severe pain with weight bearing; difficulty walking
        (2) Abnormal ROM
        (3) Swelling and local ecchymosis
        (4) Pain immediately after injury
     c. Grade 3—complete disruption of ligament
        (1) Ambulation is impossible
        (2) Resists any motion of the foot
        (3) Marked pain, edema, hemorrhage
        (4) Egg-shaped swelling within 2 hours of injury

- Differential Diagnosis
  1. Avulsion fractures of the malleoli or tarsal bones
  2. Epiphyseal fractures in young patients
  3. Fracture of the calcaneus
  4. Fracture of the fifth metatarsal base
  5. Injury to the bifurcate ligament

- Physical Findings—drawer sign determines anterior talofibular rupture—tibia is stabilized with one hand with foot in neutral and plantar flexed position, force applied to heel with other hand, positive if anterior displacement of talus occurs

- Diagnostic Tests/Findings
    1. Radiograph if fracture suspected
    2. Arthrography—determines site and extent of ligamentous injury
    3. MRI

- Management/Treatment—treatment depends upon the degree of injury
    1. General treatment
        a. Rest
        b. Ice—15–20 minutes every 1–2 hours for 72 hours, then begin contrast baths
        c. Compression
        d. Elevation
        e. Non-weight bearing
        f. NSAID for 10–14 days
        g. Begin ROM when asymptomatic
        h. Reevaluate grades 1 and 2 sprains in 7–10 days
        i. Refer grade 3 sprains for casting
    2. Rehabilitation may begin on the first day after injury and is individualized
        a. ROM
        b. Achilles tendon stretching
        c. Isometrics
        d. Manual resistance exercises
        e. Build up ankle strength after healing to prevent subsequent injury

▣ MUSCLE STRAIN

- Definition—overuse of muscle tendons, resulting in inflammation, often associated with repetitive motion; does not include disruption of tissue

- Etiology/Incidence—strains occur during mild stress by overusing muscle groups not usually used

- Signs and Symptoms—pain after overuse or injury

- Differential Diagnosis
    1. Sprain
    2. Fracture

- Physical Findings
    1. Pain on ROM
    2. Edema
    3. Ecchymosis
    4. Pain of muscle strain resolves after 1–2 days

- Diagnostic Tests/Findings—usually none indicated unless symptoms persist or to rule out suspected fracture

- Management/Treatment
    1. Rest of affected part with assistive devices, if needed
    2. Ice t.i.d. for 20 minutes
    3. Compression
    4. Elevation
    5. Analgesics
    6. NSAID
    7. Education efforts focus on prevention
    8. Increase awareness of repetitive motion
    9. Identify possible changes that will decrease stress on the extremity
    10. Emphasize warm up and stretching before any activity—occupational or sports related

▣ QUESTIONS

Select the best answer.

1. Mr. Johnson, age 55, has developed a slight limp and pain in his right knee, which is worse with weight bearing. Which other findings would be most consistent with osteoarthritis?

    a. Soft-tissue swelling on radiograph
    b. A BMI of 34
    c. A positive McMurray's test
    d. A positive serum CCP

2. Which of the following injectable therapies is used in the treatment of osteoarthritis?

    a. Methotrexate
    b. Enbrel
    c. Hyaluronic acid
    d. Anti-citrullinated antibody

3. On physical examination, enlargement of an 83-year-old patient's distal interphalangeal joints is noted. Enlargement of these joints is known as:

    a. Heberden's nodes
    b. Bouchard's nodes
    c. Tinel's sign
    d. Tenosynovitis

4. Most frequently, synovial fluid aspirate to diagnose gout reveals:

    a. WBCs
    b. RBCs
    c. Urate crystals
    d. High protein content

5. Osteoarthritis is often associated with:

    a. Systemic symptoms of disease
    b. Restricted joint motion
    c. Elevated temperature
    d. Inflammation of the proximal interphalangeal joints

6. Which of the following is not a radiological feature of osteoarthritis?

    a. Unequal loss of joint space
    b. Subchondral bone
    c. Osteophytes
    d. Osteoporosis

7. What is the primary goal of therapy for rheumatoid arthritis?

    a. Control pain
    b. Modify disease progression
    c. Reduce incidence of serious infection
    d. Maintain function with ADLs

8. Rheumatoid arthritis is often associated with:

    a. Systemic symptoms
    b. Weight-bearing joints
    c. Obesity
    d. High purine diet

9. Nonsteroidal anti-inflammatory medications are frequently used in the treatment of musculoskeletal conditions. It is important to remind a patient to:

    a. Take antacids 1 hour after taking NSAID
    b. Exercise at least ½ hour after taking medication
    c. Take the medication at least once a day
    d. Take NSAID with food

10. The onset of rheumatoid arthritis is most frequent:

    a. During 20s and 30s
    b. During 60s and 70s
    c. During 30s and 40s
    d. During 40s and 50s

11. Mrs. Franklin has been complaining of sore hands upon awakening, difficulty opening jars, and trouble holding her hairbrush. The most useful diagnostic study would be:

    a. Serum RF
    b. Anti-CCP
    c. Radiographic assessment
    d. ESR

12. Which joints are most commonly affected by rheumatoid arthritis?

    a. Proximal interphalangeal and metacarpophalangeal joints
    b. Distal interphalangeal joints
    c. Spinous processes
    d. Elbow and shoulder

13. When diagnosing rheumatoid arthritis, which of the following would not be considered a potential differential diagnosis?

    a. Reiter's syndrome
    b. Multiple sclerosis
    c. Rheumatic fever
    d. Ankylosing spondylitis

14. Primary prevention of osteoarthritis includes:

    a. Physical therapy
    b. Synvisc injections
    c. NSAIDs with H_2RA medications
    d. Weight reduction in obese patients

15. Methotrexate is included in which category of medication used to treat rheumatoid arthritis?

    a. Antimalarials
    b. Corticosteroids
    c. Nonsteroidal anti-inflammatory agents
    d. Disease-modifying antirheumatic drugs

16. Podagra is an example of:

    a. Pseudogout
    b. Gout
    c. Osteosarcoma
    d. Septic arthritis

17. Patients with rheumatoid arthritis who are on TNF inhibitors should be especially watchful for the development of:

    a. Symptoms of infection
    b. Cognitive impairment
    c. Extreme fatigue
    d. Loss of pigmentation

18. Mr. Adams, age 55, has a history of chronic exposure to lead. He presents with pain and swelling of his left foot. These facts are both associated with:

    a. Rheumatoid arthritis
    b. Gout
    c. Fracture
    d. Osteoarthritis

19. What is the most common metabolic bone disease in the United States?

    a. Rickets
    b. Scurvy
    c. Osteomyelitis
    d. Osteoporosis

20. A patient with a T-score of 1.5 has:

    a. Osteomalacia
    b. A normal bone density
    c. Osteopenia
    d. Osteoporosis

21. When a patient with gout experiences mild pain, the medication indicated is:

    a. ASA
    b. NSAID
    c. Allopurinol
    d. Probenecid

22. Mr. Jones, age 27, is complaining of acute-onset lower back pain after helping to move a refrigerator. His pain is on the right and shoots down the back of his thigh. The intervertebral space most likely affected is:

    a. L_4-L_5
    b. L_5-S_1
    c. L_3-L_4
    d. T_{10}-L_1

23. Mr. Jones's pain persists for 1 week. He has been treated with activity limitation and NSAID with minimal relief. His symptoms are worsening and you are considering specialty consultation. What is the first diagnostic test to be ordered?

    a. MRI
    b. Anteroposterior and lateral radiograph of the spine
    c. CT scan
    d. Spinal tap

24. A scan for a patient with back pain would be indicated if:

    a. Spinal nerve entrapment is suspected
    b. The history and physical exam do not suggest a cause
    c. The pain radiates to one or both legs
    d. The patient is pregnant

25. Aspirate from a joint space affected by bursitis may be indicative of a bacterial infection when:

    a. WBC is decreased
    b. Glucose is decreased
    c. RBC is increased
    d. Glucose is increased

26. Tennis elbow is a type of:

    a. Tenosynovitis
    b. Rheumatic disease
    c. Epicondylitis
    d. Osteoarthritis

27. The treatment of choice for chronic, stable bursitis is:

    a. Aspiration of fluid
    b. No intervention
    c. NSAIDs
    d. Antibiotic therapy targeting gram positive organisms

28. Positive Tinel's and Phalen's signs are associated with:

    a. Carpal tunnel syndrome
    b. Torn medial meniscus
    c. Baker's cyst
    d. Epicondylitis

29. "Loose bodies" in the knee would result in the following symptom:

    a. Inflammation
    b. "Click" on extension
    c. "Locking"
    d. Instability

30. Mrs. Abbott, age 32, "turned" her ankle when stepping off a curb. She immediately experienced pain on weight bearing and had limited range of motion on examination. What is the most likely diagnosis?

    a. Muscle strain
    b. Grade 2 ankle sprain
    c. Fractured calcaneus
    d. Grade 3 ankle sprain

Answers

1. **b**		16. **b**
2. **c**		17. **a**
3. **a**		18. **b**
4. **c**		19. **d**
5. **b**		20. **c**
6. **d**		21. **b**
7. **b**		22. **b**
8. **a**		23. **a**
9. **d**		24. **a**
10. **d**		25. **b**
11. **b**		26. **c**
12. **a**		27. **b**
13. **b**		28. **a**
14. **d**		29. **c**
15. **d**		30. **b**

◻ BIBLIOGRAPHY

American College of Rheumatology Subcommittee on Rheumatoid Arthritis Guidelines. (2002). Guidelines for the management of rheumatoid arthritis. *Arthritis & Rheumatism, 46,* 328–346.

American Pain Society. (2002). *Guideline for the management of pain in osteoarthritis, rheumatoid arthritis, and juvenile chronic arthritis.* Glenview, IL: American Pain Society.

Anders, M., Turner, L., & Wallace, L. S. (2007). Use of decision rules for osteoporosis prevention and treatment: Implications for nurse practitioners. *Journal of the American Academy of Nurse Practitioners, 19*(6), 299–305.

Anderson, B. C. (2006). *Office orthopedics for primary care* (3rd ed.). Philadelphia: Saunders.

Brigham and Women's Hospital. (2003). *Lower extremity musculoskeletal disorders: A guide to diagnosis and treatment.* Boston, MA: Brigham and Women's Hospital.

Daniels, J. M., Zook, E. G., & Lynch, J. M. (2004). Hand and wrist injuries: Part I. Nonemergent evaluation. *American Family Physician, 69*(8), 1941–1948.

Follin, S. L., & Hansen, L. B. (2003). Current approaches to the prevention and treatment of postmenopausal osteoporosis. *American Journal of Health-System Pharmacy, 60*(9), 883–901.

Holm, G. B. (2004). Office management of back and neck pain. *Advance for Nurse Practitioners, 12*(7), 38–42.

Holm, G., & Moody, L. E. (2003). Carpal tunnel syndrome: Current theory, treatment, and the use of B$_6$. *Journal of the American Academy of Nurse Practitioners, 15,* 18–22.

Klareskog, L., Catrina, A. I., & Paget, S. (2009). Rheumatoid arthritis. *Lancet, 373,* 659–672. Newsome, G. (2002). Guidelines for the management of rheumatoid arthritis: 2002 update. *Journal of the American Academy of Nurse Practitioners, 14,* 432–437.

McPhee, S., & Papadakis, M. (Eds.). (2012). *Current medical diagnosis and treatment* (51st ed.). New York: McGraw-Hill.

Peterson, E. L. (2007). Fibromyalgia—Management of a misunderstood disorder. *Journal of the American Academy of Nurse Practitioners, 19*(7), 341–348.

Saag, K. G., Teng, G. G., Patkar, N. M., Anuntiyo, J., Finney, C., Curtis, J. R . . . Furst, D. E. (2008). American College of Rheumatology 2008 recommendations for the use of nonbiologic and biologic disease-modifying antirheumatic drugs in rheumatoid arthritis. *Arthritis & Rheumatology, 59,* 762–784.

13

Neurological Disorders

Sally K. Miller

◘ HEADACHE

- Definition—very common complaint in primary care; may be actual product of a disease or syndrome (tension, migraine, cluster) or symptom of an underlying disorder (giant cell arteritis, structural lesion); since there are many types of headaches, all with varying degrees of severity, proper assessment of headache and associated symptoms is critical

- Etiology/Incidence
  1. Primary (headache is the diagnosis)
     a. Tension
     b. Migraine
        (1) Classic (occurs with aura)
        (2) Common (no aura)
     c. Cluster headaches
  2. Secondary (due to an underlying process)
     a. Toxic
        (1) Viral infection
        (2) Medication induced
     b. Subdural hematoma
     c. Subarachnoid hemorrhage—medical emergency requiring immediate hospitalization
     d. Meningeal irritation
     e. Giant cell arteritis
     f. Structural lesion—infrequently presents as headache but must be considered
     g. Referred pain from eyes, ears, sinuses, teeth
     h. Visual strain
     i. Narrow angle glaucoma
     j. Hypertensive headache
     k. Posttraumatic headache
     l. Cough headache
     m. Depression

- Components of Headache Evaluation
  1. Chronology is most important item—headache of recent onset that becomes progressively more frequent and/or severe is more ominous than extremely intense headache that has presented in same fashion over a period of time
  2. Location, duration, and quality—should be evaluated as they will provide clues to the underlying cause
  3. Associated activity—exertion, sleep, tension, relaxation
  4. Timing of menstrual cycle in women
  5. Presence of associated symptoms such as neurological symptoms, systemic symptoms of illness (rhinitis, pharyngitis), symptoms of anxiety or depression (sleep disturbance, inability to concentrate)
  6. Presence of triggers—things that seem to be associated with headache onset such as certain foods, stress, alcohol, weather changes
  7. Age and character of onset—headaches of very abrupt onset (apoplectic) are much more ominous, as are those that occur < 5 or > 50 years of age

◪ TENSION HEADACHES

- Definition—headache associated with prolonged contraction of muscles of the head

- Etiology/Incidence
  1. Physical or emotional stress
  2. Circumstances producing physical tension, prolonged muscle contraction

- Signs and Symptoms
  1. Associated complaints of poor concentration and other vague, nonspecific symptoms
  2. Usually lasts for several hours
  3. Usually described as generalized and bilateral—may be most intense about the neck or back of head
  4. Described as viselike or tight in quality
  5. Occur frequently during or following stressful circumstances
  6. No associated focal neurological symptoms
  7. No aura

- Differential Diagnosis
  1. Evaluation of social history very important in differentiating tension headache
     a. Work history
     b. Family circumstances
     c. Recent life changes—birth, death, marriage, divorce
  2. Other syndromes producing similar headache patterns
     a. Common migraine
     b. Toxic headache
     c. Hypertensive headache
     d. Referred pain from other structures in the head
     e. Meningeal irritation

- Physical Findings
  1. Often no physical findings
  2. May find cervical muscle pain/tenderness to palpation
  3. Other findings depending upon severity
     a. Tremor
     b. Disinterest in appearance

- Diagnostic Tests/Findings
  1. None specific to tension headache
  2. Radiographic imaging of head as appropriate to rule out organic disorder

- Management/Treatment
  1. Definitive management of tension headache involves determining and modifying source of tension

  2. Over-the-counter analgesics for pain control—should be taken as soon as headache begins
     a. Acetaminophen 650–1,000 mg q.i.d.
     b. Aspirin 650–1,000 mg q.i.d.
     c. Ibuprofen 400 mg q.i.d.
     d. Other NSAIDs as preferred by the patient; caution regarding GI toxicity with prolonged use
  3. Relaxation or stress-reducing techniques
     a. Biofeedback
     b. Massage
     c. Hot baths
  4. Explore underlying cause of stress/anxiety
  5. When initial measures fail, a trial of antimigraine agents is appropriate

◪ MIGRAINE HEADACHE

- Definition—an extremely painful headache syndrome that is disabling during acute attack; commonly divided into two categories
  1. Classic migraine occurring after an aura—aura precedes pain and may include visual disturbances; auditory, visual, or olfactory hallucinations; or other neurological symptoms
  2. Common migraine—not associated with an aura

- Etiology/Incidence
  1. Categorized as a neurovascular disorder
     a. Dilation and excessive pulsation of intracranial pathways stimulates trigeminal pain pathways
     b. Excess release of vasoactive peptides exacerbates pain
  2. Variety of triggers—a headache diary should be kept by the patient to identify them
     a. Emotional or physical stress
     b. Lack of or excess sleep
     c. Missed meals
     d. Specific foods
     e. Alcoholic beverages
     f. Menstruation
     g. Changes in weather
     h. Nitrate-containing foods
     i. Hormonal contraception
  3. Onset usually in adolescence or early adult years
  4. Often family history of migraine
  5. Females more often affected than males

- Signs and Symptoms
  1. Episodic unilateral, lateralized, throbbing headache
  2. Builds up gradually and lasts several hours or longer

3. Focal neurologic disturbances may precede or accompany migraines
4. Visual disturbances frequently occur
   a. Visual field defects
   b. Luminous visual hallucinations (stars, sparks, zigzag of lights)
5. Aphasia, numbness, tingling, clumsiness, or weakness
6. Nausea and vomiting
7. Photophobia
8. Phonophobia

- Differential Diagnosis
  1. Subarachnoid hemorrhage
  2. Cluster headaches
  3. Hypertensive headache
  4. Cerebrovascular accident
  5. Space-occupying lesion
  6. Giant cell arteritis
  7. Posttraumatic headache

- Physical Findings
  1. Physical examination usually normal
  2. Patient appears acutely ill during migraine
  3. Thorough neurological examination
     a. Focal deficits may accompany migraine but are usually mild and self-limiting
     b. Focal deficits may indicate tumor

- Diagnostic Tests/Findings
  1. None available specific to migraine
  2. Patients with new onset migraine require baseline studies to rule out organic cause; abnormalities may indicate organic cause of pain
     a. Blood chemistries
     b. Complete blood count
     c. Syphilis screening
     d. Erythrocyte sedimentation rate
     e. Radiographic imaging of the head
     f. Other studies indicated by history and physical examination

- Management/Treatment—prophylactic
  1. Avoidance of trigger factors very important
  2. Relaxation and stress management techniques described in management of tension headache
  3. Prophylactic pharmacologic therapy if attacks occur more than 2–3 times per month
     a. Aspirin 650–1,950 mg daily; other NSAIDs may be useful
     b. Propranolol 10–20 mg b.i.d. starting dose, gradually increase to effective dose of 80–120 mg daily—contraindicated in reactive airway disease, heart block, and severe depression

c. Clonidine 0.2–0.6 mg daily
d. Amitriptyline 10–150 mg daily
   (1) Other tricyclic antidepressants helpful
   (2) Must be taken for 2–4 weeks before improvement seen
   (3) Contraindicated in cardiac dysrhythmia, narrow angle glaucoma, and urinary difficulties
e. Selective serotonin reuptake inhibitors (SSRIs)
   (1) Better choice for geriatric patients and those with cardiac disorders
   (2) Fluoxetine, sertraline, paroxetine, and venlafaxine are common choices
      (a) Start 10 mg every day at 7:00 A.M., build to 20 mg in 7–10 days
      (b) Contraindicated in severe depression
f. Calcium channel blockers widely used but not as effective
   (1) Verapamil 40 mg t.i.d., increased to 80 mg t.i.d. over 2–3 weeks; maximum dose 160 mg t.i.d.
   (2) Contraindicated in congestive heart failure, heart block, hypotension

- Management/Treatment—acute attack
  1. Rest in dark, quiet room
  2. Serotonin (5-HT) agonists are mainstay of acute pharmacotherapy
     a. Multiple options available within the class
        (1) Sumatriptan available by injection, nasal spray, and orally
        (2) Zolmitriptan available orally and by disintegrating tablet
        (3) Rizatriptan available orally and by disintegrating tablet
        (4) Others include naratriptan, almotriptan,
     b. Contraindicated in coronary artery disease, Prinzmetal's angina, basilar and hemiplegic migraine, uncontrolled hypertension, history of anaphylaxis, and recent ergotamine use
     c. May cause chest tightness
  3. Simple analgesics (aspirin) taken immediately upon onset may provide some relief
  4. Nonsteroidal agents
     a. Naproxen 250 mg repeat in 1–4 hours as needed
     b. Ketorolac 10 mg repeat in 1–4 hours as needed
  5. Butalbital-containing medications
     a. Aspirin, caffeine, butalbital combination
     b. Acetaminophen, caffeine, butalbital combination

6. Opiates—may be effective but should be used with caution
   a. Butorphanol 1 mg every 4 hours
   b. Meperidine 75–100 mg with hydroxyzine 50 mg IM every 4 hours
7. Ergot alkaloids orally or as suppository—contraindicated in pregnancy, uncontrolled hypertension, peripheral vascular disease, coronary artery disease, liver and kidney disease, and concomitant use of sumatriptan
8. Migranal 2 mg intranasal spray
9. Medicate for nausea as indicated
10. Acetaminophen, aspirin, and caffeine preparation (oral)

◘ CLUSTER HEADACHES

- Definition—among the most painful of all pain-inducing conditions

- Etiology/Incidence
  1. Intrinsic histamine-mediated dilation of external carotid artery
  2. Decreased oxygen saturation due to intrinsic hypothalamic abnormality stimulates brainstem causing pain
  3. Episodic (90%); chronic (10%)
  4. Cycles occur the same time each year—most often during fall and spring
  5. Males more often affected than females at 5:1 ratio
  6. Most common in middle age but affects all age groups
  7. May be precipitated by alcohol ingestion

- Signs and Symptoms
  1. Severe unilateral, orbital, supraorbital, and/or temporal pain occurring in clusters of days or weeks with pain-free period in between
  2. Pain lasts 15 minutes to 2 hours
  3. Attacks occur 1–8 times daily
  4. May rock, pace, or put fist against the painful eye

- Differential Diagnosis
  1. Migraine headache
  2. Narrow angle glaucoma
  3. Structural lesions

- Physical Findings
  1. May be none
  2. Conjunctival injection
  3. Ipsilateral nasal congestion
  4. Rhinorrhea
  5. Forehead or facial sweating
  6. Miosis
  7. Ptosis
  8. Eyelid edema

- Diagnostic Tests/Findings
  1. None diagnostic of cluster headache
  2. As indicated to rule out organic disorders
     a. Computerized axial tomography (CT) scan of the head
     b. Magnetic resonance imaging (MRI) of the head
     c. Complete blood count
     d. Serum chemistries
     e. Erythrocyte sedimentation rate
     f. Electroencephalogram (EEG)

- Management/Treatment—prophylaxis
  1. Ergotamine tartrate 2 mg every day, 0.5–1.0 mg per rectum, or 0.25 mg SQ t.i.d. 5 days weekly
  2. Prednisone 20–40 mg daily or q.o.d. for 2 weeks, then taper
  3. Verapamil 240–480 mg every day
  4. Methysergide 4–6 mg every day
  5. Lithium 300–600 mg every day

- Management/Treatment—acute attack
  1. As described for acute migraine
  2. Inhalation of 100% oxygen—typically only effective in case of cluster headache

◘ TRANSIENT ISCHEMIC ATTACK (TIA)

- Definition—interruption in the cerebral vascular flow, causing ischemia and resultant temporary focal neurologic deficits; two types of TIA—carotid and vertebrobasilar; treatments are same for either type but presenting signs and symptoms differ; by definition attacks are transient, typically lasting < 1 hour but in all cases < 24 hours

- Etiology/Incidence
  1. Embolization is an important cause
     a. Cardiac dysrhythmia
     b. Rheumatic heart disease
     c. Mitral valve disease
     d. Ulcerated plaque on a major artery
     e. Infective endocarditis
     f. Mural thrombus following myocardial infarction
  2. Fibromuscular dysplasia
  3. Inflammatory disorders
     a. Giant cell arteritis
     b. Systemic lupus erythematosus
  4. Hypotension in clients with extracranial artery stenosis
  5. Hematologic disorders
     a. Polycythemia
     b. Sickle cell disease
     c. Severe anemia
  6. Risk factors for vascular disease are often present
     a. Diabetes mellitus
     b. Tobacco use

    c.   Hypertension
    d.   Elevated serum cholesterol
7. Patients with acquired immune deficiency syndrome (AIDS) at increased risk
8. 30,000–150,000 occur annually (may be underreported)

- Signs and Symptoms (Carotid TIA)
  1. Weakness of the contralateral arm, leg, or face, singly or in combination
  2. Numbness or paresthesia of the contralateral side may occur alone or in combination with motor deficits
  3. Homonymous hemianopsia
  4. Ipsilateral monocular vision loss
  5. Symptoms usually disappear within 1 hour and must resolve completely within 24 hours for a diagnosis of TIA
  6. Any of the above symptoms may occur singly or in combination with other symptoms

- Signs and Symptoms (Vertebrobasilar TIA)
  1. Unilateral or bilateral weakness
  2. Vertigo
  3. Ataxia
  4. Diplopia
  5. Dysarthria
  6. Perioral numbness
  7. Drop attacks may occur due to bilateral leg weakness
  8. Dysphasia
  9. Hearing loss
  10. Symptoms may occur singly or in any combination

- Differential Diagnosis
  1. Focal seizures
  2. Classic migraine
  3. Hypoglycemia
  4. Cerebral vascular attack
  5. Vitamin B_{12} deficiency
  6. Drug toxicities
  7. Electrolyte imbalance

- Physical Findings
  1. Physical findings present only during event
  2. Hyperactive deep tendon reflexes
  3. Slowness of movement
  4. Flaccid weakness with pyramidal distribution
  5. May identify sensory impairment
  6. May see atherosclerotic changes on funduscopic examination
  7. Carotid artery bruit
  8. Cardiac examination may suggest source
     a. Murmur
     b. Dysrhythmia
  9. Physical findings absent if patient examined after resolution of symptoms

- Diagnostic Tests/Findings
  1. Clinical and laboratory evaluation must include assessment of risk factors for vascular disease
     a. Complete blood count
     b. Serum glucose
     c. Serum cholesterol
     d. Syphilis screening
     e. Electrocardiogram
     f. Chest radiograph
  2. Echocardiography if cardiac emboli suspected
  3. Evaluate for hypertension
  4. Holter monitor if transient disturbance in cardiac rhythm suspected
  5. CT scan of the head to rule out small hemorrhage, infarct, or tumor
  6. Ultrasound to evaluate cerebral circulation and major vessels to head
  7. Arteriography is definitive study of vasculature—should be considered if patient is good operative risk, CT scan is normal, and no apparent source of cardiac emboli present

- Management/Treatment
  1. Medical management aimed toward preventing further attacks as 30% of patients with cerebrovascular accident have history of TIA
     a. Cessation of tobacco use
     b. Control of underlying medical conditions with emphasis to thromboembolic disease
        (1) Hyperlipidemia
        (2) Diabetes mellitus
        (3) Hypertension
        (4) Arteritis
        (5) Hematologic disorders
     c. Immediate anticoagulation when cardiac emboli is strong possibility—intravenous heparin followed by oral warfarin sodium
     d. Aspirin 325 mg daily when cardiac emboli not strong possibility
     e. Platelet inhibitors in those intolerant of aspirin
        (1) Dipyridamole/ASA 50 mg daily for patients who have had a TIA or cerebrovascular accident (CVA) while taking aspirin
        (2) Clopidogrel bisulfate 75 mg daily for patients with aspirin allergy or intolerance—caution with severe liver disease
        (3) Ticlopidine 250 mg b.i.d. for patients who cannot tolerate first-line choices—monitor for neutropenia or agranulocytosis
  2. Carotid thromboendarterectomy considered when
     a. Arteriography reveals a surgically accessible stenosis > 70%
     b. Relatively little atherosclerosis elsewhere
     c. Patient is a good surgical candidate

■ SEIZURE DISORDER

- Definition
  1. A disorder characterized by transient disturbance of cerebral function due to an abnormal paroxysmal neuronal hyperexcitability and discharge in the brain
  2. Two main classifications of seizure
     a. Partial seizures
        (1) Simple partial seizure
        (2) Complex partial seizure
        (3) Secondarily generalized tonic-clonic seizures
     b. Generalized seizures
        (1) Absence (petit mal) seizure
        (2) Tonic seizure
        (3) Clonic seizure
        (4) Myoclonic seizure
        (5) Atonic seizure
        (6) Tonic-clonic (grand mal) seizure
  3. Partial seizures result from an activation of part of one hemisphere (unilaterally)
  4. Generalized seizures result from a generalized activation of the brain (bilateral)

- Etiology/Incidence
  1. Congenital abnormalities and perinatal injuries may result in seizures presenting in infancy and early childhood
  2. Metabolic disorders
     a. Hypocalcemia
     b. Hypoglycemia
     c. Hyponatremia
     d. Pyridoxine deficiency
     e. Renal failure
     f. Acidosis
     g. Alcohol withdrawal
  3. Infectious diseases
     a. Bacterial meningitis
     b. Herpes encephalitis
     c. Neurosyphilis
  4. Trauma an important cause in young adults
  5. Tumors and other space-occupying lesions
  6. Vascular disease, an increasingly frequent cause in the older population—most common cause when seizure onset is after age 60
  7. May be due to unknown cause
  8. Overall affects approximately 0.5% of the population in the United States

- Signs and Symptoms—simple partial seizure
  1. No loss of consciousness
  2. Lasts approximately 1 minute
  3. Focal motor symptoms (convulsive jerking)
  4. Speech arrest or vocalizations
  5. Jacksonian march

  6. Special sensory symptoms
     a. Light flashes
     b. Buzzing
  7. Paresthesias
  8. Autonomic symptoms
     a. Flushing
     b. Diaphoresis
     c. Pupillary dilation
  9. Dysmnesic symptoms (déjà vu)

- Signs and Symptoms—complex partial seizures—any symptoms of simple partial seizure accompanied by a period of impaired consciousness before, during, or after episode

- Signs and Symptoms—absence (petit mal) seizures
  1. Impairment of consciousness
  2. Mild tonic, clonic, or atonic components
  3. Occasional autonomic components
     a. Flushing
     b. Diaphoresis
     c. Enuresis
  4. Onset and termination very brief, lasting seconds—individual may break off in mid-sentence for a few seconds
  5. Almost always begin in childhood
  6. Frequently cease by age 20, occasionally replaced by other forms of generalized seizure

- Signs and Symptoms—myoclonic seizures
  1. Single or multiple myoclonic jerks
  2. No loss of consciousness

- Signs and Symptoms—tonic-clonic (grand mal) seizures
  1. Sudden loss of consciousness
  2. Patient becomes rigid, falls to the ground
  3. Respiration is arrested
  4. Clonic phase follows tonic phase—jerking of body musculature lasting 2–3 minutes followed by stage of flaccid coma
  5. Urinary and/or fecal incontinence may occur
  6. Lips or tongue may be bitten
  7. After one tonic-clonic cycle, patient may
     a. Recover consciousness
     b. Fall into deep sleep (postictal state)—headache, disorientation, soreness, nausea, and drowsiness common upon awakening
     c. More attacks after recovering consciousness (serial seizures)
     d. More attacks without recovering consciousness (status epilepticus)
     e. Display postepileptic automatism
        (1) Behave in an abnormal fashion in immediate postictal period
        (2) No subsequent memory of events

** AN EYEWITNESS ACCOUNT OF SEIZURE ACTIVITY IS EXTREMELY VALUABLE AND SHOULD BE OBTAINED IF AT ALL POSSIBLE **

- Differential Diagnosis—partial seizures
  1. Transient ischemic attacks
  2. Rage attacks
  3. Panic attacks

- Differential Diagnosis—generalized seizures
  1. Syncope
  2. Cardiac dysrhythmia
  3. Brain stem ischemia
  4. Pseudoseizures

- Physical Findings
  1. May be none
  2. May show evidence of underlying disorder
     a. Trauma
     b. Focal neurological deficits (brain lesion)
     c. Hyperactive reflexes
  3. Muscle soreness following grand mal seizure
  4. Tongue trauma

- Diagnostic Tests/Findings
  1. As indicated to investigate underlying cause and as indicated by history and age of patient
  2. Initial evaluation in patients over 10 years of age should include the following tests in order to investigate cause and provide a baseline for subsequent monitoring of long-term treatment
     a. Complete blood count
     b. Serum glucose
     c. Liver function tests
     d. Renal function tests
     e. Serologic test for syphilis
     f. Head imaging
  3. EEG for paroxysmal abnormalities containing spikes or sharp waves
     a. May help classify disorder
     b. Support clinical diagnosis of seizure
     c. Evaluate candidates for surgical treatment by localizing epileptogenic source
  4. CT scan or MRI to rule out lesion or neoplasm when
     a. Focal neurological signs and symptoms present
     b. EEG findings suggestive of focal disturbance
     c. Onset after age 30
     d. Seizure disorder is progressive
  5. Chest radiograph to rule out primary or secondary neoplasms
  6. Lumbar puncture (LP)—rule out infectious process

- Management/Treatment—acute seizures
  1. Diazepam 5–10 mg slow IV
  2. Lorazepam 4 mg slow IV

- Management/Treatment—preventive
  1. May need to be reported to Department of Motor Vehicles
  2. Treat underlying problem as appropriate
     a. Infectious process
     b. Metabolic disturbance
  3. Pharmacologic choice depends upon type of seizure
  4. Pharmacologic options for generalized tonic-clonic or partial seizures
     a. Levetiracitam 1,000–3,000 mg daily in divided doses—does not require serum level monitoring
     b. Phenytoin 200–400 mg daily or in divided doses
        (1) Maintain serum level 10–20 μg/mL
        (2) Contraindicated in patients with sino-atrial or atrioventricular block
     c. Carbamazepine 600–1,200 mg in 2 divided doses daily
        (1) Maintain serum level 4–12 μg/mL
        (2) Contraindicated in patients with known hypersensitivity to tricyclic antidepressants, patients with past or present bone marrow depression, and patients on monoamine oxidase inhibitors
     d. Valproic acid 1,500–2,000 mg in 3 divided doses daily
        (1) Maintain serum level 50–100 μg/mL
        (2) Contraindicated in patients with known hepatic disease
  5. Pharmacologic choices for petit mal seizures
     a. Ethosuximide 1,000–1,500 mg in 2 divided doses daily
        (1) Maintain serum level 40–100 μg/mL
        (2) Use with extreme caution in patients with hepatic or renal disease
     b. Valproic acid at doses indicated for tonic-clonic seizure
     c. Clonazepam 0.05–0.2 mg/kg in 2 divided doses daily
        (1) Maintain serum level 20–80 ng/mL
        (2) Contraindicated in patients with known hypersensitivity to benzodiazepines, hepatic disease, chronic respiratory disorders, and untreated glaucoma
  6. Pharmacologic choice for myoclonic seizures
     a. Valproic acid at doses indicated for tonic-clonic seizure
     b. Clonazepam at doses indicated for petit mal seizure

7. Newer antiseizure medications for adjunctive therapy of partial or secondary generalized seizures
    a. Gabapentin 900–1,800 mg daily in divided doses
    b. Lamotrigine 100–500 mg daily in divided doses
    c. Topiramate 200–400 mg daily in divided doses
8. Patients should be advised to avoid dangerous situations
9. When first drug choice does not provide control, add second drug until therapeutic levels obtained, then first drug gradually withdrawn
10. Prophylactic medication not generally indicated based on one seizure unless further attacks occur or investigation identifies untreatable pathology
11. Withdrawal of medication should only be considered when patient has been free of seizure activity for at least 4 years
    a. Dose reduction over a period of weeks/months
    b. Reinstitution of same drug(s) if seizure recurs

◘ PARKINSON'S DISEASE

- Definition—degenerative central nervous system disorder characterized by any combination of tremor, rigidity, bradykinesia, or progressive postural instability

- Etiology/Incidence
  1. Degeneration of the dopaminergic nigro-striatal system leads to dopamine depletion and consequently a dopamine/acetylcholine imbalance
  2. Most commonly idiopathic, but causes may include
     a. Exposure to toxins
        (1) Manganese dust
        (2) Carbon disulfide
        (3) Carbon monoxide
     b. Postencephalitic parkinsonism
  3. Onset usually between 45 and 65 years of age
  4. Approximately equal gender distribution
  5. Occurs in all ethnic groups

- Signs and Symptoms
  1. Any combination of
     a. Tremor
     b. Rigidity
     c. Bradykinesia
     d. Progressive postural instability
  2. Wooden facies
  3. Impaired swallowing

  4. Decreased automatic movement
  5. Seborrhea of scalp and face

- Differential Diagnosis
  1. Side effects of high-potency neuroleptics
  2. Brain tumor
  3. Depression
  4. Benign essential tremor
  5. Dementia
  6. Huntington's disease
  7. Creutzfeldt-Jakob disease

- Physical Findings
  1. Relatively immobile face with wide palpebral fissures
  2. Infrequent blinking
  3. Seborrhea
  4. Myerson's response—repetitive tapping over bridge of nose produces sustained blinking response
  5. Drooling
  6. Bradykinesia
  7. Slow cycle tremor—most conspicuous at rest
  8. No muscle weakness
  9. No alteration in deep tendon reflexes or plantar response
  10. Slow shuffling steps; loss of automatic arm swing

- Diagnostic Tests/Findings
  1. None specific to Parkinson's disease
  2. As indicated to rule out toxins
  3. As indicated to rule out differential diagnoses

- Management/Treatment
  1. Levodopa/carbidopa 25/100 or sustained release form 50/200 t.i.d.
     a. Initial drug of choice in more progressive disease
     b. Improves all clinical features but does not halt progression
     c. Contraindicated in
        (1) Narrow angle glaucoma
        (2) Psychotic illness
        (3) Patients taking monoamine oxidase A inhibitors
     d. Use caution with malignant melanoma or active ulcer disease
     e. Generally loses effectiveness after several years of treatment; generally 5 years therapeutic efficacy anticipated
  2. Dopamine agonists—stimulate dopamine receptors in brain; may be used as monotherapy early in disease or in combination with levodopa/carbidopa
     a. Ropinirole 0.25–3 mg t.i.d.—adverse effects include orthostatic hypotension, syncope, hallucinations

b. Pramipexole 1.5–6 mg daily—adverse effects include orthostatic hypotension, hallucinations, somnolence, nausea, vomiting

c. Bromocriptine 1.25 mg b.i.d. titrate to symptom improvement—contraindicated in
   (1) History of mental illness
   (2) Recent myocardial infarction
   (3) Peripheral vascular disease
   (4) Bleeding ulcers

d. May delay need to initiate levodopa, subsequently prolonging the therapeutic lifespan of pharmacotherapy

e. Adverse effects similar to those of levodopa but typically more pronounced

f. May be preferred initial treatment for younger patients

3. Catechol-o-methyl transferase (COMT) inhibitors

   a. Used as an adjunct to levadopa/carbidopa for those with unsatisfactory clinical response

   b. All agents in this class have black box warning; require close monitoring for hepatic toxicity

   c. Tolcapone 100–200 mg t.i.d.

   d. Entacapone 200 mg with each dose levadopa/carbidopa to maximum 1,600 mg daily

   e. Due to risk of hepatocellular injury, tolcapone should be discontinued in 3 weeks if no clinical response noted

4. Selegiline 5 mg b.i.d. with breakfast and lunch with levodopa

   a. Clinical responses not consistent

   b. Evidence that it arrests the progression of disease requires it be considered for patients with early disease or mild forms

5. Anticholinergics to alleviate tremor and rigidity

   a. Benztropine mesylate 1–6 mg daily

   b. Trihexyphenidyl 6–20 mg daily

   c. Biperiden 2–12 mg daily

   d. Poorly tolerated by elderly; side effects include
      (1) Urinary retention
      (2) Increased intraocular pressure
      (3) Dysrhythmia
      (4) Constipation

   e. Contraindicated in
      (1) Narrow angle glaucoma
      (2) Prostatic hypertrophy
      (3) Obstructive gastrointestinal disease

6. Amantadine 100 mg b.i.d.

   a. Mode of action unclear

   b. Improves clinical features in mild disease

   c. Side effects include confusion, depression, restlessness, hypotension, and cardiac abnormalities

7. Clozapine 6.25 mg; titrate to 25–100 mg for confusion, psychosis, and dyskinesias; monitor CBC

8. Physical therapy and speech therapy may be helpful

9. Surgical thalamotomy or pallidotomy a consideration for those with severe disease and medication intolerance

◘ MULTIPLE SCLEROSIS

- Definition
  1. Pathological focal areas of demyelination with reactive gliosis scattered in white matter of brain and in optic nerve; single lesions cannot explain clinical findings
  2. Months or years may pass between initial symptom appearance and recurrence or exacerbation, but eventually progressive disability usually results (relapsing, remitting)
  3. Less commonly, symptoms worsen steadily from onset and disability occurs early (primary progressive)

- Etiology/Incidence
  1. Cause unknown
  2. May be familial incidence
  3. Association with HLA-DR2 antigen suggests genetic predisposition
  4. Immunological basis suspected
  5. Greatest incidence in young adults—onset usually < 55 years of age
  6. More common in persons of Western European descent who live in temperate climates through adolescence
  7. Certain factors may trigger exacerbation
     a. Pregnancy and postpartum period
     b. Infection
     c. Trauma
  8. 300,000 cases in the United States
  9. Female to male ration 2.5:1
  10. Family history with first-degree relative increases risk by 15%

- Signs and Symptoms
  1. Weakness, numbness, tingling, or unsteadiness in a limb
  2. Spastic paraparesis
  3. Diplopia
  4. Disequilibrium
  5. Urinary urgency or hesitancy
  6. Vertigo
  7. Sphincter disturbance

- Differential Diagnosis
  1. Anxiety
  2. Brain tumor

3. Spinal cord lesion
4. Neurosyphilis
5. Systemic lupus erythematosus
6. Metastatic carcinoma

- Physical Findings
  1. Optic atrophy
  2. Nystagmus
  3. Ataxia
  4. Dysarthria
  5. Muscle weakness
  6. Decreased vibratory sense
  7. Hyperactive deep tendon reflexes
  8. Positive Babinski with clonus
  9. Sensory deficits in some or all limbs

- Diagnostic Tests/Findings
  1. Definitive diagnosis cannot be based on laboratory findings alone
  2. Diagnostic tests as indicated to rule out other causes of symptoms
     a. Serum B_{12}
     b. Syphilis screening
     c. Serum antinuclear antibody (ANA)
  3. Mild lymphocytosis
  4. Cerebrospinal fluid abnormalities
     a. Slightly elevated protein
     b. Elevated IgG
     c. Discrete bands of IgG called oligoclonal bands—presence of oligoclonal bands not specific but supportive
  5. MRI preferred to CT scan
     a. Demonstrates multiplicity of lesions
     b. Rule out surgically treatable lesions
     c. Visualize foramen magnum to rule out Arnold-Chiari malformation
     d. Neurophysiological assessment of electrocerebral responses to evaluate subclinical involvement of cerebral pathways

- Management/Treatment
  1. No definitive method of arresting disease process, but areas of investigation include
     a. Immunosuppressive therapy
     b. Plasmapheresis
     c. Beta interferon used in relapsing-remitting form of disease
     d. Cop 1 (a random polymer-stimulating myelin basic protein) may be helpful to patients with relapsing-remitting form
  2. Methylprednisolone 1 g intravenously for 3 days followed by prednisone 80 mg daily for 1 week then tapered for 2–3 weeks
     a. May hasten recovery from acute exacerbation
     b. Does not improve the extent of recovery
     c. Does not slow progression of disease

3. Treatment of urinary retention
   a. Various pharmacologic options to stimulate urination
   b. Intermittent self-catheterization
   c. Indwelling foley catheter last option
4. Diazepam and carbamazepine may relieve paresthesias
5. Medications to relieve fatigue
   a. Antidepressants
   b. Amantadine
   c. Modafinil
6. Rest/activity balance
7. Treatment of constipation
   a. High-fiber diet
   b. Stool softeners/laxatives as indicated
8. Emotional support, patient education
   a. Sexual dysfunction may be a problem
   b. Other social/intimacy issues
      (1) Questions regarding marriage
      (2) Questions regarding having children
9. Avoidance of triggers

▣ QUESTIONS

Select the best answer.

1. All of the following are considered primary headache syndromes except:
   a. Hypertension
   b. Common migraine
   c. Classic migraine
   d. Tension

2. Which of the following causes of headache is a medical emergency?
   a. Toxic headache
   b. Classic migraine
   c. Subarachnoid hemorrhage
   d. Subdural hematoma

3. A systematic and thorough assessment of the headache is important in making the appropriate diagnosis. Which of the following components of headache assessment is the most important?
   a. Presence of associated symptoms
   b. Chronology of headache
   c. Presence of triggers
   d. Age of onset

4. Your patient describes a headache that is quite painful and vise-like in quality. The pain is generalized about the head and lasts for several hours at a time. There does not appear to be an aura, and the patient does not report any symptoms suggestive of focal neurological deficits. Based

upon your knowledge of headache evaluation, you know that the most likely diagnosis is:

a. Cluster headache
b. Common migraine
c. Tension headache
d. Hypertensive headache

5. Migraine and cluster headaches are both extremely painful headache syndromes that may be difficult to differentiate. Based on known epidemiological patterns, who is most likely to suffer from migraines?

a. A 45-year-old male with history of excess alcohol use
b. A 35-year-old female with history of excess alcohol use
c. A 19-year-old female with family history of migraine
d. A 24-year-old male with family history of migraine

6. Excess release of serotonin is proposed as possible etiological factor in:

a. Migraine headache
b. Seizure disorder
c. Parkinson's disease
d. Multiple sclerosis

7. Which of the following is not typically a trigger of migraine headache?

a. Menstruation
b. Excess sleep
c. Changes in weather
d. Loud noise

8. 5HT agonists are considered primary therapy for acute migraine headache. Which of the following is a contraindication to their administration?

a. A history of serotonin syndrome
b. Current treatment with beta adrenergic antagonists
c. Current treatment with calcium channel antagonists
d. A history of angina

9. Cluster headaches are different from other headache syndromes in that they are sometimes responsive to therapy with:

a. NSAIDs
b. Inhaled oxygen
c. 5HT agonists
d. Clonidine

10. Propranolol is a pharmacologic agent used in the prophylactic management of migraine, but there are several contraindications to its use. In which of the following patients is propranolol not contraindicated?

a. A 40-year-old man with asthma
b. A 39-year-old woman with Grave's disease
c. A 32-year-old woman with type 1 heart block
d. A 24-year-old man with severe depression

11. Amitriptyline is an antidepressant medication that can be useful in the prophylactic management of migraine headache. Which of the following statements is true regarding amitriptyline therapy for migraine prophylaxis?

a. It is the only antidepressant that is useful in migraine prophylaxis
b. Improvement is usually seen in 2–4 weeks
c. It is contraindicated in severe depression
d. It has fewer side effects than paroxetine

12. Possible organic causes of cluster headache include:

a. Histamine release
b. Constriction and rebound dilation of arteries
c. Physical tension of muscle tissue
d. Chronic alcohol ingestion

13. Many headache-inducing conditions are difficult to diagnose because there are no associated physical exam findings. Ptosis, eyelid edema, conjunctival injection, and ipsilateral nasal congestion are findings associated with:

a. Classic migraine
b. Toxic headache
c. Narrow angle glaucoma
d. Cluster headache

14. Tapered corticosteroids are a recommended prophylactic regimen in the treatment of:

a. Cluster headache
b. Tension headache
c. Migraine headache
d. Subdural hematoma

15. Which of the following is a diagnostic criterion for transient ischemic attack?

a. Numbness or parasthesia with motor deficits
b. Symptoms resolve in < 24 hours
c. Symptoms include homonymous hemianopsia
d. Lacunar infarct on CT scan

16. Medical management of transient ischemic attack (TIA) is aimed toward preventing further attacks and subsequent cerebrovascular accident (CVA). When atrial fibrillation is discovered during the clinical examination, therapy of TIA should include:

a. Aspirin
b. Coumadin
c. Ticlopidine
d. Verapamil

17. When is ticlopidine preferred in the management of TIA?

    a. When the patient is intolerant of aspirin
    b. When cardiac emboli is suspected
    c. When heparin has been administered for 5–7 days
    d. When the patient is dysrhythmic

18. What is the most common cause of seizure disorder in the elderly population?

    a. Congenital abnormalities
    b. Renal failure
    c. Neurosyphilis
    d. Vascular disease

19. What is the primary difference between a simple partial seizure and complex partial seizure?

    a. There are no EEG changes
    b. They do not require chronic medication therapy
    c. There is no loss of consciousness
    d. There is no postictal state

20. Which type of seizure is almost exclusively found in children and young adults?

    a. Myoclonic
    b. Simple partial
    c. Absence
    d. Tonic-clonic

21. Postepileptic automatism is characterized by:

    a. More tonic-clonic attacks with periods of consciousness in between
    b. Headache, disorientation, and nausea
    c. More tonic-clonic attacks without periods of consciousness in between
    d. Abnormal behavior in the immediate postictal period

22. The most important information in seizure assessment is usually provided by

    a. An eyewitness
    b. An electroencephalogram (EEG)
    c. A CT scan
    d. Magnetic resonance imaging (MRI)

23. Which form of seizure disorder does not require antiepileptic drug (AED) therapy?

    a. Simple partial
    b. Complex partial
    c. Absence
    d. Alcohol withdrawal

24. An EEG is helpful in the evaluation of seizure disorder for several reasons. Which of the following is not accomplished with an EEG?

    a. Classification of the disorder
    b. Etiology of the disorder
    c. Localization of the epileptogenic source
    d. Support of clinical diagnosis

25. What is the drug of choice for acute seizure management?

    a. Phenytoin
    b. Clonazepam
    c. Lorazepam
    d. Valproic acid

26. Several antiepileptic drugs are characterized by:

    a. A tendency to promote tolerance requiring progressively higher doses
    b. A narrow range of effectiveness to safety requiring periodic assessment of serum levels
    c. The potential risk for clotting abnormalities and subsequent bleeding disorders
    d. Potentially dangerous interactions with benzodiazepines, which are required for acute seizure suppression

27. When is it appropriate to withdraw seizure medication?

    a. When the patient is pregnant
    b. When the patient has been seizure free for 4 years
    c. When the patient is an alcoholic
    d. When the patient has untreatable pathology

28. What is the most common cause of parkinsonism?

    a. Postencephalitic
    b. Manganese dust
    c. Exposure to toxins
    d. Idiopathic

29. Immobile face with wide palpebral fissures is a common physical finding in the patient with:

    a. Absence seizure
    b. Depression
    c. Multiple sclerosis
    d. Parkinson's disease

30. When are dopamine agonists preferred for initial management of Parkinson's disease?

    a. In the younger patient
    b. In a patient no longer responsive to levodopa
    c. When liver function abnormalities prohibit use of COMT inhibitors
    d. When there is comorbid schizophrenia

31. Which of the following is true regarding the use of corticosteroids in treating multiple sclerosis?

    a. It hastens recovery from exacerbation
    b. It improves the extent of recovery
    c. It slows progression of the disease
    d. It relieves paresthesias

◻ ANSWERS

1.	**a**	17.	**a**
2.	**c**	18.	**d**
3.	**b**	19.	**c**
4.	**c**	20.	**c**
5.	**c**	21.	**d**
6.	**a**	22.	**a**
7.	**d**	23.	**d**
8.	**d**	24.	**b**
9.	**b**	25.	**c**
10.	**b**	26.	**b**
11.	**b**	27.	**b**
12.	**a**	28.	**d**
13.	**d**	29.	**d**
14.	**a**	30.	**a**
15.	**b**	31.	**a**
16.	**b**		

◻ BIBLIOGRAPHY

Aminoff, M. J., & Kerchner, G. A. (2012). Nervous system. In S. J. McPhee & M. A. Papadakis (Eds.), *Current medical diagnosis and treatment* (51st ed., pp. 936–1009). New York: McGraw-Hill.

Cavasoz, J. E., & Spitz, M. (2009). Seizures and epilepsy, overview & classification: Treatment and medication. Emedicine. Retrieved from http://emedicine.medscape.com/article/1184846-treatment

Dangond, F. (2006). Multiple sclerosis. Emedicine. Retrieved from http://www.emedicine.com/neuro/TOPIC 228.htm

Fenstermacher, K., & Hudson, B. (2003). *Practice guidelines for family nurse practitioners* (3rd ed.). Philadelphia: Saunders.

French, J. A., Kanner, A. M., Bautista, J., Abou-Khalil, B., Browne, T., Harden, C. L . . . Glauser, T. A. (2004). Efficacy and tolerability of the new antiepileptic drugs I: Treatment of new onset epilepsy: Report of the Therapeutics and Technology Assessment Subcommittee and Quality Standards Subcommittee of the American Academy of Neurology and the AES. *Neurology, 62*(8), 1252–1260.

Goolsby, M. J., (2003). Migraine headaches. *Journal of the American Academy of Nurse Practitioners, 15*(12), 536–538.

Scott, B. L., & Stacy, M. A. (2009). The management of Parkinson's disease in the primary care setting. Clinician Reviews, 19(6, supp), 3–11.

14

Psychosocial Disorders

Sister Maria Salerno

◘ DEPRESSION (MAJOR)

- Definition—a complex clinical syndrome consisting of physical, affective, and cognitive symptoms that range from mild to severe; it is attributable to a variety of organic, environmental, and developmental causes and is diagnosed according to defined clinical criteria—commonly used subtypes include
  1. Adjustment disorder with depressed mood
     a. Occurring within 3 months of an identifiable stressor
     b. Depressed mood and impairment of function or symptoms in excess of those normally expected
     c. Symptoms ease as stressor passes
     d. Often self-limiting but can lead to major depression
  2. Major depression (MD)
     a. Five of nine symptoms are present continuously during the same 2-week period
        (1) Presence of depressed mood, OR
        (2) Anhedonia (loss of interest or pleasure in most all activities most of the day) with
            (a) Increased or decreased appetite or significant weight loss or gain—more than 5% of body weight in a month
            (b) Sleep disturbance—hypersomnia or insomnia
            (c) Psychomotor agitation or retardation
            (d) Fatigue or loss of energy
            (e) Feelings of worthlessness or inappropriate guilt or low self-esteem
            (f) Decreased ability to think, concentrate, or make decisions
            (g) Recurrent thoughts of death, suicidal ideation without an attempt or specific plan
     b. The symptoms represent a change from previous functioning and are severe and disabling
     c. The onset is variable and may be superimposed on dysthymia
  3. Dysthymia (chronic depression)
     a. Milder than MD
        (1) Depressed mood
        (2) At least two other symptoms
        (3) Loss of self-esteem prominent
     b. Poor coping skills
     c. Often associated with chronic drug use
     d. More chronic—symptoms present for 2 years or more
     e. No clear onset
  4. Depressive disorder not otherwise specified (NOS)
     a. Depressed mood and two to four moderate to severe symptoms
     b. Does not meet criteria for MD or dysthymia
     c. Includes several subcategories
        (1) Atypical depression—characterized by
            (a) Hypersomnia
            (b) Hyperphagia
            (c) Lethargy
            (d) Rejection sensitivity

(2) Seasonal affective disorder
  (a) Disturbance of circadian rhythm
  (b) Related to light spectrum exposure
  (c) Carbohydrate craving, lethargy, hyperphagia, and hypersomnia are characteristic
(3) Premenstrual dysphoric disorder—symptoms occur year round during the late luteal phase of the cycle and resolve when menses begins
  (a) More disabling than premenstrual syndrome
  (b) Cardinal feature is irritability; a variety of additional symptoms produce emotional and physical disability
(4) Prenatal depression and postpartum depression
  (a) 10–15% accompanied by obsessive concerns about ability to care for infant or fear of doing harm to the infant
  (b) Usually occurs 2 months to 1 year postpartum
  (c) Occurs in approximately 20% of the population
  (d) Is *not* postpartum psychosis—no recognized danger to infant

5. Bipolar disorder—recurrent episodes of depression interspersed with bouts of mania
  a. Heredity a strong factor
  b. Tricyclic antidepressants (TCA) often precipitate a manic response called "hypomania"
  c. Early onset, usually before age 30
  d. Incidence in African-Americans and whites similar
  e. Incidence is similar in males and females
6. Organic mood syndrome—major depressive episode associated with a general medical condition or medications
  a. Substance abuse (alcoholism is a common cause)
  b. Endocrinopathy, e.g., hypothyroidism, Cushing's disease, Addison's disease
  c. Neurological disorders—left-sided stroke, parkinsonism
  d. Pancreatic cancer
  e. Antihypertensives

- Etiology/Incidence
1. Psychosocial and/or biochemical causes for depression have been theorized
  a. Psychosocial
    (1) Psychoanalytical
      (a) Anger turned inward
      (b) Regression to a less mature stage of functioning
    (2) Environmental
      (a) Stressful life events
      (b) Changes or inadequacies in social support
    (3) Psychodynamic
      (a) Personality development
        (i) Passive/dependent
        (ii) Obsessive/compulsive
      (b) Effects of past relationships and developmental task on coping styles, particularly use of defense mechanisms
        (i) Denial
        (ii) Suppression
        (iii) Sublimation
    (4) Cognitive
      (a) Self-reinforcing habit of unrealistic negative ideas
      (b) Recent or past style of thinking and relating
      (c) Learned "helplessness"
  b. Biochemical
    (1) Catecholamine
      (a) Poorly functioning neurotransmitter
      (b) Primarily dopamine, norepinephrine, epinephrine, and serotonin
    (2) Endocrine
      (a) Cortisol
      (b) Thyroid releasing hormone
2. Incidence
  a. Depressive illness most common mental health problem seen in general practice
  b. Estimated 13–20% of the general population suffer from depressive illness, yet fewer than a third will receive treatment
  c. Twice as many women as men with major depression worldwide
  d. Lifetime risk for developing depressive illness
    (1) 20% for females
    (2) 10% for males
  e. Major depression can occur in any age group
    (1) Adolescents and the elderly at higher risk
    (2) Peak incidence 55–65 years old
    (3) Other risk factors
      (a) Family history of depressive illness, chemical dependency, substance abuse, or major medical illness
      (b) Prior depressive episode or suicide attempt
      (c) Recent childbirth (postpartum)
      (d) Unanticipated or prolonged stress
      (e) Lack of social support

f. Bipolar disorder occurs equally among the genders

g. Race is not a factor; prevalence is equal among ethnic groups

h. Major depression has a 50–85% recurrence rate within 3–9 years

i. 15% of patients with depression successfully commit suicide

j. Only one-half of patients with depression receive treatment

- Signs and Symptoms
  1. None specific
      a. Aggravation of any physical pathology
      b. Pains of undetermined etiology in a variety of anatomical sites
  2. Mnemonic device to recall major symptoms— IN SAD CAGES
      a. *IN*terest—loss of interest or pleasure in just about any activity
      b. *S*leep disturbances
          (1) Hypersomnia or insomnia
          (2) Early morning awakenings with painful ruminations
      c. *A*ppetite and/or weight change
      d. *D*epressed mood
          (1) Tends to be most pervasive symptom
          (2) May manifest as crying spells
      e. *C*oncentration poor; indecisiveness, inability to act, procrastination
      f. *A*ctivity—agitation or retardation
      g. *G*uilt, low self-esteem
      h. *E*nergy loss, fatigue
      i. *S*uicidal ideation, thoughts of death, suicide attempts

- Differential Diagnosis
  1. Since depression may be a manifestation of many illnesses the differential diagnosis must include a thorough search for factors or organic diseases that may be responsible for symptom manifestation including
      a. Infections, inflammation
      b. Neurological neoplasms, stroke, trauma
      c. Endocrine disorders
      d. Nutritional deficiencies
      e. Electrolyte disturbances
  2. Differentiate major depression from other mental disorders, e.g., schizophrenia, dementia, adjustment disorder with depressed mood
  3. Currently the trend is to address the signs and symptoms of major depression; if criteria presented previously are met the diagnosis is made regardless of comorbidity

- Physical Findings
  1. General—may show lack of personal grooming and hygiene, inattention to dress, slouched posture, slowed speech and movements, long pauses in response to questions, tearfulness; weight may be less than or more than ideal for body size, may appear dehydrated
  2. Mental status—poor concentration, decreased memory, indecision, pessimism

- Diagnostic Tests/Findings
  1. Initial tests
      a. CBC—normal
      b. Chemical profile including liver function— normal
      c. Urinalysis and urine toxicology screen— normal
      d. Thyroid function—normal
      e. VDRL—normal
      f. B_{12} level—normal
      g. EKG—normal
      h. Chest radiograph—normal
      i. In first or second episode
          (1) Computer tomography (CT) scan or magnetic resonance imaging (MRI) of the brain—normal
          (2) HIV screen—normal
  2. Depression screening instruments—scores indicative of depression
      a. Beck Depression Inventory
      b. Yesavage Geriatric Depression Scale
      c. Zung Self-Rating Depression Scale
  3. Special tests (primarily used in psychiatric and research settings)
      a. Thyroid stimulating hormone (TSH) response to thyroid releasing hormone (TRH) may be decreased
      b. Dexamethasone suppression test (DST) used to distinguish between major and minor depression
      c. EEG sleep profile—may show reduction in REM sleep
      d. Platelet monoamine oxidase (MAO) activity—increased
      e. Biogenic amines (norepinephrine, serotonin)—increased levels
      f. Dementia screening test in at-risk populations

- Management/Treatment
  1. General considerations
      a. Assess degree of problem related to daily functioning
      b. Refer those with evidence of
          (1) Hallucinations, delusions
          (2) Loss of contact with reality
          (3) Suicidal thoughts, wishes, tendencies (see section on Suicide)

2. Mild depression (no clear criteria but general functional status tends to be high)
   a. Cognitive behavioral intervention (CBI) is the mainstay of therapy for mild depression and should be a component of all depression management
   b. Structured monitoring with weekly appointments with phone contact for backup
   c. Use therapeutic communication skills to
      (1) Encourage verbalization, clarification of feelings and fears, as well as relationship of feelings to specific events if known
      (2) Assess and discuss losses that have occurred and their meaning
      (3) Help correct cognitive errors in thinking
   d. Use crisis or social skills models to teach and promote more effective coping strategies
      (1) Help patient recognize need for and identify alternative coping methods
      (2) Encourage interaction with other people
      (3) Encourage planned, regular physical activity
      (4) Teach relaxation techniques
      (5) Provide patient with anticipatory guidance regarding feelings and usual course of the problem, e.g., gradual improvement and abatement of symptoms
   e. Provide consistency and caring, avoiding a judgmental or blaming attitude
   f. Reinforce positive behaviors
   g. Avoid actions or response that could be interpreted as punishment
   h. Consult with physician or psychiatrist regarding psychotherapy and use of antidepressants; both have been shown to be of help in mild depression; see **Tables 14-1** and **14-2**
3. Moderate to severe depression
   a. Consultation with psychiatry regarding patients who may
      (1) Be a potential danger to self or others; unable to meet basic needs; suicidal ideation or behavior
      (2) Have impaired cognition or judgment
      (3) Need skilled observation for diagnosis, assessment, or monitoring of therapy
      (4) Have inadequate social supports for outpatient treatment
   b. Antidepressant and/or antianxiety medications; most appropriate initial therapy for reasonably healthy individual; see Tables 14-1 and 14-2; refer to pharmacology references for more complete information
      (1) SSRI is the initial drug of choice for patients with functional depression
         (a) Initial choice based upon predominant symptom (hypersomnia, depressed mood, agitation, etc.), potential for drug interaction, and half life
         (b) Fluoxetine should be avoided in the elderly due to its prolonged half life as compared to other SSRI options
         (c) Fluoxetine and paroxetine are most CNS activating and sedating respectively; also have the greatest potential for CYP-450-mediated drug interaction
         (d) Excellent safety profile—no cardiovascular effects, may have undesirable adverse sexual effects, weight gain, and nausea
      (2) SNRI indicated for those with SSRI-resistant depression or comorbid neuropathic pain
         (a) Consider risk of hypertension in higher doses
         (b) Safety profile much better than TCA
      (3) TCA drugs very effective but adverse effect profile prohibitive; not used routinely by primary care providers
         (a) Potentially cardiotoxic with impact on conduction system
         (b) Powerful anticholinergic properties
         (c) Among the most efficacious drugs for endogenous depression
         (d) Patients who require TCA for depression management should be comanaged with psychiatry
      (4) Only 65% have complete remission with any one drug
      (5) No concrete evidence that any specific drug in one class is more efficacious than any other
      (6) Choice based on predominant symptoms, side effects, cost, and complexity of dosing—affect compliance
      (7) Most will demonstrate some response within 4–6 weeks of beginning treatment
      (8) Cannot assess therapeutic efficacy before 3 months of treatment
      (9) Continue medication full 6–12 months after complete remission of symptoms
      (10) When drugs are discontinued taper over 6–8 weeks
      (11) Long-term prophylaxis—full treatment dosage for those with recurrent episodes (at least three)

(12) Some controversy regarding efficacy in minor depression, dysthymia, and adjustment disorder

c. Electroconvulsive therapy (ECT)

(1) More rapid improvement than with pharmacologic agents

(2) Indicated for severely depressed or suicidal persons for whom pharmacologic agents are contraindicated or ineffective

(3) Barbiturates and muscle relaxants used prior to the procedure

■ **Table 14-1**   Examples of Antidepressants

Drug Name	Anticholinergic Effect	Sedative Effect	Orthostatic Hypotension	Cardiac Conduction	Adult Dose Range per Day (mg)[a]
Tertiary Tricydics					
Amitriptyline	+4	+4	+4	+4	25–300
Clomipramine	+3	+2	+3	+3	25–250
Doxepin	+3	+4	+4	+2	25–300
Imipramine	+3	+2	+4	+4	25–300
Trimipramine	+3	+4	+3	+4	25–300
Secondary Tricydics					
Amoxapine	+3	+2	+1	+2	50–600
Desipramine	+2	+2	+2	+3	25–300
Nortriptyline	+2	+3	+1	+3	25–250
Protriptyline	+2	+1	+4	+4	15–60
Tetracyclics					
Maprotiline	+2	+4	+2	+3	50–225
Mirtazapine	+3	+2	+2	+2	15–45
Others					
Alprazolam[b]	0	0	0	0	5–6
Bupropion	0	0	0	+1	100–450
Nefazodone	0	+3	+2	0/+1	200–600
Trazadone	0	+4	+4	+1	50–600
Venlafaxine	+1	0	0	+1	75–375
Selective Serotonin Reuptake Inhibitors (SSRI)					
Citalopram	0	0	0	0	20–40
Escitalopram	0	0	0	0	10–20
Fluoxetine	0	0	0	0	20–80
Fluvoxamine	0	0	0	0	50–300
Paroxetine	+1	0	0	0	20–50
Sertraline	0/+1	0	0	0	50–200
Selective Serotonin Reuptake Inhibitor (SSRI) + 5-hydroxytryptamine 1A (5-HT 1A) receptor agonist					
Vilazodone	0	0	0	0	10–40
Serotonin Norepinephrine Reuptake Inhibitors (SNRI)					
Desvenlafaxine	0/+1	0/+1	0	0	50–400
Duloxetine	0/+1	0/+1	0	0	40–60
Milnacipran	0	0	0	0	100–150
Venlafaxine	0/+1	0/+1	0/+1	0	75–375
Monoamine Oxidase Inhibitors (MAO)					
Phenelzine	+1	+1	+1	+3	45–90
Tranylcypromine	0	+1	+1	+2	30–60

Note: Data derived from Eisendrath & Lichtmacher, 2012; [a]Generally lower doses are recommended for adolescents and the elderly. [b]Only benzodiazepine approved for depression.

■ **Table 14-2** Antidepressants and Antianxiety Medications: Contraindications and Precautions

Drug Group	Contraindications	Precautions
Antidepressants		
Tricyclics	Acute MI, hypersensitivity; concurrent administration of MAO inhibitors	In patients with urinary retention; prostatic hypertrophy; narrow angle glaucoma, convulsive disorders; cardiovascular disease; thyroid disease; pregnant patients
MAO inhibitors	Hypertension, cardiovascular disease, headaches, liver disease or advanced renal disease, concurrent use of a tricyclic; schizophrenia	Safety during pregnancy not established; avoid fermented foods, pickles, cheeses, red wine, beer, fava beans, raisins, chocolate; cold remedies, weight-reduction meds, e.g., anything with tyramine
Lithium carbonate	Significant renal disease, dietary salt restriction; cardiovascular disease; brain damage	Use caution with pregnant patients; elderly; patient who is breastfeeding; persons with thyroid disease; mild renal and cardiovascular disease; epilepsy
Antianxiety Drugs		
Benzodiazepines	Glaucoma, hypersensitivity	Use caution if hx of allergies; psychological addiction to these drugs; hepatic or renal impairment; lower dose for elderly or for breastfeeding mothers
Carbamazepine	Severe renal, cardiovascular, or liver disease	Use with caution if liver, renal disease, or blood dyscrasias
SSRI[a]	Do not administer with MAO inhibitors or with tryptophan supplements	Caution in persons with history of seizures; impaired renal or hepatic function; mania or hypomania; in pregnant or nursing women; in the elderly

[a]Selective serotinin uptake inhibitors

     (4) Confusion, headache, temporary amnesia lasting 1–2 weeks are common side effects in about 40%; may be clinically apparent up to 1 month

     (5) Avoided in persons with brain tumor, recent (3 months) MI, CVA, or perforated viscus repair

  d. Other options include exercise and light therapy

4. Patient education

  a. Disease course, expected outcomes, and usual treatment modalities

  b. Purpose, dosage, side effects of medication

     (1) Improvement in symptoms not evident for 3–4 weeks

     (2) Importance of adhering to prescribed pharmacologic regimen; avoid abrupt discontinuation of medications

     (3) Caution against concomitant use of over-the-counter preparations

     (4) Interactions with food or other medications; see Table 14-2

5. Secondary prevention

  a. Screening those populations who have the means for treatment is recommended

  b. Asking the patient one of two questions is considered a highly sensitive screening tool

     (1) Over the last 2 weeks have you felt depressed?

     (2) Over the last 2 weeks have you felt disinterested in your activities of living?

6. Persons with major depression should be followed at least weekly for first 6–8 weeks, preferably by a mental health professional for medication adjustment and brief psychotherapeutic support

7. Persons known to be on antidepressants or receiving care for depression, who are being seen for other reasons, should be routinely checked for

  a. Suicidal feelings, plans, intentions, risks

  b. Tremor, blurred vision, dry mouth, tachycardia, postural hypotension

◻ SUICIDE

- Definition
  1. The intentional taking of one's own life
  2. Usually described as
     a. Attempted—unsuccessful conscious attempt to take one's own life
     b. Threatened—verbal or physical indication of intent for self-destruction
     c. Ideation—thoughts or behaviors indicating conscious intent for self-destruction; ominous when it includes the development of a viable plan

- Etiology/Incidence
  1. Often a manifestation or complication of depressive illness or anxiety states
  2. Approximately 2–9% of depressed patients commit suicide
  3. Eleventh leading cause of death in United States
  4. Risk factors include
     a. Sudden crisis or loss
     b. Destructive coping mechanisms
     c. Few or no significant others
     d. Poor social or personal resources
     e. Past suicide attempts or family history of suicide
     f. Previous psychotic problems
     g. Unstable lifestyle
     h. Specific plan
     i. Substance abuse
     j. Recent initiation of pharmacotherapy for depression
  5. Eight of 10 persons who state an intent to commit suicide do so; risk for depressed patients is greatest during the first month of treatment when the individual begins to feel better and has more energy
  6. In the United States women attempt suicide more often, but men are three times as likely to succeed; in elderly, suicide among males outnumber those among women at a rate of 4:1
     a. Female rates peak at age 55
     b. Male rates peak at age 75
  7. Adolescents and white males over the age of 75 have a higher incidence rate; second leading cause of death in adolescent
  8. In adolescents increased risk has been associated with
     a. Extreme parental control or permissiveness
     b. Loss of communication with parents and teachers
     c. Hostility and difficulty in school or with the law
     d. Lack of social supports (peers, social, work, and school)

- Signs and Symptoms
  1. Feelings of worthlessness and/or helplessness
  2. Preoccupation with a dead relative or friend
  3. Excessive denial, indignation, or anger in response to being questioned about suicide
  4. Verbalization or rehearsal of a realistic plan
  5. Sudden mood elevation in a depressed patient often accompanied by more energy and calmer, more placid manner
  6. Giving possessions away
  7. Setting affairs in order
  8. Making a will
  9. Presence of hallucinations or delusions
  10. Intuition on the part of the health professional
  11. In adolescents these may be more prominent
      a. Taking excessive risks
      b. Self-destructive behaviors, e.g., drug abuse, accident proneness
      c. Negative self-concept
      d. Expression of wish to die
      e. Withdrawal from family and people
      f. Increased interest and companionship with animal/pets
  12. All depressed patients need to be asked about suicide. If patient does not volunteer information, ask directly about thoughts of taking their own life. Also ask direct questions to elicit information about a plan, its lethality, and any mental or actual rehearsals of the plan. Risk is highest if planned in 24 hours; low or moderate if planned for a later time
      a. Presence of five or more risk factors constitutes high risk
      b. Mnemonic device to recall risk factors—SAD PERSONS
         (1) *S*ex
         (2) *A*ge
         (3) *D*epression
         (4) *P*revious attempt
         (5) *E*thanol abuse
         (6) *R*ational thinking diminished
         (7) *S*ocial support loss or absence
         (8) *O*rganized plan
         (9) *N*o spouse
         (10) *S*ick

- Differential Diagnosis
  1. Depression with melancholic features
  2. Depression with seasonal pattern (seasonal affective disorder)
  3. Nonfatal self-inflicted injury
  4. Organic disease

- Physical Findings
  1. No specific physical findings, however those of depression may be evident
     a. General appearance—unkempt, slumped or stooped posture, slow speech pattern, lack of expression or dejected look or agitation, hostility, tremulousness
     b. Mental status—disorientation, poor concentration, agitation, hallucinations, or delusions
  2. Old scars or evidence of injury from past attempts or high-risk behaviors

- Diagnostic Tests/Findings—there are no specific laboratory tests. See Diagnostic Tests/Findings in section on Depression

- Management/Treatment
  1. Treatment usually includes hospitalization with psychotherapy, antidepressant medications, and/or ECT; see previous section on Management/Treatment in section on Depression
  2. If a patient is deemed suicidal or if there is concern about the patient's potential for suicide, do not leave the patient alone but obtain immediate psychiatric consultation
  3. There is no evidence that suicide screening reduces mortality

☐ ANXIETY

- Definition
  1. An unpleasant feeling of dread, apprehension, foreboding, or tension resulting from an unexpected threat to one's feelings of self-esteem or well-being
  2. Major categories
     a. Generalized anxiety disorder—unrealistic or excessive anxiety and worry about life circumstance
     b. Panic disorders—unfounded morbid dread of seemingly harmless object or situation often leads to agoraphobia
     c. Obsessive compulsive disorder (OCD)—repetitive thoughts (obsession) that a person is unable to control and/or urge to perform an act that cannot be resisted without great difficulty (compulsion), and which interferes with functional abilities
     d. Posttraumatic stress disorder (PTSD)—delayed (at least 6 months) anxiety after a severe trauma often perceived as a threat to physical integrity or self-concept; intrusive thoughts, flashbacks, and nightmares form the symptomatic triad

     e. Other categories include adjustment disorder with anxious mood, simple and social phobias; refer to psychiatric or major primary care text for detailed discussion

- Etiology/Incidence
  1. Various theories related to etiology include
     a. Psychodynamic
        (1) Freudian—conflict between id and superego; ego not strong enough to resolve the conflict
        (2) Sullivanian—fear of disapproval from mother figure; conditional love leads to fragile ego, lack of self-confidence, lack of self-esteem, fear of failure
        (3) Dollar and Miller—learned response to innate drive to avoid pain; anxiety the result of two competing drives or goals
     b. Biologic
        (1) Genetic influence with high family incidence
        (2) Autonomic nervous system response—fight or flight mechanism
        (3) Biologic abnormalities of neurotransmitter receptors in the central nervous system, particularly gamma aminobutyric acid (GABA) receptors
     c. Family dynamics
        (1) Individual with dysfunctional behavior is representative of family system problems
        (2) Carrier of problems resulting from disrupted interrelationships
  2. Incidence
     a. Anxiety disorders occur in 10–15% of patients seen in healthcare settings
        (1) Only 1 in 4 diagnosed and treated
        (2) 3% of Americans will experience an anxiety disorder in their lifetime
        (3) Slight preponderance in woman
        (4) Lower incidence in the elderly
        (5) Often associated with depression in the elderly
     b. Panic disorders
        (1) Occur more frequently in women than in men
        (2) Onset usually in late teens or early adulthood
        (3) More common in those who have had an early traumatic event, e.g., the death of a parent
     c. Obsessive compulsive disorder
        (1) Most often seen in adolescence and early adulthood
        (2) Males and females affected equally

(3) More frequent in upper middle class and in persons with higher levels of intellectual functioning

- Signs and Symptoms
  1. Generalized anxiety and panic attacks
     a. A feeling of tightness in the throat
     b. Difficulty breathing; feelings of suffocation
     c. Palpitations
     d. Chest tightness or pain
     e. Tachypnea, tachycardia
     f. Gastric distress or discomfort
     g. Nausea
     h. Diarrhea
     i. Feeling of weakness in lower limbs
     j. Tingling, numbness of extremities
     k. Feeling of light-headedness
     l. Dryness of the mouth
     m. Feeling of something caught in the throat
     n. Cold, sweaty hands
     o. Feelings of loss of control; irritability; impatience
     p. Motor tension—shakiness, jitteriness, trembling, restlessness
     q. Anxiety insomnia, difficulty falling asleep
     r. Symptoms of panic generally develop suddenly and have been related to mitral valve prolapse
  2. OCD
     a. Recurrent, persistent thoughts, ideas, or images experienced as intrusive
     b. Repetitious, purposeful, intentional behaviors that are distressing, time consuming, or interfere with functioning
  3. PTSD
     a. Intrusive thoughts, flashbacks, nightmares related to the traumatic event
     b. Poor impulse control, unpredictability, and/or aggressiveness
     c. Avoidance symptoms
        (1) Avoids reminders of event
        (2) Memory difficulty
        (3) Detachment and restricted affect
     d. Hyperarousal symptoms
        (1) Hypervigilance
        (2) Insomnia
        (3) Irritability, poor concentration

- Differential Diagnosis
  1. Drug abuse, withdrawal, or intoxication
  2. Thyrotoxicosis
  3. Hypoglycemia
  4. Acute hypoxia
  5. Myocardial infarction
  6. Pheochromocytoma
  7. Seizure disorder
  8. Side effects of chemical agents or medications, e.g., caffeine, nicotine, beta adrenergic agonists

- Physical Findings
  1. Between attacks may all be within normal limits
  2. During an attack
     a. General appearance—looks worried, frightened, restless
     b. Vital signs—tachycardia, increased respirations, elevated BP
     c. Integumentary—pallor, flushed face, cold clammy hands
     d. Gastrointestinal—possible loss of bowel or bladder control
     e. Mental status—hypervigilance, easy distractibility, poor concentration
     f. Motor tension—tremulous

- Diagnostic Tests/Findings
  1. Serum drug analysis—negative
  2. Thyroid function tests—normal
  3. Serum glucose—normal
  4. ECG—normal

- Management/Treatment
  1. Depends on careful workup and identified anxiety subtype
  2. Obtain consult regarding testing for other emotional or physical disorders
  3. Cognitive behavioral therapy more effective for generalized anxiety than for panic attacks
     a. Assess usual coping mechanisms, lifestyle, social supports
     b. Establish a trusting, warm, empathetic, respectful relationship
     c. Assist patient to identify and describe emotional and physical feelings and to identify the relationship between them
     d. Identify patient behaviors that cause anxiety to the healthcare provider
     e. Use supportive confrontation as needed
     f. Keep focus of responsibility on the patient
     g. Encourage use of and teach or refer for relaxation techniques, biofeedback, and meditation
  4. Antianxiety medications (see Table 14-2 and **Table 14-3**)
     a. For chronic anxiety management
        (1) SSRIs are drug of choice for most anxiety syndromes
        (2) Doses may need to be higher than those for depression
        (3) Consider those that are most sedating, e.g., paroxetine, citalopram

■ **Table 14-3** Antianxiety Medication

Generic	Average Daily Dose*
Benzodiazepines (Longer acting; preferred in generalized anxiety disorder)	
Chlordiazepoxide	15–40 mg
Clorazepate dipotassium	15–60 mg
Diazepam	4–40 mg
Halazepam	60–160 mg
Benzodiazepines (Shorter acting; indicated in elderly or decreased clearance)	
Alprazolam	0.75–1.5 mg
Lorazepam	2–6 mg
Oxazepam	30–60 mg
Nonbenzodiazepines	
Buspirone	20–30 mg
Hydroxyzine	30–300 mg
Meprobamate	400–2,000 mg
Paroxetine	40 mg
For control of aggression and mania	
Carbamazepine	100–200 mg initially; increase to 400–1500 mg until serum level is 8–12 μg/ml

*Most divided in 2–4 portions per day. Elderly would have lower averages and treatment-resistant patients might have much higher averages than those shown.

    (4) SNRIs may be considered for those unresponsive to SSRI, those with chronic neuropathic pain, or those in whom symptoms are more severe at time of diagnosis

  b. For acute anxiety management

    (1) Benzodiazepines drug of choice for acute, short-term management

      (a) Not intended for long-term use

      (b) May result in fatal withdrawal syndrome if discontinued abruptly after extended use

    (2) Benzodiazepines may provide short-term symptom control until SSRI reaches therapeutic efficacy

    (3) Most have behavioral profile similar to alcohol

    (4) All have hypnotic properties

    (5) Antihistamines for those with COPD or potential for abuse of benzodiazepines

  c. Beta adrenergic blockers, e.g., propranolol more effective in reducing marked autonomic symptoms (tachycardia, palpations, breathlessness)

  d. Tricyclics and MAO inhibitors good for panic attacks but not for generalized anxiety; safety profile limits their utility as first-line agents

  e. Buspirone only anxiolytic not classified as a tranquilizer

    (1) Not linked to dependence or depressant effects

    (2) Does not impair motor skills

    (3) Does not potentiate alcohol effects

  f. Optimal duration of treatment not well established

5. Refer to psychiatric mental health professional for counseling and more specific therapy

6. Obtain consult regarding testing for other physical or emotional disorders

7. Patient education

  a. Disease course, expected outcome

    (1) Reassurance that anxiety rarely evolves into a more serious disorder

    (2) Reassurance that symptoms can be alleviated with appropriate therapy

    (3) Condition is temporary and with appropriate therapy and time, anxiety may be alleviated

    (4) Dosage, side effects, expected action of pharmacologic agents

  b. Chart attacks—date, time, situation, level of anxiety or symptoms on a scale of 0 to 10

■ ALCOHOLISM

- Definition
  1. Recurrent use of alcohol to the extent it significantly interferes with the individual's physical, social, and/or emotional life
  2. Characterized by preoccupation with the drug, loss of control over its use, physical dependence, and tolerance

- Etiology/Incidence
  1. Multifactorial and poorly understood; several etiologic theories have been developed
     a. Psychological
        (1) Retarded ego, weak superego
        (2) Fixed in lower level of psychosocial development
            (a) Dependent personality with poor impulse control
            (b) Low frustration tolerance
            (c) Low self-esteem
        (3) No evidence to support distinct personality predisposition
     b. Biologic
        (1) Physiologic changes in enzymes, genes, brain chemistry, hormones cause the disorder
        (2) May be familial, inherited, or acquired
  2. About 1 in 12 persons have serious problems related to alcohol use
     a. Children of alcoholics are four times as likely to develop alcoholism as children of nonalcoholics
     b. Three times as many men as women are alcoholics and they are more likely to develop the problem early in life
     c. Highest prevalence of drinking problems in 18–29 year olds
  3. Risk factors include
     a. Use of alcohol or other psychoactive substance
     b. Family history of alcohol abuse
     c. Being a young single male
     d. Heavy drinking—five or more drinks in one sitting or getting drunk once a week
     e. Family or social background that accepts or promotes intoxication
     f. Ready accessibility
     g. Comorbid psychiatric disease or disorder
     h. Cultural or environmental conditioning

- Signs and Symptoms
  1. Definite (Level I)
     a. Blackouts
     b. Alcoholic hepatitis
     c. Withdrawal symptoms—hallucinations; fine tremors of face, tongue, and hands; disorientation; seizures
     d. Memory loss, confabulation
     e. Nystagmus
     f. Prior exhibition of signs and symptoms of levels II and III
  2. Probable (Level II)
     a. Previous diagnosis of
        (1) Cirrhosis
        (2) Pancreatitis without cholelithiasis
     b. Loss of control over alcohol intake, increased alcohol tolerance
     c. Numbness of hands and feet
     d. Increased incidence of infection
     e. Weight loss
     f. Forgetfulness
     g. Trauma from accidents or altercations—cigarette burns, healed fractures
     h. Hypothermic injuries
     i. Attempted suicide
     j. Symptoms of associated diseases; see **Table 14-4**
  3. Possible (Level III)
     a. Blurred or dim vision
     b. Nocturnal diuresis
     c. Anxiety or depression
     d. Impotence
     e. Symptoms of associated diseases; see Table 14-4
     f. History of chronic gastritis, anemia, clotting disorders, marital discord, or loss of significant relationships (job, family, friends)
     g. Preoccupation with alcohol; thinking about it when not drinking

- Differential Diagnosis
  1. Distinguish from a wide variety of medical and psychiatric problems that may account for

■ **Table 14-4** Conditions Commonly Associated with Substance Abuse

1. Frequent upper respiratory infection
2. Slowly healing skin ulcers
3. Recurrent vaginal infections
4. Hepatitis
5. Sexually transmitted disease
6. Mononucleosis
7. Malnutrition
8. HIV infection
9. Pancreatitis
10. Tuberculosis

signs and symptoms, e.g., depression, anxiety, endocrinopathies, viral hepatitis

2. Determine level of alcoholism and look for concurrent abuse of other substances; see **Table 14-5**
   a. Use history and physical evidence to determine stage and further testing
   b. Use of CAGE screening test
      (1) Four questions related to drinking patterns
          (a) **C**ut—Ever felt you ought to cut down on your drinking?
          (b) **A**nnoyed—Have people annoyed you by criticizing your drinking?
          (c) **G**uilt—Ever felt bad or guilty about your drinking?
          (d) **E**ye-opener—Ever had an eye-opener to steady nerves in the A.M.?
      (2) Scores > 2 indicate alcoholism
   c. Alternately use modified CAGE or two-item conjoint screen for alcohol and other drug problems (Brown, Leonard, Saunders, & Papasouliotis, 2001)
      (1) Used substances more than intended this year?
      (2) Have you ever felt the need to cut down?
      (3) Yes to both is 80% sensitive and specific
   d. Use of an addiction severity tool such as the Michigan Alcohol Screening Test (MAST)
      (1) 25-item questionnaire with 90% sensitivity and 74% specificity
      (2) Scores > 5 indicative of alcoholism
   e. Short MAST (SMAST) (Pokorny, Miller, & Kaplan, 1972)
      (1) 13 questions
      (2) Score > 3 indicative of alcoholism
      (3) Sensitivity 70%, specificity 74%
   f. Refer to DSM-IV criteria for alcohol abuse and alcohol

■ **Table 14-5** Commonly Abused Drugs

Generic or Trade Name	Street/Slang Name
Depressants	
Codeine	School boy
Meperidine HCL (Demerol)	Demies
Gamma Hydroxybutyrate (GHB)	Liquid E, liquid ecstasy, liquid X, grievous bodily harm, easy lay
Hydromorphone HCL (Dilaudid)	Little D
Heroin	H, horse, junk, downtown, hard stuff, scag, white stuff
Methadone HCL	Meth, dollies
Morphine	M, Miss Emma, morph
Opium	Black stuff, blue velvet
Methaqualone (Qualude)	Ludes, 714s, Qs, soapers
Pentobarbital	Downers, yellow jackets
Amobarbital/secobarbital (comb.), Phenobarbital	Blues, red hearts, purple hearts, reds, F40s, rainbows
Benzodiazepines (Librium, Valium)	Tanks, downs
Stimulants	
Cocaine	Coke, snow, flake, toot, uptown, crack, blow
Dextroamphetamines,	Bennies, black beauties, copilots
Methamphetamines (Benzedrine)	Dexies, speed, meth, crank
Biphetamine (Desoxyn, Dexedrine)	Crystal, uppers
Hallucinogens	
Lysergic acid diethylamide	LSD, acid
Mescaline (peyote)	Buttons, cactus, mesc.
Myristicin	Nutmeg
Dimethyltryptamine	DMT, STP
Psilocybin	Magic mushroom
Phencyclidine HCL	PCP, angel dust, DOA, peace pill, hog
Marijuana	Pot, maryjane, chronic

- Physical Findings
  1. Definite (Level I)
     a. General appearance—fearful, anxious, stuporous, hyperactive, or incoherent
     b. Vital signs—mild fever, tachycardia, increased or labile blood pressure
     c. Integumentary—flushed face and/or palms, spider nevi, angiomas on face, numerous scars, ecchymotic areas; generalized tissue edema, and dry, dull hair
     d. Head, Ear, Eye, Nose, Throat (HEENT)—pupil constriction, nystagmus, parotid adenopathy, inflamed buccal cavity, alcoholic odor to breath, fissures at corners of mouth
     e. Cardiovascular—tachycardia; dysrhythmias; weak, irregular peripheral pulses
     f. Abdomen—gastric distention, ascites, enlarged liver, tenderness
     g. Musculoskeletal—muscle wasting, healed or new fractures
     h. Neurological—memory loss, confabulation, hallucinations, disorientation, fine motor tremors, unsteady ataxic gait, gaps in word-finding, conversation
  2. Probable (Level II) and possible (Level III)
     a. General appearance—no major abnormalities
     b. Vital signs—normal or possible tachycardia, hypertension, and cardiac dysrhythmias
     c. Integumentary—unexplained ecchymosis
     d. HEENT—parotid adenopathy, angiomas
     e. Abdomen—hepatomegaly, tenderness
     f. Neurological—hyperreflexia; unsteady walk, ataxia (Wernicke-Korsakoff syndrome)

- Diagnostic Tests/Findings
  1. Blood alcohol/drug levels—may or may not be severely elevated depending on amount and time of consumption
     a. 300 mg/100 mL at anytime = definite diagnosis
     b. 100 mg/mL on routine exam = definite diagnosis
     c. 150 mg/mL without evidence of intoxication = alcohol tolerance
  2. CBC—increased or depressed white count; macrocytosis with or without anemia; decreased platelets
  3. Blood glucose—hyper or hypoglycemia
  4. Electrolytes—hypokalemia and hypomagnesemia
  5. Liver function—all may be increased
     a. Gamma glutamyl transferase (GGT)— > 30 units/L suggests recent episode heavy drinking, not sensitive to chronicity
     b. Alanine aminotransferase (ALT) elevated to 3 times normal
     c. Aspartate aminotransferase (AST) elevated to 3 times normal with a level above that of ALT
     d. Lactate dehydrogenase (LDH)
  6. Total bilirubin and amylase—increased
  7. Hypertriglyceridemia without elevations in other cholesterol indices
  8. Prothrombin time—prolonged in severe disease
  9. Urinalysis—infection, ketones
  10. Nutritional—albumin and total protein decreased, folic acid low
  11. Chest radiograph—enlarged heart, right lower lobe pneumonia
  12. ECG—dysrhythmias, cardiac myopathies, ischemic heart disease

- Management/Treatment
  1. Consult with physician regarding treatment and possible need for detoxification—will need acute pharmacologic management in acute withdrawal phase
     a. Benzodiazepines for seizure suppression
     b. Blood pressure management; significant hypertension possible
     c. May need management of psychosis
  2. Confront patient with diagnosis "alcoholism"
  3. Do not use nebulous statements, e.g., "We think you might have a drinking problem" or "You need to cut down on your drinking"
  4. Tell the patient it is a disease and treatable
  5. Tell the patient it is not his/her fault but he/she IS responsible for accepting treatment and the goal of therapy is abstinence
  6. Describe treatment options; many treatment programs will not accept pregnant women
  7. Make appropriate referral for treatment and follow-up
     a. Alcoholics Anonymous (most successful)
     b. Behavioral approaches
     c. Rational emotive psychotherapy
     d. Psychodrama
  8. Provide family members with information on alcoholism and encourage involvement in Al-Anon (for families of alcoholics) and/or Ala-Teen and Ala-Tots (for teenagers and young children of alcoholics)
  9. General considerations
     a. Alcoholic women have a higher incidence of suicide attempts than both alcoholic men and the female population as a whole; see section on Suicide
     b. Females, even with less alcohol consumption, are more likely to develop liver disease than males

c. Alcohol use by pregnant women is the leading cause of mental retardation

d. Women's drinking and drug problems are often viewed as less serious than men's and are more frequently misdiagnosed

e. If seeing a patient who was referred for treatment of alcoholism, reinforce participation in treatment and use of any agreed upon treatment aids

f. Avoid compounding the problems or hindering recovery by prescribing sedatives or other depressants (cross tolerance)

◻ PSYCHOACTIVE SUBSTANCE ABUSE

- Definition
  1. Misuse of any substance capable of producing altered state of consciousness and/or euphoria
  2. Addiction or compulsive use includes
     a. Psychologic craving
     b. Physiologic dependence (withdrawal symptoms with discontinuance)
     c. Tolerance (need for larger and larger doses to produce desired effect)

- Etiology/Incidence
  1. As with alcohol abuse, several theories have been developed to explain the cause of substance abuse, which include
     a. Psychologic
        (1) Failure to complete developmental tasks
        (2) Underdeveloped ego
        (3) Dependent personality
        (4) Poor impulse control
        (5) Ego breakdown with subsequent drug use as a coping mechanism
     b. Biologic hereditary/genetic factors
        (1) Neurotransmitter deficiency
        (2) Enzyme deficiency
     c. Family dynamics
        (1) Dysfunctional family system
        (2) Absent parent
        (3) Tyrannical or weak ineffective parent
        (4) Negative role models
        (5) Drugs used for stress relief
        (6) Cultural perceptions of drug abuse
  2. Incidence
     a. 26% of females and 24% of males between the age of 12 and 17 years have used an illicit drug
     b. More than 1 million women on legal psychoactive drugs
     c. 66% of psychoactive drugs are prescribed for women
     d. Most commonly used substances alone or in combination (see Table 14-5)
        (1) Depressants—benzodiazepines, barbiturates, opiates, morphine, heroin, alcohol, sedatives, hypnotics, and minor tranquilizers
           (a) Most widely used and abused drugs
           (b) Often prescribed for anxiety, depression, or sleep disorders
        (2) Stimulants (amphetamines, cocaine, caffeine, tobacco)
           (a) Most commonly abused stimulants other than caffeine and nicotine are amphetamine and cocaine
           (b) Twice as many males as females use stimulants, primarily in the 21- to 44-year age range
        (3) Hallucinogens (lysergic acid diethylamide, LSD; myristicin, nutmeg; dimethyltryptamine, DMT; psilocybin, magic mushroom; phencyclidine, PCP or angel dust; mescaline, peyote; cannabis, hashish and marijuana; and chemically related substances)
     e. Solvents/gases
        (1) Used to reproduce effects of depressants, stimulants, hallucinogenics
        (2) Produce inebriation similar to volatile anesthetics
        (3) Examples include gasoline, paint thinners, correction fluid

- Signs and Symptoms
  1. Depressants
     a. Nausea/vomiting
     b. Myalgia, deep bone or muscle pain (methadone abusers)
     c. Rhinorrhea, sneezing, excessive lacrimation
     d. Headache
     e. Miosis
     f. Euphoria
     g. Apathy, dysphoria, depression
     h. Drowsiness, psychomotor retardation, slurred speech
     i. Impaired attention, memory, social judgment (disinhibition)
     j. Ataxia, tremors, lack of coordination
     k. Mood swings, aggression, combativeness; loss of impulse control
     l. Auditory hallucinations, paranoia
     m. Bradycardia/respiratory depression
     n. Fever, perspiration (with withdrawal)
     o. Altered level of consciousness
  2. Stimulants
     a. Restlessness, irritability, anxiety, confusion, aggression
     b. Tachycardia, cardiac dysrhythmia, chest pain (cocaine), increased blood pressure
     c. Elation, grandiosity

d. Perspiration or chills

e. Hyper or hypothermia

f. Abdominal pain, nausea/vomiting, diarrhea, frequent urination

g. Insomnia

h. Paranoia, hallucinations (visual and tactile with cocaine)

i. Dilated pupils

3. Hallucinogenics

a. Dilated pupils, vertical and horizontal nystagmus

b. Flushed skin

c. Increased pulse and BP

d. Marked anxiety; panic paranoia, hypomania

e. Hallucinations, visual and sensory distortions

f. Rapid, severe mood changes, hostility, aggression, violence

g. Depression, suicidal thoughts

h. Grandiosity, euphoria

i. Tremors

j. Flashbacks

k. Insensitivity to pain

4. Solvents/gases (inhaled)

a. Euphoria

b. Slurred speech

c. Hallucinations/confusion

d. Unconsciousness

e. Cardiopulmonary depression or failure

- Differential Diagnosis

1. Poly abuse is common and may present with intoxication, overdose, and/or in various stages of withdrawal

2. Rule out other disorders that may account for presenting signs and symptoms, for example

a. Seizure disorders

b. Hypo or hyperthyroidism, thyroid storm

c. Hyper or hypoglycemia

d. Schizophrenia, mania

e. Head injury

- Physical Findings—in addition to drug-specific signs, some general physical findings might include

1. General appearance—unkempt, poor hygiene

2. Vital signs—temperature elevation, increased or decreased BP, tachycardia, tachypnea

3. Integumentary—bruises, burns, needle marks, infections, cellulitis, ulcerations, abscesses

4. HEENT—changes in pupil size, reaction to light, and extraocular movements; poor oral hygiene, puncture wounds under the tongue, pharyngitis, inflammation and or erosion of the nasal mucosa

5. Abdomen—tenderness, organomegaly

6. Cardiovascular—dysrhythmia

7. Neuromuscular—incoordination; decreased pain perception (PCP); alterations and distortions in consciousness, attention, sensory perceptions

- Diagnostic Tests/Findings

1. CBC—leukocytosis; anemia

2. Urine and drug screens—positive for abused substance(s)

3. If associated diseases are present other alterations will be noted, e.g., abnormal liver enzymes, thyroid function tests, or glucose levels; positive HIV test

- Management/Treatment

1. Depressant abuse

a. Identify drugs taken, when taken, and route of administration if possible

b. Assess level of consciousness

c. Evaluate for evidence of head trauma

d. Refer to physician, emergency room, or drug detoxification unit if acute overdose or intoxication is noted

e. In the meantime provide quiet, lighted room and do not leave patient alone

f. Monitor vital signs

g. In consultation with physician determine need for starting an IV

2. Stimulant abuse

a. In cases of intoxication, overdose, or withdrawal refer to physician or emergency room

b. In the meantime provide quiet area with reduced stimuli and high staff profile; aggressive behavior is associated with amphetamine use

c. Monitor cardiac rate and rhythm; ventricular arrhythmia and/or cardiac arrest may occur with toxic levels of cocaine

d. Persons experiencing stimulant withdrawal may be suicidal as a result of profound CNS rebound depression; use suicide precautions until patient is transferred to emergency room or detoxification unit

e. For nonemergency cases refer to drug rehabilitation unit

3. Hallucinogenic abuse

a. Hallucinogenics do not have a withdrawal syndrome and do not require detoxification as such

b. Refer patients with psychotic symptoms to the psychiatric unit

c. Protect patient and others from injury

(1) Darkened, quiet, nonthreatening environment to decrease the likelihood of confusion, fear, and violent behavior

(2) Speak in a soft, nonthreatening voice
  (a) If LSD has been taken provide reassurance verbally and by touch and orient the individual ("talking down")
  (b) If PCP intoxication is present do not attempt "talking down" it will increase the patient's agitation and tendency for violent behavior
(3) Suspiciousness and paranoia, visual and auditory hallucinations, and agitation make suicide or accidental injury a likely possibility; take precautions early
(4) If frightened and hallucinating avoid the use of physical restraints, however, use of restraints with PCP users may be necessary for the safety of self and others; PCP is an anesthetic and alters thinking; persons on PCP are a danger to themselves as well as to others

4. General considerations
  a. Primary role is diagnosis and referral
  b. Consult with physician on medication use
    (1) Period of drug-free observation usually recommended
    (2) Haloperidol may be given to control psychotic and assaultive behaviors
    (3) Diazepam is used to reduce muscle spasm and restlessness
    (4) Phenothiazine neuroleptics should be avoided in patients on PCP because of the possibility of potentiating the anticholinergic effects of PCP
    (5) Vitamin C tablets (ascorbic acid) or cranberry juice may be used to acidify the urine and promote excretion of PCP
  c. Many treatment programs will not accept pregnant women
  d. Many treatment programs do not provide child care or other alternatives for woman, which can be a significant barrier to help
  e. Alcoholics Anonymous, Al-Anon will also accept other substance abusers; family members should be given information on Al-Anon and Ala-Teen even if patient refuses treatment
  f. Narcotics Anonymous (substance abusers) and Nar-Anon (families of substance abusers) groups are available in some areas

◘ DELIRIUM (ACUTE CONFUSION)

- Definition—a transient global disorder of attention, with clouding of consciousness and cognitive impairment; considered a symptom of underlying abnormality rather than a disease entity

- Etiology/Incidence
  1. Usually the result of systemic problems, e.g., infection, medications, hypoxia, dehydration, or electrolyte imbalance—examples include
    a. Intoxication—alcohol, analgesics, bromides, sedatives, psychedelics
    b. Withdrawal from alcohol, sedatives, hypnotics, or corticosteroids
    c. Infections—urinary, respiratory, meningitis, encephalitis, septicemia, syphilis—most common cause of delirium in the elderly population
    d. Endocrine disorders—diabetes, hyper or hypothyroidism, Addison's disease, Cushing's syndrome
    e. Nutritional deficiencies especially of B_1, B_6, B_{12}
    f. Medications—anticholinergics, antidepressants, digoxin, H_2 blockers, overdose of recreational drugs
    g. May be related to sensory deprivation or overload
    h. Sleep deprivation
    i. Psychological stress
  2. Can occur in any age group but the elderly are particularly vulnerable
  3. Estimated that 40–80% of elderly patients hospitalized for acute physical illness exhibit delirium at time of admission or soon after
  4. Prolongs hospital length of stay by an average of 6 days

- Signs and Symptoms
  1. Symptom onset is acute and global
  2. Cognitive impairment
    a. Inability to focus attention/short attention span
    b. Impaired recent memory and recall
    c. Problems in perceptual processing
    d. Disorientation
    e. Impaired judgment
  3. Emotional lability
  4. Impaired impulse control
  5. Anxiety/irritability
  6. Mild to moderate depression
  7. Visual and auditory hallucinations
  8. Confabulation
  9. Fluctuating mental status; worse in the evening "sundowning," more common in those with preexisting dementia
  10. Psychomotor restlessness with insomnia
  11. Tachycardia, dilated pupils, sweating

- Differential Diagnosis
  1. Dementia
  2. Pseudodementia
  3. Amnestic syndrome

4. Substance-induced hallucinosis
5. Schizophrenia
6. Other psychoses

- Physical Findings—varies according to the underlying cause
    1. General appearance—may be restless, hyper or hypovigilant; dazed expression
    2. Tachycardia, elevated blood pressure, increased temperature, tachypnea
    3. Focal neurological symptoms may be present
    4. Additional symptoms depending upon underlying cause
        a. Fever
        b. Poor skin turgor
        c. Pale skin and mucosa
        d. Muscle twitch; hyperactive deep tendon reflexes (DTR)
        e. Seizure
        f. Cyanosis of nail beds or extremities

- Diagnostic Tests/Findings
    1. Thorough history and physical examination with mental status and neurological examination—may reveal clues to etiology
    2. Basic laboratory workup may include
        a. CBC with differential, chemical screen, blood gas analysis
        b. Electrocardiogram
        c. Chest radiograph
        d. Urinalysis and urine toxicology screen
    3. Special tests as needed
        a. EEG—tends to show general slowing in delirium
        b. CT scan or MRI of the brain—expect to be normal
        c. Blood levels for medications

- Management/Treatment
    1. Diagnostic consult with physician
    2. Identify suspected cause
    3. Remove or modify etiology when possible, e.g., treat infections with antimicrobials, discontinue or simplify medication regimens
    4. Nonpharmacologic interventions
        a. Provide adequate nutrition, hydration, oxygenation
        b. Institute environmental controls to control stimuli levels
        c. Provide reassurance and institute safety measures
        d. Institute reorientation measures; provide patient and family with sensitive reassurance
    5. Pharmacologic intervention
        a. Judicious use of sedation to promote rest, reduce anxiety, decrease agitation and restlessness

b. No ideal drug
c. Short-acting anxiolytics without active metabolites
    (1) Oxazepam 10–50 mg/day
    (2) Lorazepam 0.5–2 mg/day
    (3) Alprazolam 0.5–4 mg/day
d. For immediate calming of acute agitation—haloperidol 0.5 mg IV combined with 0.5–1 mg lorazepam, repeated in 30 minutes
    (1) Repeat every hour until calming achieved
    (2) Once delirium cycle is broken sedation may be continued particularly in evening and night hours

6. General considerations
    a. Anticipate delirium when risk factors are present
        (1) Being > 80 years of age
        (2) Having visual or hearing impairments
        (3) Pain
        (4) Multiple medications
        (5) Urine elimination problems
        (6) Fracture injury
        (7) Multiple chronic diseases
        (8) Previous history of acute confusion
        (9) Immobilized
        (10) Low scores on mental status examinations
        (11) Being hospitalized or experiencing a change in environment
        (12) Drug or alcohol withdrawal
    b. Prevention strategies
        (1) Avoid polypharmacy
        (2) Monitor medication intake and monitor for side effects, interactions, toxicity
        (3) Maintain adequate hydration and oxygenation
        (4) Maintain adequate nutrition
        (5) Assess for adequate pain control
        (6) Control environmental stimuli to avoid sensory deprivation or overload
        (7) Provide assistive devices to supplement sensory alterations, e.g., glasses, hearing aids, controlled lighting

❑ QUESTIONS

Select the best answer.

1. Which of the following is one of the two conditions required for a diagnosis of major depression?

    a. Contemplating a plan for suicide
    b. Unplanned weight loss > 10% body weight
    c. Unresponsive to cognitive-behavioral therapy
    d. Loss of interest or pleasure in activities

2. Which is true of major depression?

   a. Majority of patients will have a reoccurrence
   b. It may be a normal grief reaction
   c. It is often self-limiting
   d. Strongly associated with chronic drug use

3. What class of drug represents the first choice for the management of both depression and chronic anxiety?

   a. SNRI
   b. TCA
   c. SSRI
   d. MAO-B inhibitors

4. Posttraumatic stress disorder is marked by which triad of findings?

   a. Intrusive thoughts, nightmares, flashbacks
   b. Tendency to globalize, psychomotor retardation, hypersomnia
   c. Weight loss, feelings of helplessness, irritability
   d. Indifference, decreased concentration, hyperphagia

5. Contraindications to SSRI therapy do not include:

   a. Coronary artery disease controlled with beta adrenergic blockade
   b. Unmedicated hypertension
   c. Chest tightness that may represent acute anxiety
   d. An eating disorder characterized by a BMI < 19

6. Therapy for depression should always include:

   a. A trial of SSRIs
   b. Short-term benzodiazepines when anxiety component present
   c. Cognitive-behavioral intervention
   d. Quantification of symptoms with a depression rating scale

7. Premenstrual dysphoric disorder (PMDD):

   a. Is disabling in some way
   b. Is an exacerbation of PMS
   c. Improves in the luteal phase
   d. Is not recognized by DSM-IV TR as a distinct diagnosis

8. Which population has the highest rate of completed suicides?

   a. Single Caucasian men > 75 years old
   b. Latina girls ages 15–19
   c. Persons of all ages with a history of substance abuse
   d. Persons who were recently treated for depression with pharmacologic therapy

9. Who among the following is the most appropriate candidate for benzodiazepine initial therapy for anxiety?

   a. A 65-year-old male whose wife just died of colon cancer
   b. A 29-year-old female who is unable to work because of her excessive anxiety
   c. A 33-year-old female who has been in recovery for alcoholism for 1 year and is having anxiety related to a new relationship
   d. A 49-year-old male who is having flashbacks from a severe motorcycle accident

Questions 10–13 refer to the following scenario:

A 17-year-old male student comes into the student health service complaining of weight loss, fatigue, anorexia. He states that the symptoms began about a month ago after he broke up with his girlfriend. He has difficulty sleeping and says he wakes up thinking about her. He says that since she left him he just doesn't enjoy going out anymore and has been spending most of his free time in his room. His affect is flat and he shows little expression as he relates his problem. The physical examination is within normal limits.

10. You suspect depression to be his problem. Your next step would be to:

    a. Prescribe an antianxiety medication
    b. Find out how he has coped with losses in the past
    c. Explain that this is a temporary situation and will probably clear up in another couple of weeks
    d. Ask him directly about feelings or thoughts of harming himself

11. Which factors in the available data might lead you to suspect that he might be suicidal?

    a. Weight loss, fatigue, anorexia
    b. Insomnia, loss of pleasure, social withdrawal
    c. Gender, emotional loss, signs of depression
    d. Intrusive thoughts, flat affect, with normal physical exam

12. Upon further questioning he admits to suicidal ideation. Knowing which of the following would be most helpful in assessing his suicide risk?

    a. Whether there have been any suicides in his family
    b. If he rooms alone or has a roommate
    c. If his family lives nearby
    d. If he has a viable plan for suicide in the next 24 hours

13. This patient has a roommate, but his family lives in another state. He denies substance abuse or definite plan or time for suicide. What would be the least useful action at this point?

    a. Consult with a physician regarding psychotherapy and antidepressants
    b. Assess him with a structured suicide screening tool
    c. Contract with him to not harm or kill himself until he talks with you at a defined point in the near future
    d. Consult with psychiatry to evaluate need for hospitalization

Questions 14 and 15 refer to the following scenario:

A 38-year-old married male comes to the clinic asking for an AIDS test. He has been awakening at night with sweating and his heart pounding. He has read in *Time* magazine that night sweats were a sign of AIDS and a few years ago he had to have a transfusion after a car accident. He would also like to have a radiograph of his throat as he feels like there's something stuck in it and wonders if it might be cancer. At times he feels like he's losing control. He denies IV drug use or high-risk sexual activities. He denies marital or work problems. In fact, he just got a promotion 2 weeks ago and he and his wife have bought a new home.

14. What other information would be most helpful to you in your diagnosis?

    a. The duration of symptoms
    b. The presence of nightmares
    c. A family history of major mental health problems
    d. Past medical history significant for mitral valve prolapse

15. If he denies nightmares, has had symptoms for about 2 weeks, and the physical findings are normal, you should:

    a. Order a barium swallow
    b. Refer to a gastroenterologist
    c. Consider a posttraumatic stress syndrome as the probable diagnosis
    d. Consider situational anxiety as the probable diagnosis

16. Benzodiazepines are used in anxiety disorders. They are:

    a. Contraindicated in narrow angle glaucoma
    b. Not helpful for short-term use in situational anxiety
    c. Usually physiologically addicting
    d. As effective as beta blockers for control of palpitations

17. The most common mental health problem seen in general practice is:

    a. Anxiety
    b. Depression
    c. Alcoholism
    d. Schizophrenia

18. Which of the following symptoms is least characteristic of anxiety?

    a. Sleep disorder
    b. Decreased concentration
    c. Irritability
    d. Indifference

19. All of the following organic conditions may produce anxiety-like symptoms except:

    a. Thyrotoxicosis
    b. Hyperglycemia
    c. Hormone-releasing tumor
    d. Prolapsed mitral valve

20. A potential consequence of prescribing antidepressants in undiagnosed bipolar disorder is:

    a. Precipitating a manic episode
    b. Desensitizing the patient to serotonin reuptake inhibition
    c. Producing physiologic dependence
    d. Contributing to serotonin syndrome

21. Mrs. J. is a 65-year-old widow who completed a series of ECT treatments 1 week ago with positive results. Both she and her daughter are concerned that she continues to experience significant memory loss. It is most appropriate to tell Mrs. J. that:

    a. She may need to take memory-enhancing agents for 4–6 months
    b. This is an unfortunate but common adverse effect of ECT
    c. The loss is temporary and full memory will return
    d. Memory will improve as her mood stabilizes

22. Mr. P. is a 45-year-old divorced male who presents for a physical exam required by his employer. During the interview he reveals previous hospitalization for pancreatitis and long-term self-medication for gastritis. His physical exam is normal except for slight tenderness in the RUQ. A CBC reveals macrocytic, megaloblastic anemia. Which diagnostic test would be most helpful at this point?

    a. ECG and electrolytes
    b. Liver function, B_{12} and folic acid levels, and triglycerides
    c. Chest radiograph and ultrasound of the gallbladder
    d. Blood albumin levels and bone marrow studies

23. Ms. Z., a 35-year-old female, comes into the clinic demanding to be seen immediately. She is agitated and complaining loudly of police brutality. She states that she was unjustly jailed overnight because of a misunderstanding and that she was shackled for more than 3 hours causing bruises on her wrists and ankles. Upon further elaboration she states the police altered a blood test and said her blood alcohol level was 300. This information alone indicates:

    a. Paranoid ideation
    b. Alcoholism
    c. Need for legal services referral
    d. The patient may have a drinking problem

24. Noncompliance with medication is a concern in outpatient treatment of patients with mental health problems. Which of the following would be least helpful in promoting medication regimen compliance?

    a. Patient involvement in treatment decision making
    b. Providing the patient with information about expected action and side effects of the medications
    c. Arranging follow-up visits with whatever staff are available
    d. Maintaining telephone communication with the patient to monitor effects and response to medication

25. One of the most effective treatments for alcoholism is:

    a. Psychoanalysis
    b. Active participation in AA
    c. Aversion therapy with Antabuse (disulfiram)
    d. Active participation in Al-Anon

26. Ms. C. is brought to the emergency room from a party by her friends. She is stuporous, confused, and has pinpoint pupils. These signs are consistent with:

    a. PCP intoxication
    b. Heroin use
    c. LSD
    d. Amphetamine withdrawal

27. A 23-year-old male comes to the clinic to obtain treatment for a cut on his arm he received in a street fight. His face is badly bruised from a previous fight. He is unkempt and shows evidence of poor personal hygiene. He has a history of alcohol abuse. At present he is tachycardic and has an elevated blood pressure. His pupils are dilated and he is slightly diaphoretic. He complains of chest pain. These signs are consistent with:

    a. Acute alcohol intoxication
    b. Chronic heroin use
    c. Recent use of hallucinogenics
    d. Recent use of cocaine

28. A young male adult is brought into the emergency room by the police. He is highly agitated, hostile, verbally abusive, and threatening. He has several lacerations and bruises he sustained in a fight at a local club where he "tore the place apart." You should:

    a. Suspect police brutality
    b. Suspect heroin use
    c. Try to talk the patient down and keep him oriented
    d. Be prepared to administer a chemical restraint

29. Which of the following IS NOT associated with physiologic dependence?

    a. Heroin
    b. Phenobarbital
    c. LSD
    d. Amphetamines

30. A cocaine overdose may typically present with all of the following symptoms except:

    a. Extreme anxiety
    b. Bleeding
    c. Angina or MI
    d. Stupor

31. Your first action in a suspected cocaine overdose should be to:

    a. Administer antipsychotics
    b. Prepare for cardiopulmonary support
    c. Prepare for mechanical restraint
    d. Administer reversal agents

32. To enhance the excretion of PCP from the body give:

    a. Haloperidol
    b. Ascorbic acid
    c. Valium
    d. A phenothiazine

33. Withdrawal from opiates is often characterized by:

    a. Palpitations and anginal chest pain
    b. Abdominal cramping and diarrhea
    c. Tonic-clonic seizures and delirium
    d. Progressive, deteriorating consciousness

34. CNS rebound is seen in withdrawal of:

    a. Depressants
    b. Stimulants
    c. Hallucinogenics
    d. Alcohol

35. Aggressive behavior can be seen with abuse of which of the following?

    a. Amphetamines
    b. Depressants
    c. Hallucinogenics
    d. Any psychoactive substance

Answers

1. **d**		19. **b**	
2. **a**		20. **a**	
3. **c**		21. **c**	
4. **a**		22. **b**	
5. **d**		23. **c**	
6. **c**		24. **c**	
7. **a**		25. **b**	
8. **a**		26. **b**	
9. **b**		27. **d**	
10. **d**		28. **d**	
11. **c**		29. **c**	
12. **d**		30. **d**	
13. **b**		31. **b**	
14. **a**		32. **b**	
15. **d**		33. **b**	
16. **a**		34. **b**	
17. **b**		35. **d**	
18. **d**			

◘ BIBLIOGRAPHY

American Psychiatric Association. (2000). *Diagnostic and statistical manual of mental disorders, text revision (TR)* (4th ed.). Washington, DC: Author.

Brown, M. N., Lapane, K. L., & Luisi, A. F. (2002). The management of depression in older nursing home residents. *Journal of the American Geriatric Society, 50*(1):69–76.

Brown, R. L., Leonard T., Saunders, L. A., & Papasouliotis, O. (2001). Two-item conjoint screen for alcohol and other drug problems. *Journal of the American Board of Family Practice, 14*(2):95–106.

Burke, W. J., Schultz, S. K., & Smith, M. (2004). Management of anxiety in late life. *Annals of Long-Term Care, 12*(8) 28–33.

Centers for Disease Control and Prevention (CDC). (2005). Web-based Injury Statistics Query and Reporting System (WISQARS). National Center for Injury Prevention and Control, CDC (producer). Retrieved from www.cdc.gov/ncipc/wisqars/default.htm

Chychula, N. M., & Sciamanna, C. (2002). Help substance abusers attain and sustain abstinence. *The Nurse Practitioner, 27*(11), 30–47.

Davis, B. D. (2004). Assessing adults with mental disorders in primary care. *The Nurse Practitioner, 29*(5), 19–29.

Eisendrath, S. J., & Lichtmacher, J. E. (2012). Psychiatric disorders. In S. J. McPhee, & M. A. Papadakis (Eds.). *Current medical diagnosis and treatment* (51st ed., pp. 1010–1064.). New York: Lange Medical Publishing/McGraw-Hill.

Enoch, M. A., & Goldman, D. (2002). Problem drinking and alcoholism: Diagnosis and treatment. *American Family Physician, 65*, 441–448.

Gerhardt, A. M. (2004). Identifying the drug seeker: The advanced practice nurse's role in managing prescription drug abuse. *Journal of the American Academy of Nurse Practitioners, 16*(6), 239–243.

Hollander, E., & Wong, C. M. (2000). *Contemporary diagnosis and management of common psychiatric disorders* (2nd ed.). Newtown, PA: Handbooks in Health Care.

Kosten, T. R., & O'Connor, P. G. (2003). Management of drug and alcohol withdrawal. *New England Journal of Medicine, 348*, 1786–1795.

Longo, L. P., & Johnson, B. (2000) Addiction: Part I. Benzodiazepines—side effects, abuse risk, and alternatives. *American Family Physician, 6*(7), 2121–2128.

Lyon, D. E., Chase, L. S., & Farrell, S. P. (2002). Using an interview guide to assess suicidal ideation. *The Nurse Practitioner, 27*(8), 26–31.

Pokorny, A. D., Miller, B. A., & Kaplan, H. B. (1972). The brief MAST: A shortened version of the Michigan Alcoholism Screening Test. *American Journal of Psychiatry, 129*, 342–345.

Sekula, L. K., DeSantis, J., & Gianetti, V. (2003). Considerations in the management of the patient with comorbid depression and anxiety. *Journal of the American Academy of Nurse Practitioners, 15*(1), 23–33.

Sobczak, J. A. (2009). Managing high-acuity depressed adults in primary care. *Journal of the American Academy of Nurse Practitioners, 21*(7), 362–370.

15

Care of the Aging Adult

Debbie Gilbert Kramer

◻ DEMOGRAPHICS OF OLDER ADULTS

The elderly population in America is increasing rapidly. The rates are significantly higher than for other segments of the population. A greater number of aged persons are living longer and healthier due to improved health care and a healthier lifestyle. The average U.S. life span has increased appreciably since the beginning of the century. The average life expectancy at birth increased by almost 2 years during the past decade. The term *elderly* is generally accepted as referring to persons 65 years and older; however with respect to nurse practitioner certification, the American Nurses Credentialing Center (ANCC) regards any person over the age of 55 as geriatric; the American Academy of Nurse Practitioners (AANP) considers any person over the age of 65 as geriatric.

- Definitions of Late Adulthood
  1. Age 65–74 years—the young-old
  2. Age 75–84 years—the middle-old
  3. Age 85 and over—the oldest-old

- Population Statistics (CDC, 2007)
  1. In 1900, individuals aged 65 and over numbered 3.1 million persons—1 in every 25 Americans
  2. In 2002, the elderly comprised 1 in 8 (35.6 million), an elevenfold increase
  3. The Census Bureau projects the elderly population will more than double to 80 million, 1 in 4 persons, between now and 2050
  4. Fastest growing subgroup is the oldest-old, also referred to as the frail elderly—4.6 million persons in 2002 and up to 9.6 million in 2030

  5. The elderly population is estimated at 12.3% while utilizing 25% of total healthcare expenditures and prescription drugs
  6. Greatest growth spurt will be seen when the "baby-boomers" enter the 65-and-over group, between the years of 2010 and 2030
  7. The "baby-boomers" will number 19 million in 2050 when they become the oldest-old, making them 24% of elderly Americans and 5% of all Americans
  8. The leading causes of death age 65 and over are heart disease, cancer, stroke, chronic obstructive pulmonary disease, and pneumonia/influenza

- Gender Statistics
  1. Elderly women outnumber elderly men with a ratio of 100 to 80 between ages 65 and 74; ratio widens to 100 to 42 by age 85
  2. In 2001, persons reaching age 65 years of age will have a life expectancy of 83
  3. Men have higher death rates at each age

- Gender Statistics
  1. Caucasians comprise the highest percentage of the U.S. population > 65 years of age at 83% but this trend is narrowing
  2. Representation by other ethnic groups is on the rise; by 2030 it is projected that
     a. Percentage of African-Americans will increase from 8 to 11%
     b. Percentage of Latinos will increase from 4.5 to 17%
     c. Percentage of Asians and Pacific Islanders will increase from 2.3 to 7.4%

- Marital Status and Living Arrangements
  1. In 2002, over half of the older noninstitutionalized persons were living with a spouse
  2. The likelihood of living alone or in a residential care facility increases with age
     a. 73% of noninstitutionalized elderly men were married and living with their spouses; 41% of their female counterparts were married and living with their spouses
     b. 10% of the older population were divorced or separated
     c. 31% of noninstitutionalized elderly live alone; half of women over 75 lived alone
     d. Older women were four times more likely than men to be widowed—46% versus 14%; 8 out of 10 elderly persons living alone are women
  3. Only 9% of noninstitutionalized persons aged 65–69 years needed assistance with their activities of daily living (ADL), whereas 50% of the 85-and-over age group required such assistance
  4. While a small number of the over-65-year-old population lived in nursing homes in 2000, the percentage increases dramatically with age from 1.1% at ages 65–74 to 18.2% for persons over 85
  5. In 2000, almost 400,000 grandparents over 65 years old were the persons with primary responsibilities for their grandchildren who lived with them
  6. Most persons over 65 years live in metropolitan areas
  7. In 2002, about half (52%) of persons 65 years or older lived in nine states: California, Florida, New York, Pennsylvania, Texas, Ohio, Illinois, Michigan, and New Jersey

- Income and Poverty
  1. Likelihood of living below the government-defined poverty level increases with age
  2. Older persons living alone are much more likely to be poor than those living with families
  3. Older women (12.4%) have higher poverty rate than older men (7.7%), and, in 2002, 10.4% of married couples were living below the poverty line
  4. Elderly African-Americans (23.8%) and Hispanics (21.4%) outnumber Caucasians (8.3%) with low income levels
  5. Within each race/ethnic group, poverty is more prevalent in women than men; income varies with differences in age, gender, race, ethnicity, marital status, living arrangements, education, former occupation, and work history

  6. In 2002, the median income of elderly men was $19,436 and $11,406 for women

- Educational Status
  1. Better education is correlated with a healthier, longer life
  2. In 2002, 70% of noninstitutionalized elderly had completed high school, a statistic that varied considerably by race and ethnicity
  3. The oldest-old were more likely to have only an eighth grade education or less (24% versus 6%); the level of education decreases with increase in age
  4. 17% of the elderly have college degrees versus 20% of those aged 55–59 and 27% of persons 45–49

☐ THEORIES OF AGING

Aging is a process that occurs to an organism with the passage of time, eventually resulting in death. Understanding by scientists of the mechanisms of the theories of aging may show an interaction and interrelatedness among the theories in the future (Spirduso, 1995).

- Genetic Theories
  1. Genes—process of aging is dictated by preprogrammed genetic components influenced by biological markers such as puberty and menopause; one or more genes control the cellular aging process, and specific genes may influence longevity; these are activated and the organism dies
  2. Error-catastrophe—an early theory suggesting errors occur through somatic mutations, chromosomal rearrangements, or genetic material transcriptions, and as the errors accumulate the cell cannot survive
  3. DNA—mutations occur in the mitochondria of DNA and continually mount upwards throughout an individual's lifetime, causing aging
  4. Hayflick limit or cell aging—cells will multiply and divide only a finite number of times; genetically preprogrammed
  5. Programmed—a senescence or aging factor accumulates in cells and dominates cellular function

- Damage Theories
  1. Chemical—chemical reactions occur naturally and result in irreversible molecular defects; may occur from air, food, smoking, and the like; if insults and injuries outweigh the repairing process, the system fails
  2. Cross-linkage—atoms or molecules have chemical sites that may link to DNA in the cell; damaged DNA is repaired by body's defense

mechanism; if cross-linkage impedes transport of nutrients and information, the damage cannot be repaired

3. Free-radical—free radicals are oxygen metabolites produced by one-electron reduction of oxygen that can produce damage and lead to cell death

- Gradual Imbalance Theories
  1. Autoimmune—immune system loses its ability to distinguish normal material from foreign antigens and begins to destroy its host
  2. Gradual imbalance—brain, endocrine, or immune system begins to fail, possibly at different rates, causing an imbalance and decreased effectiveness
  3. Neuroendocrine regulatory system—enables body to adapt to real or perceived challenges such as changes in workload, temperature, or psychological threats

- Wear and Tear—mechanical and biological features of aging; irreversible damage occurs over time

- Social Theory—activity theory—maintenance of activity, social roles, and social supports directly related to satisfaction with life and self-concept; quality of activities more important than quantity

- Developmental Theories
  1. Erik Erickson's resolution of psychological conflict—ego integrity vs. despair
  2. Robert Peck expanded upon Erickson's conflict of aging
     a. Ego differentiation vs. work role preoccupation
     b. Body transcendence vs. body preoccupation
     c. Ego transcendence vs. ego preoccupation
  3. Daniel Levinson's Seasons of Life—individual must ultimately come to terms with the inevitability of death; focus is on the relationship of physical changes to personality
  4. Developmental tasks theory
     a. Adjust to decreasing physical strength and health
     b. Adjust to retirement and reduced income
     c. Adjust to death of partner
     d. Establish affiliation with peers
     e. Adapt to social rules
     f. Establish satisfactory physical living arrangements

◘ INTERVIEW AND HEALTH HISTORY

Geriatric intervention goals include care and cure, improvement and maintenance of function, and quality of life. The goal of the interview is to obtain a complete and accurate health history. It is a subjective account of the individual's status. Much of the information obtained will be utilized to formulate diagnoses and a plan of care.

- Develop a Relationship
  1. Develop a climate of trust
  2. Establish a caring relationship
  3. Identify the chief complaint
  4. Maintain a goal-directed interview, as older adults may have long and complex histories
     a. Direct flow of conversation—avoid a "positive" review of systems, answering "yes" to all questions
     b. Ask specific questions, but allow individual to elaborate
     c. Design questions to address one issue at a time
  5. Be aware that gender and age can influence the patient-provider relationship
  6. Family may be present to assist in the evaluation. The patient may rely on the family for answers to interview questions
  7. Sensitive issues such as incontinence, abuse, failing cognition, sexual dysfunction, and alcohol abuse need to be addressed. It is critical that the patient not feel trust or confidence is betrayed

- Communication
  1. Speak slowly; do not shout; lower octaves are generally heard more clearly as bilateral, symmetrical, high-frequency hearing loss is a common age-related change
  2. Help interpret patient's feelings; ask for clarification
  3. Convey warmth and concern through listening, appropriate touch
  4. Observe for signs of anxiety, exhaustion, nervousness
  5. Understand social mores, cultural differences, language barriers, personal biases

- Environment
  1. Provide a quiet, private setting
  2. Set time limit, as the elderly may tire
  3. Sit face-to-face to ensure eye contact; exhibit a relaxed, but concerned, atmosphere
  4. Provide good lighting and ventilation; avoid light source shining from behind you as it creates shadows and glares

- Values Assessment
  1. Elderly patients may have different goals and values from those traditionally assumed during a health-related encounter

2. Assessing values and goals for care will determine the direction of the remainder of the encounter
   a. Will the patient consider primary prevention strategies?
      (1) Sometimes elderly patients feel that quality of life is more important, e.g., an 80-year-old patient will not discuss smoking cessation
      (2) Short-term comfort strategies may be more valuable to the patient than actions that promote long-term survival
   b. Will the patient pursue secondary prevention activities?
      (1) Elderly patients may not be willing to discuss or consider vascular and cancer screenings
      (2) May not return for care if the provider pursues this agenda
   c. Will the patient consider tertiary prevention, e.g., medication and other disease control activities?
      (1) Often elderly patients have a very specific agenda
      (2) Prioritize short-term comfort over improved long-term outcomes, e.g., antihypertensives make them feel unwell, so they prefer to risk target organ damage rather than take medication
3. The primary goal of care for elderly patients may be conservative, short-term peace or comfort; recognizing goals should direct the care encounter

- Health History—format (assess reliability of historian)
  1. Biographical data—important to obtain name and phone number of closest relative
  2. Family history
     a. Parents' health history; cause of death (if applicable)
     b. History of diabetes, heart and kidney disease, cancer, alcoholism, drug abuse, mental illness, and other major medical problems in family
     c. Special attention should be given to neurodegenerative or mood disorders
  3. Occupation—any environmental or occupational exposure to pulmonary toxins; adjustment to retirement; source of income
  4. Medications—prescriptions, over-the-counter, nontraditional modalities, home remedies, herbal medications, use of medications prescribed to spouse and friends
  5. Smoking history, illegal drug use history
  6. Alcohol use or abuse
  7. Allergies, drug sensitivities, foods

8. Mental health problems
9. Nutrition evaluation
   a. General
      (1) Attitude towards eating—alone, with family or caregiver
      (2) Appetite
      (3) Change in ability to taste
      (4) Consumption, special dietary restrictions
      (5) Meal preparation
      (6) Shopping
   b. Significant weight loss (at least 5% of usual body weight)—sudden (days to weeks) vs. gradual weight loss
   c. Common causes of weight loss
      (1) Cancer (lung, GI, lymphoma, GU)—up to 36% of cases
      (2) Diabetes and hyperthyroidism
      (3) Depression, anxiety, and dementia
      (4) AIDS—do not rule out high-risk behaviors in elderly such as homosexuality, IV drug abuse, history of blood transfusion, infected spouse, multiple sexual partners, paid sexual partners
10. Sleep
    a. Note patterns—hour of bedtime/sleep, daytime fatigue/naps, insomnia
    b. Sleep aids—pharmacological and nonpharmacological
    c. Normal changes of sleep patterns with aging
       (1) Longer stage 1, light sleep
       (2) Shorter stages 3 and 4, decreased 20%—deep sleep shorter, therefore less restful nights
       (3) Increased sleep apnea of 10 seconds or more without awakening
       (4) Increased time awake during night
11. Exercise patterns, recreational profile
12. Review of systems
    a. Systematic review of elderly individual
    b. Subjective data collected
    c. Diseases may present atypically
13. Preventive health practices—check frequency of screening tests such as Papanicolaou smear, testicular and prostate exams, stool guaiac test, sigmoidoscopy, cholesterol level, mammograms

- Past Medical History
  1. Hospitalization and operations
  2. Vaccinations—influenza, pneumonia, hepatitis, tetanus
  3. Accidents, injuries, falls
  4. Childhood and adult illnesses
  5. Communicable disease history
     a. Tuberculosis
     b. Influenza

    c. HIV status

    d. Sexually transmitted diseases

    e. Streptococcal infections

    f. Hepatitis

- Health Practices, Religious Implications
  1. Blood transfusion acceptance/denial
  2. Dietary restrictions
  3. Fasting on certain holidays
  4. Sabbath restrictions for procedures, activities

- Safety Assessment
  1. Environment
     a. Home—stairs, scatter rugs, electrical wires, telephone cords, locks on doors and windows
     b. Neighborhood—sidewalks, location of stores, banks, post office, pharmacy
     c. Community services
     d. Crime
  2. Driving—loss of independence if taken away (difficult decision); must weigh the risks versus benefits of action
     a. Assessment of driver safety may be indicated
     b. Specific driving safety test not available
     c. American Medical Association makes some recommendations for driver safety assessment—see the *Physician's Guide to Assessing and Counseling Older Drivers*
        (1) Clock draw test
        (2) Clinical Dementia Rating (CDR)— AMA advocates on-road testing for those who score > 0.5
  3. Elder abuse—recent and increasingly common form of domestic violence
     a. Estimated to be approximately 1 million persons
     b. Abuser frequently is caregiver or family
     c. Physical or psychological abuse, neglect, financial abuse, or sexual abuse

- Patient Self-Determination Act (1990)—encourage patient to discuss this with family and healthcare provider and act upon wishes
  1. Advance directives—indicates intent of patient based on his/her wishes with right to refuse any or all interventions of medical care
  2. Living will—a contract specifying the patient's wishes concerning the end of his/her life; varies according to state in which he/she resides; a copy should be given to the healthcare provider and family member
  3. Durable power of attorney for health care— authorizes an agent to make medical decisions on behalf of the patient when the patient is unable

    4. Physician-assisted suicide may become an issue

◻ LIVING SITUATIONS AND INCOME STATUS

1. Socialization
2. Support systems in place such as family and friends
3. Available resources in the community
4. Effect of change in financial resources upon retirement or disability
5. Effect of change when spouse or important family member is institutionalized or dies
6. Assess role and status of caregiver; care of the caregiver

◻ FUNCTIONAL ASSESSMENT

- Definition—method used to measure an individual's ability to perform activities ADL and instrumental activities of daily living (IADL) through physical, emotional, cognitive, and social parameters
  1. Physical function identifies sensorimotor ability, gait, and mobility
  2. Emotional function focuses on coping mechanisms
  3. Cognitive function identifies intellectual and reasoning capabilities
  4. Social function evaluates ability to maintain social roles

- Certain deficits affect functional status
  1. Visual and auditory deficits may precipitate or worsen confusion; eye and ear examination should be performed when deteriorating function is the chief complaint
  2. Unfamiliar surroundings may cause confusion, sleep disturbances
  3. Musculoskeletal injury resulting in mobility impairment, dependence, loss of control, and sleep disturbances

- Determine ability to perform ADL and self-care activities independently using the Index of Independence in Activities of Daily Living Scale (Katz, 1983)
  1. Elderly tend to overrate abilities; underrate disabilities
  2. Family members tend to underrate abilities
  3. Index ranks ability to perform basic functions such as bathing, dressing, feeding, and continence

- Determine ability to perform IADL (Katz, 1983)
  1. More complex personal tasks such as cooking and shopping

2. More complex independent functions such as taking care of finances, banking, and managing medications

- Cognitive status assessments are used to detect causes of cognitive impairment
  1. Short Portable Mental Status Questionnaire (SPMSQ) is used to identify the presence and degree of intellectual impairment by testing orientation, memory concerning self-care, remote memory, and math (Pfeiffer, 1975)
  2. The Mini-Mental State Exam (MMSE) is used to identify cognitive aspects of mental functions such as orientation, attention, recall, and language (Folstein, Folstein, & McHugh, 1975)

- Other functional issues may be assessed such as medical conditions, communication, senses, resources, and behavior problems

◻ PHYSICAL ASSESSMENT

An essential component of the evaluation from which valuable information can be obtained; an organized, systematic approach such as head-to-toe or major organ system should be utilized

- General Inspection
  1. Provide initial assessment of health status
  2. Identify specific characteristics—posture, gait, appearance
  3. Determine if exhibiting altered concentration due to pain, memory loss, agitation, and other signs of focusing deficits
  4. Identify strengths, disabilities, and limitations
  5. Evaluate skin changes consistent with frequent accidental or purposeful injury that may provide information about declining functional abilities or abuse

- Normal Aging Changes in the Elderly: General Appearance
  1. Fat increases by 30% and water decreases by 53% by age 70; fat distribution shifts from extremities to trunk
  2. Weight increases until about age 50 and then begins to fall; longevity favors individuals who are "ideal" weight or slightly above
  3. Anatomic size and height—elderly lose 1–2 inches due to thinning of cartilage between vertebrae and poor posture; kyphosis; males and females lose approximately $\frac{1}{16}$ inch each year beginning around age 30

- Integumentary System
  1. Anatomical and physiological changes
     a. Decreased elasticity—increased wrinkles, folds, sagging, dry skin resulting in poor turgor
     b. Decreased perspiration—increased heat tolerance, poor temperature regulation; tendency towards hypo/hyperthermia
     c. Body and facial hair thins and grays; increased facial hair on women
     d. Nail growth slows, thickens; hypertrophy common
     e. Eyebrows coarse, bristlelike
     f. Cell regeneration slower
     g. Thinning of epithelial cells and subcutaneous fat layers
  2. Clinical implications
     a. Increased risk of infection
     b. Decreased wound healing
     c. Pruritus
     d. Poorly supported blood vessels rupture easily causing purpura
     e. Common benign skin lesions
        (1) Seborrheic/senile keratosis—macular-papular, dark, warty areas seen on face, neck, and trunk
        (2) Cherry angioma—small, round, red, domed papules seen on trunk and proximal extremities
        (3) Cutaneous skin tags—pedunculated papillomas seen on neck, chest, and intriginous sites
        (4) Common blue nevus—benign, firm, dark-blue/gray/black, well-defined papule, usually seen on hands and feet
     f. Sun exposure changes
        (1) Solar lentigo—flat, brown, pigmented macule on exposed areas only
        (2) Solar keratosis—single or multiple discreet, dry, rough, scaly lesions on face, neck, and hands
  3. Abnormal changes and disease
     a. Infections—viral, bacterial, fungal
     b. Skin ulcerations
     c. Ingrown toenails
     d. Bunions, corns, calluses
     e. Onychomycosis—fungal infection of nails
     f. Abnormal skin lesions
        (1) Actinic keratosis—precancerous macular, irregular, scaly lesions seen on sun-exposed areas, e.g., hands, arms, neck, and face; small (1:1000) but present risk of progression to squamous cell carcinoma
        (2) Squamous cell carcinoma—malignant soft, red-brown lesion of skin and mucous membrane arises as result of exogenous carcinogens such as sunlight or x-rays; seen on exposed areas, especially face, ears, scalp, arms, lips, and genitalia; low but present risk of metastasis

(3) Basal cell carcinoma—most common type of skin cancer; hard pearly-gray or pink, round, oval lesion with depressed center; usually on forehead, eyelids, nose, and lips—no risk of metastasis but may produce significant local, invasive damage

(4) Malignant melanoma—round, oval, brown, or tan irregular macular lesions seen mostly on trunk, arms, legs; familial tendency, not as common in older population, high risk of metastasis with lung as most common site

- Cardiovascular System
  1. Anatomical and physiological changes
     a. Slight decrease in heart size
     b. Decreased cardiac output by up to 30%; heart fills and expels blood less efficiently
     c. Increased peripheral vascular resistance due to arteriosclerotic calcification of the vascular endothelium
     d. Increased ectopic activity due to decreased threshold for cellular excitability
     e. Decreased resting heart rate; increased with exercise/stress, takes longer to return to baseline; decreased exercise tolerance
     f. Increased rigidity and thickness of valves—development of aortic stenosis may occur
     g. Decreased sensitivity of baroreceptors
  2. Clinical implications
     a. Hypertension leads to a significant increase in the risk of heart attack, stroke, and heart failure
     b. Orthostatic hypotension; near syncope with sudden position change
     c. Increased narrow or wide pulse pressure
     d. Unilateral or bilateral pain or swelling in lower extremities
     e. Varicosities—tortuous peripheral vessels
     f. Functional systolic murmurs increase with age; systolic heart murmurs are reported in one-third of 80 years olds; assess to determine etiology
     g. S_4 commonly heard
     h. Heart rate < 60 or > 90 beats per minute may be diagnostically significant
     i. Blood pressure of < 120/< 80 is classified as "Normal"; 120–139 systolic or 80–89 diastolic is "Prehypertension"; 140–159 systolic or 90–99 diastolic is "Hypertension, Stage 1"; and ≥ 160 or ≥ 100 is "Hypertension, Stage 2"
     j. Prehypertension readings indicate a 1.5–2.5% greater risk of heart attack, stroke, or heart failure over 10 years than optimal blood pressures

3. Abnormal changes and disease
   a. Hypertension or isolated systolic hypertension
   b. Coronary artery disease—may present with fatigue, confusion, dizziness, dyspnea, palpitations; may *not* present with pain
   c. Cerebrovascular disease—may present as confusion, headache
   d. Congestive heart failure—may present as confusion/delirium, anxiety, shortness of breath, cough, and/or palpitations
   e. Arrhythmias (atrial fibrillation common)—may present with restlessness, diaphoresis, syncope
   f. Peripheral vascular disease
      (1) Arterial—claudication
      (2) Venous—stasis
      (3) Trophic changes with decreased peripheral hair distribution
   g. Valvular pathology and cardiac dysfunction are most common causes of murmurs

- Respiratory System
  1. Anatomical and physiological changes
     a. Decreased vital capacity, decreased tissue elasticity, loss of elastic recoil of alveolar tissue
     b. Increased residual volume, decrease in functional alveoli
     c. Increased diameter of the chest
     d. Decreased ability to clear lungs, less efficient cough
     e. Decreased diffusion of gases
     f. Decreased strength of expiratory muscles, more rigid intercostal muscles
     g. Decreased clearance of congestion
     h. Kyphosis may be present
  2. Clinical implications
     a. Increased antero-posterior diameter
     b. Barrel chest, retraction
     c. Decreased ventilation at lung bases
     d. Pallor, cyanosis
     e. Nail clubbing
     f. Vesicular breath sounds, bilateral basilar crackles
     g. Decreased reserve
     h. Decreased response to exercise, stress, and disease
  3. Abnormal changes and disease
     a. Bronchitis, emphysema
     b. Tumor, lung cancer
     c. Pleural effusion
     d. Pneumonia—atypical presentation of tachypnea, confusion, chest pain, dyspnea, and often no fever or low-grade fever
     e. Tuberculosis

f. Atelectasis

g. Infection

h. Adventitious sounds—bronchi, crackles, wheezing, pleural friction rub

i. Tachypnea, irregular breathing, labored breathing

j. No breath sounds

- Breasts
  1. Anatomical and physiological changes
     a. Atrophy of fatty tissue and glands, pendulous breasts
     b. May appear nodular
     c. Increased sagging
     d. Nipples are lower
     e. Elderly men may have increased breast size
  2. Clinical implications
     a. Wide variation of size, symmetry, contour, texture, pigmentation
     b. Development of fibrocystic breasts
     c. Gynecomastia for men
  3. Abnormal changes and disease
     a. Unilateral mass, pain, tenderness, cancer
     b. Grossly unequal
     c. Redness, bloody discharge
     d. Dimpling
     e. Fixed inversion or retraction of nipple

- Gastrointestinal System
  1. Anatomical and physiological changes
     a. Loss of taste-functional taste buds
     b. Loss of or "softening" of teeth
     c. Decreased saliva
     d. Decreased mastication
     e. Decreased peristalsis
     f. Weakening of lower esophageal sphincter
     g. Lower esophageal sphincter often fails to relax
     h. Decreased gastric acid secretion
     i. Decreased hepatic metabolism
     j. Decreased pancreatic secretion
     k. Decreased insulin release
     l. Decreased smooth muscle motility
     m. Decreased function of rectal stretch receptors
  2. Clinical implications
     a. Constipation, fecal impaction
     b. Indigestion
     c. Increased sensitivity to medication in GI tract
     d. Increased response to alcohol, nicotine, chocolate, peppermint, and caffeine
     e. Periodontal disease
     f. Malnutrition
  3. Abnormal changes and disease
     a. Diabetes
     b. Nutritional deficiencies
     c. Gastroesophageal reflux disease

d. Hiatal hernia

e. Intestinal obstruction, jaundice

f. Stool changes—black, tarry; blood; mucus; light tan or gray color

- Genitourinary and Reproductive Systems
  1. Anatomical and physiological changes
     a. Renal changes
        (1) Decreased kidney function, number of nephrons and glomerular filtration rate (GFR)
        (2) Decreased bladder capacity and muscle tone
        (3) Decreased sphincter control
        (4) Increased frequency, urgency, nocturia
     b. Hormonal changes
        (1) Decreased estrogen in females
        (2) Decreased testosterone in males
        (3) Atrophy of ovaries, uterus, and vagina
        (4) Development of firmer testes, may be smaller
        (5) Sclerosis of penile arteries and veins
        (6) Decreased seminal fluid, sperm number, motility
        (7) Pubic hair thins and grays
        (8) Prostate gland enlargement
        (9) Decreased vaginal secretions
  2. Clinical implications
     a. Asymptomatic urinary tract infections
     b. Urinary incontinence
     c. Atrophic vaginitis, foul-smelling vaginal discharge
     d. Dyspareunia
     e. Pelvic prolapse
     f. Benign prostatic hypertrophy
     g. Drug toxicity
     h. Urinary retention
     i. Impotency
     j. Testicular enlargement, nodules
  3. Abnormal changes and disease
     a. Cervical, ovarian cancer/disease/nodules
     b. Testicular, penile cancer/lesions/nodules
     c. Bladder, kidney cancer/disease/lesions

- Endocrine System
  1. Anatomical and physiological changes
     a. Decreased size, number, and activity of sweat glands
     b. Decline in body's cooling mechanism
     c. Decreased ability to perspire
     d. Decreased ability to metabolize glucose
     e. Reduced insulin secretion
     f. Delayed insulin response
     g. Increased insulin resistance
  2. Clinical implications
     a. Dehydration
     b. Hyperthermia
     c. Hyperglycemia

3. Abnormal changes and disease
   a. Diabetes mellitus
   b. Tumors
   c. Thyroid disease

- Musculoskeletal System
  1. Anatomical and physiological changes
     a. Bone demineralization
     b. Decreased strength and endurance, range of motion
     c. Joint and cartilage erosion
     d. Loss of flexibility in the joints
     e. Bony growths at joints
     f. Decreased muscle mass
     g. Bony prominences develop
  2. Clinical implications
     a. Gait disturbances
     b. Falls
     c. Loss of height
     d. Hallux valgus—bunions
     e. Hammer toes
     f. Valgus, varus deformities
     g. Lordosis, scoliosis, kyphosis
     h. Stiffness and decreased range of motion of joints
  3. Abnormal changes and disease
     a. Osteoporosis
     b. Degenerative joint disease
     c. Fractures—vertebrae, hip, colles' (fracture of lower end of radius)
     d. Extra-articular pathologic changes—bursitis, fibrositis
     e. Swelling, tenderness, pain in joints
     f. Neuropathy and ischemia

- Sensory System
  1. Vision
     a. Anatomical and physiological changes
        (1) Lens yellows and clouds
        (2) Pupils smaller, but remain equal
        (3) Decreased tear production
        (4) Lens stiffens
        (5) Decreased peripheral vision
        (6) Difficulty in color discrimination
        (7) Eyelids thinning, increased stretching, poor fit; entropion and ectropion
        (8) Conjunctiva pale and less white
        (9) Arcus senilis
     b. Clinical implications
        (1) Decreased visual acuity
        (2) Decreased adaptation to darkness
        (3) Corneal irritation
        (4) Decreased peripheral vision
        (5) Dry appearance
        (6) Progressive eyelid relaxation
     c. Abnormal changes and disease
        (1) Macular degeneration
        (2) Blindness

        (3) Retinal detachment
        (4) Glaucoma
        (5) Cataracts
  2. Hearing
     a. Anatomical and physiological changes
        (1) Decreased discrimination of pitch and acuity
        (2) Decreased sensitivity to higher frequency sounds
        (3) Excessive cerumen, drying of cerumen, hair growth in canal
        (4) Tympanic membranes may lose mobility
     b. Clinical implications
        (1) Vertigo, tinnitus
        (2) Diminished hearing
        (3) Auricle loses elasticity, lobe elongates
        (4) Conductive hearing loss
     c. Abnormal changes and disease
        (1) Tumors
        (2) Deafness
        (3) Presbycusis
        (4) Otosclerosis
        (5) Impacted cerumen
        (6) Tophi, pain
  3. Head/throat/neck/nose
     a. Anatomical and physiological changes
        (1) Decreased sense of smell; difficulty distinguishing specific odors
        (2) Decreased size of thyroid gland
        (3) Atrophy of pharynx, larynx
        (4) Nose sags, appears longer
        (5) Lymph nodes may be noted—less than 1 cm in size, soft discrete and mobile considered normal variation
     b. Clinical implications
        (1) Marked asymmetry of face
        (2) Increased size of lymph nodes
        (3) Soft voice
        (4) Difficulty swallowing
        (5) Postnasal drip
     c. Abnormal changes and disease
        (1) Anosmia (loss of smell)
        (2) Allergic rhinitis
        (3) Cracks, fissures of lips
        (4) Head, neck, throat nodules/cancer
  4. Taste
     a. Anatomical and physiological changes
        (1) Decreased number of taste buds, papillary atrophy
        (2) Difficulty distinguishing specific tastes
        (3) Teeth yellow, increased space between teeth
        (4) Decreased ability to chew
     b. Clinical implications
        (1) Loss of interest in eating
        (2) Poor fitting dentures, loose or broken teeth

(3) Dental caries, gingival disease or decay

(4) Dehydration

c. Abnormal changes and disease

(1) Oral cancer

(2) Ulcerations

5. Touch

a. Anatomical and physiological changes

(1) Decreased receptors

(2) Lower ability to distinguish temperature and pain

(3) Increased pain tolerance

b. Clinical implications

(1) Decreased sensation

(2) Numbness, tingling

(3) Potential for burns, injury

c. Abnormal changes and disease

(1) Loss of feeling

(2) Scalding, frostbite

- Neurological system
  1. Anatomical and physiological changes
     a. General decrease in cerebral blood flow
     b. Global brain atrophy
     c. Slowed response to heat and cold
     d. General slowing of reaction time
     e. Sluggish deep tendon reflexes
     f. Loss of vibratory sensation
  2. Clinical implications
     a. Benign senile tremors
     b. Decreased coordination and balance
     c. Wide-based gait
     d. Nystagmus
     e. Decreased response to pain
     f. Loss of balance
  3. Abnormal changes and disease
     a. Ataxia
     b. Dysphasia, aphasia
     c. Dysarthria
     d. Parkinson's disease
     e. Senile dementia, Alzheimer's disease
     f. Delirium
     g. Cerebrovascular accident (CVA)
     h. Vertigo

❏ COMMON NEUROLOGICAL DISORDERS AND MENTAL HEALTH ISSUES

- Delirium—acute change of mental status with disturbance of attention and cognition due to an organic cause; common problem of hospitalized elderly, indicates an acute abnormality that must be addressed for resolution of delirium
  1. Definitive diagnostic features
     a. Acute onset; may be worse at night; "sundowning"
     b. Varying course

c. Psychotic symptoms

(1) Often iatrogenic—related to infection, medications, fluid and electrolyte imbalance, or hypoxia

(2) Initial presentation of many serious and treatable medical disorders

(3) Initial presentation in many common disorders, for example

(a) Urinary tract infection

(b) Long history of alcohol abuse combined with an anticholinergic or narcotic

d. Visual and auditory hallucinations

e. Frequent disorientation

2. Common medications causing delirium

a. Narcotics

b. Benzodiazepines

c. Anticholinergics

d. Antidepressants

e. Barbiturates

f. Antihypertensives

g. Digoxin

h. Antibiotics such as cephalosporins, fluoroquinolones, aminoglycosides, and metronidazole

i. H_2 blockers such as cimetidine

3. Conditions predisposing the elderly to development of delirium

a. Head injury

b. Dementia

c. History of significant substance abuse

d. Advanced medical illness or organ failure

e. Chronic subdural hematoma

4. Effective treatment

a. Treating the underlying cause is definitive intervention

b. May be difficult; interventions that help orientation may be helpful

c. Keep out of bed during waking hours

d. Presence of family members or familiar possessions

e. Bedroom lights kept on at night; use of clock and calendar

f. Regular schedule

g. Trial of low-dose neuroleptic medication or high-potency antipsychotic

- Dementia—defined by DSM-IV TR as a mental disorder that involves deterioration in mental, behavioral, and emotional function; typically includes gradual regression and loss of intellectual functioning, such as thinking, remembering, and reasoning, of sufficient severity to interfere with daily functioning
  1. Definitive diagnostic features
     a. Cognitive impairment
     b. Change in personality

    c.   Mood swings

    d.   Erratic behavior

    e.   Significant short-term memory impairment

    f.   Impairment in abstract thinking

    g.   Aphasia, apraxia, agnosia

2.   Major causes of dementia

    a.   Alzheimer's disease (AD)

       (1) Affects 4.5 million Americans; 10% of people ages 65 and over; the prevalence doubles every 10 years thereafter; half the population 85 and over may have AD

       (2) Most common type of dementia; 16% of women and 6% of men who survive to an average life expectancy will develop Alzheimer's disease

       (3) Gradual onset

       (4) Senile plaques and neurofibrillary tangles seen on autopsy

       (5) Proven risk factors are age and a positive family history; especially for early onset prior to age 65

    b.   Vascular dementia (VaD)

       (1) Onset may be sudden; deterioration is more stepwise, less insidious as with AD

       (2) Generalized symptoms of disorientation, confusion, behavior change

       (3) Depression more common in VaD

       (4) VaD coexists in 15–20% of AD

       (5) Risk factors include high blood pressure, vascular disease, diabetes, or previous stroke

    c.   Parkinson's disease (PD)

       (1) Lack of dopamine, which controls muscle activity

       (2) Symptoms include tremors, stiffness, and slow speech

       (3) Late in the course, some individuals develop dementia

    d.   Other related disorders include Huntington's disease, Creutzfeldt-Jakob disease, Pick's disease, Lewy body dementia, and normal pressure hydrocephalus

    e.   Other causes of dementia are alcohol, drugs, nutritional and metabolic disorders; rarely a tumor

3.   Effective treatment

    a.   Good preventive health practices may impact the risk of developing dementia

    b.   Use of lists to assist with memory impairment

    c.   Correct vision and hearing deficits

    d.   Use of day hospital and outpatient day care centers

    e.   Make few environmental changes to avoid confusion

    f.   Pharmacologic treatment has demonstrated improved short-term memory, delayed long-term care placement, and maintenance of function

       (1) Combination therapy with acetylcholinesterase inhibitors and NMDA inhibitors is standard of care; should be instituted in mild-moderate Alzheimer's disease

          (a) Acetylcholinesterase inhibitors

             (i)   Donepezil 5–10 mg daily

             (ii) Rivastigmine 3–6 mg b.i.d.; also available as transdermal patch

             (iii) Galantamine 8–24 mg daily

          (b) NMDA inhibitor

             (i)   Memantine 5–20 mg daily

       (2) Both classes of drug ultimately attempt to preserve/protect acetylcholine-producing neurons in the midbrain

    g.   Dietary recommendations focus on neuroprotection and the effect of dietary fat composition on the risk of AD; some evidence suggests that elevated blood cholesterol is related to the development of AD; some studies report dietary intake of fish, nuts, seeds, and eggs may protect against AD; while it is generally advised that individuals should limit intake of foods high in saturated and transunsaturated fats such as red meat, butter, ice cream, commercially baked products, and partially hydrogenated oils, there is no direct evidence that this will improve risk for dementing disorders

- Depression—psychiatric condition that is an affective disorder characterized by physical, cognitive, and emotional symptoms; frequently underdiagnosed in the elderly and less likely to be treated than in younger adults; decrease in cognitive functioning may be falsely attributed to dementia when the underlying cause is actually depression

1.   Definitive diagnostic features

    a.   Regular markedly depressed mood

    b.   Cognitive symptoms worsen; inability to concentrate

    c.   Loss of interest in life, vegetative symptoms

    d.   Lack of pleasure in almost all activities

    e.   General feeling of worthlessness

    f.   Significant unintentional weight loss or weight gain

    g.   Insomnia or hypersomnia

    h.   Improvement in mentation seen with treatment

    i.   Past and family history more likely

    j.   Diagnosis of depressive disorders based upon DSM-IV TR is described in the psychosocial disorders

2. Marked depressive symptoms noted with the following medical conditions
    a. Endocrine/metabolic disorders (thyroid disease, diabetes mellitus, hypokalemia, anemia)
    b. Brain tumors
    c. Chronic obstructive pulmonary disease (COPD)
    d. Vitamin deficiencies
    e. Neurological disorders (Parkinson's disease, stroke, multiple sclerosis, seizure disorder)
    f. Drug therapy used to treat medical conditions
    g. Alcohol abuse
    h. Chronic pain
    i. Cancer
3. Complications in diagnosing in the elderly
    a. Behavioral and cognitive changes of the aging central nervous system (CNS) make the differential diagnosis of depression versus dementia challenging
    b. Presence of other major medical conditions
    c. Common complaints of insomnia, awakening during sleep or sleepy during day
4. Effective treatment
    a. Counseling, psychotherapy is the treatment of choice in mild dementia
    b. Exercise, diet, rest
    c. SSRI therapy is the drug of choice when pharmacologic intervention required
        (1) Excellent safety profile in older adults
        (2) Avoid fluoxetine due to long half life
    d. Tricyclic antidepressants (TCA) avoided in the elderly population due to cardiovascular safety concerns and anticholinergic effects

- Suicide—increasing rates in this population, higher than at younger ages; highest incidence of successful suicide is in Caucasian males > 75 years old; multiple losses and decreased internal and external resources contribute to incidence; perceived intolerable psychological distress, frustration, and unmet needs
    1. Risk factors
        a. Sex (male rate is seven times higher than for same-age women)
        b. Race (white)
        c. Marital status (divorced, separated, or single)
        d. Economic status (low, unemployed)
        e. Mental illness (depression, schizophrenia, and individuals in early stages of dementia who are aware of their deficits are at highest risk)
        f. Health, pain (cancer, AIDS, dialysis patients)
        g. Alcohol abuse, dependence
        h. Bereavement (especially within 1 year of a loss, retirement)
        i. Social isolation
        j. Previous attempts
    2. Types
        a. Overt suicide—specific act that terminated life (weapon, hanging, poison, toxic fumes)
        b. Covert suicide—destructive behaviors that erode health and lead to death
            (1) Alcohol abuse, drug abuse
            (2) Medication misuse (overdosage or omission)
            (3) Smoking
            (4) Poor dietary habits, self-starvation
            (5) Ignoring disease symptoms
    3. Treatment—prevention depends on prompt recognition of signs; autonomy and confidentiality do not take priority over one's safety
        a. May be difficult
        b. Close observation during acute phase
        c. Identify and treat underlying depression
        d. Excellent listening skills and willingness to listen
        e. Ensure safe environment; determine if hospitalization is indicated

▣ PHARMACOTHERAPY AND THE ELDERLY

Age-related physiological changes result in elderly being at high risk for side effects and toxic effects; compounded when chronic diseases are present.

- Important Issues
    1. The average older adult is on six prescription medications and eight total medications
    2. Approximately one-third of drug-related hospitalizations and one-half of all drug-related deaths occur in persons 60 years and older
    3. Thirty percent of all U.S. dollars spent on prescription medication annually and 40–50% of all U.S. dollars spent on over-the-counter medications annually is for elderly patients
    4. More than $3 billion a year is spent by elderly on prescription and nonprescription drugs
    5. Majority of elderly have one or more chronic conditions such as arthritis, hypertension, heart disease, and diabetes that are treated with multiple medications
    6. Drug therapy for one condition may adversely impact another medical condition
    7. Increased number of adverse drug reactions (ADR); ADR have occurred in 30% of elderly outpatients and account for up to 10% of hospital admissions

a. Reflective of number and type of medications taken

b. Frequent use of over-the-counter, self-prescribed medication, home remedies

c. Multiple healthcare providers with lack of coordination of care

d. Multiple pharmacies used with lack of ability to identify potential drug interactions

e. Do not assume that behavior change is age-related

8. Common ADR in the elderly include edema, nausea, vomiting, anorexia, dizziness, diarrhea, constipation, confusion, and urinary retention or incontinence; should not be misinterpreted as signs and symptoms of illness or due to the aging process

- Physiological Changes—may lead to increased plasma concentrations of drugs

1. Decreased tolerance of standard dosages; toxic reactions occur at lower doses

2. Decreased metabolism—usually occurs in the liver, which is decreased in sized with decreased blood flow

3. Decreased absorption—decreased liver enzyme activity and gastric emptying time; gastric pH and transit time increased

4. Variable distribution—lean muscle mass decreases and fat tissue increases; fat soluble drugs have longer duration; water soluble drugs have smaller volume of distribution and higher plasma concentrations; increased adipose tissue can cause increased storage of lipid-soluble drugs

5. Decreased ability to excrete drugs due to decreased GFR; results in decreased excretion time for medication; GFR declines 50% between third and ninth decades of life

- Potential Side Effects of Commonly Prescribed Drugs

1. Confusion—digoxin, cimetidine, dopamine agents, antihistamines, hypnotics, sedatives, anticholinergics, anticonvulsants, fluoroquinolones

2. Anorexia—digoxin

3. Fatigue/weakness—diuretics, antidepressants, antihypertensives

4. Ataxia—sedatives, hypnotics, anticonvulsants, antipsychotics

5. Forgetfulness—benzodiazepines

6. Constipation—anticholinergics, calcium channel blockers

7. Diarrhea—oral antacids

8. GI upset—iron, nonsteroidal anti-inflammatory drugs (NSAIDs), salicylates, corticosteroids, estrogens

9. Tinnitus—analgesics, NSAIDs, some antibiotics

10. Urinary retention—anticholinergics, alpha-agonists, antihistamines

11. Orthostatic hypotension—antihypertensives, sedatives, diuretics, antidepressants

12. Depression—benzodiazepines, beta adrenergic antagonists

13. Delirium—corticosteroids, sedatives, antihistamines

14. Dizziness—sedatives, antihypertensives, anticonvulsants, diuretics

- Problems with Use of Medication

1. Overuse—elderly feel when they seek care from a healthcare provider they should receive a prescription

2. Misuse—self-prescribing habits, changing dosages, use of old prescriptions, use of friend's medication, poor history given to provider, outdated prescriptions

3. Knowledge deficit—difficulty understanding due to educational level, *or* misunderstanding due to hearing deficits, *or* inadequate information provided by healthcare professional

4. Memory deficit—forget purpose, dosage, frequency of taking medication, may accidentally repeat dosage

5. Cost—may not purchase medication due to limited financial resources

6. Visual deficit—inability to properly read label, may take wrong medication

7. Mobility problems—difficulty opening bottles, small tablets hard to handle, splitting pills in half is sometimes necessary, difficulty manipulating inhalers

8. Multiple providers, multiple pharmacies—conflicting/duplicate medications prescribed by various healthcare practitioners; generic and brand name prescriptions being taken concurrently

- Recommendations for drug use in the elderly—identify factors that predispose the elderly to ADR, e.g., multisystem disease, greater severity of disease, female gender, small body size, hepatic or renal disease, previous drug reactions; proceed cautiously with the following

1. Clear indication for use

2. Reliably effective drug

3. Shortest duration appropriate

4. Lowest dosage, "start low, go slow"

5. Cost effective

6. Likeliness to enhance quality of life

7. Avoid adverse outcomes

8. Evaluate patient compliance

9. Identify resource person to assist in administering if necessary

10. Use calendars, pill boxes, and large print to assist
11. Use of devices to aid administration such as spacers for inhalers

◘ PREVENTIVE HEALTH CARE RECOMMENDATIONS

The focus is to prevent disease or injury and promote health. Life expectancy has improved, but chronic diseases remain the major causes of death. The elderly have a greater absolute risk of disease and respond positively to preventive measures. Implement the following by using a tracking system such as a checklist or flowsheet.

- History—annual review and recommendations for persons over age 65
  1. Dietary intake—protein-calorie malnutrition is common
  2. Functional status—identify issues
  3. Substance abuse
     a. Tobacco—directly and negatively affects both health and financial status
     b. Alcohol—heavy use is more than two drinks/day
     c. Illegal drug use
     d. Abuse of prescription medications
  4. Physical activity—exercise and physical fitness improve multiple physiological functions such as cardiorespiratory capacity, muscle strength, endurance, range of motion, sleep, and cognitive function; reduces falls and injury

- Physical Examination
  1. Height and weight, blood pressure
  2. Clinical breast exam
  3. Complete skin exam
  4. Thyroid nodules (if history of irradiation), auscultation for carotid bruits (if risk factors for cerebrovascular, cardiovascular, or neurological disease)
  5. Oral cavity examination

- *Recommended* screening tests by U.S. Preventive Services
  1. Fasting glucose if marginally obese or family history of type 2 diabetes
  2. Papanicolaou smear—perform if no previously documented screen is consistently negative or hysterectomy was performed because of cervical cancer or its precursors; otherwise there is insufficient evidence for routine Pap testing over age 70
  3. Dipstick urinalysis
  4. Mammography—every 1–2 years—there are no studies supporting the utility of mammography after age 74 in patients with no risk factors and a history of negative screening

5. Purified protein derivative (PPD)—if at high risk for close/personal contact with disease
6. Fecal occult blood/sigmoidoscopy—annual fecal occult blood and flexible sigmoidoscopy every 3–5 years beginning at age 50
7. Electrocardiogram with two or more risk factors (high blood cholesterol, hypertension, smoking, diabetes mellitus, family history of coronary artery disease)
8. Thyroid function tests
9. Glaucoma and visual acuity testing annually
10. Hearing impairment testing
11. Total cholesterol in older persons with major coronary heart disease risk factors (smoking, hypertension, diabetes)
12. Prostate cancer screening by digital rectal examination (DRE) in men over age 50 (high-risk patients over age 45) presuming a life expectancy of at least 10 years

- Immunizations
  1. Influenza vaccine—annually
  2. Pneumococcal vaccine
     a. Once
     b. Revaccination is not recommended for healthy persons 65 years and older
     c. A one-time revaccination is recommended by the Centers for Disease Control and Prevention (CDC) for adults at highest risk for serious pneumococcal infection
        (1) As long as a minimum of 5 years has passed since first vaccinated
        (2) Were less than 65 years old at the time
        (3) Risk groups include, but are not limited to, adults with leukemia, lymphoma, Hodgkin's disease, malignancy, HIV infection, chronic renal failure, nephrotic syndrome, asplenia, and other conditions associated with immunosuppression and immunosuppressive chemotherapy
  3. Tetanus-diphtheria toxoids (Td) should be completed for adults who have not received the primary series; periodic Td boosters

- Routine screening—data does **not** yet indicate *for or against* routine screening for the following
  1. Depression in asymptomatic patients
  2. Dementia in asymptomatic patients
  3. Osteoporosis with bone densitometry in postmenopausal women, but women should be counseled about hormone prophylaxis
  4. Controversy over whom and how to screen for colon and prostate cancers; digital rectal exams and serum tumor markers such as prostate specific antigen (PSA) are not routinely recommended for prostate cancer screening;

should be limited to males with a greater than 10 years life expectancy

5. Total cholesterol in asymptomatic patient

6. Zostavax vaccine for those over 60 years old for prevention of shingles

◻ QUESTIONS

Select the best answer.

1. The greatest increase in ethnic representation in the elderly population by 2030 will be:

    a. African-American
    b. Caucasian
    c. Latino
    d. Asian Pacific Islander

2. By the year 2050, the elderly population will:

    a. Begin to decrease
    b. Level off at 50 million persons
    c. Include those persons 55 and over
    d. More than double to 80 million

3. Elderly women outnumber elderly men:

    a. Three to two
    b. 20 million to 10 million
    c. Five to two
    d. Two to one

4. Which of the following is a true statement with regard to elderly men?

    a. They comprise the poorest subgroup of the elderly population
    b. They are much more likely to live with a spouse than elderly women
    c. They have the greatest incidence of nonsuccessful suicides
    d. They are more likely to be institutionalized than elderly women

5. Better education has been proven to improve one's life. The following statement is true about noninstitutionalized adults:

    a. 70% of the elderly have completed high school
    b. The elderly are as likely to have only completed eighth grade as persons under 75 years old
    c. Middle-old have the highest percentage of college degrees
    d. Lack of education increases with age

6. What percentage of the over-85-year-old population lives in long-term care?

    a. Less than 5%
    b. More than 50%
    c. Almost 20%
    d. Between 30% and 35%

7. When performing a health history on the elderly, which of the following should the nurse practitioner avoid?

    a. Standing near the window so the patient can see the interviewer more clearly
    b. Implications of cultural differences and social mores
    c. Asking open-ended questions, but keeping conversation focused
    d. Observing for signs of fatigue

8. Which of the following is not a normal age-related physical change?

    a. Short-term memory loss
    b. Urinary incontinence
    c. Loss of 30% ejection fraction
    d. Joint degeneration

9. Which statement is most accurate about the sleep patterns of older persons?

    a. Sleep apnea of 10 seconds or more may occur, awakening the elderly
    b. The elderly fall asleep quickly but awaken frequently during the night
    c. The elderly have difficulty falling asleep, but then sleep soundly
    d. There are shorter stages 3 and 4 and longer stage 1 sleep cycles

10. Elder abuse is presently a problem in the United States. Which of the following statements regarding elder abuse is not true?

    a. The most common abusers are the family or caregivers
    b. Physical abuse is four times more common than psychological abuse
    c. It is a common form of domestic violence
    d. Up to 10% of the elderly may be subjected to one type of abuse

11. Which of the following is not included in the Patient Self-Determination Act of 1990?

    a. Durable power of attorney for health care
    b. Living will
    c. Organ donation
    d. Indication of patient's intent for medical care

12. In performing activities of daily living:

    a. The elderly overrate their own abilities
    b. The family members overrate the elder's ability
    c. The elderly cannot manage their finances well
    d. The elderly frequently pay for services such as cooking and cleaning

13. When observing general physical findings, the nurse practitioner is aware that:

    a. The elderly lose 1–2 inches in height due to the thickening of the cartilage
    b. The fat distribution shifts from the trunk to the extremities
    c. Fat decreases as body water decreases
    d. An increased AP chest diameter is a normal finding

14. The elderly are at increased risk for some skin cancers because they have been exposed to the sun for many decades. Which of the following is considered a precancerous skin condition?

    a. Solar lentigo
    b. Actinic keratoses
    c. Cherry angiomas
    d. Seborrheic keratoses

15. A decrease in threshold for cellular membrane excitability increases the elderly patient's risk for:

    a. Atrial fibrillation
    b. Orthostatic hypotension
    c. Constipation
    d. Thinning hair

16. Normal age-related changes of the cardiovascular system increase the elderly patient's risk for all of the following except:

    a. Isolated systolic hypertension
    b. Hyperdynamic precordium
    c. Atrial fibrillation
    d. Orthostatic hypotension

17. Which of the following is not a normal age-related change of the head and neck?

    a. Hypertrophy of taste buds
    b. Bilateral high-frequency hearing loss
    c. Decreased saliva production
    d. Optic disk opacity

18. Which of the following age-related changes of the respiratory system is not typically found in the elderly?

    a. Decreased vital capacity and tissue elasticity
    b. Increased residual volume
    c. Decreased anterior-posterior diameter of the chest
    d. Less efficient cough and clearance of congestion

19. Normal age-related changes frequently result in atypical presentation of illness in the elderly client. Which of the following signs and symptoms of pneumonia is frequently not found in the elderly?

    a. High fever
    b. Tachypnea
    c. Confusion
    d. Chest pain

20. The elderly have breast-related variations. Which statement is true?

    a. Elderly men have a decrease in breast size
    b. There is atrophy of the fatty tissue and a nodular appearance
    c. Significantly unequal breast size is a normal variation
    d. Dimpling and milky discharge are not uncommon

21. Which of the following is not a normal age-related change of the GI tract?

    a. Decreased gastric acid secretions
    b. Decreased response to alcohol, caffeine, and nicotine
    c. Constipation and indigestion
    d. Weakening of the esophageal sphincter

22. Which of the following is a typical consequence of normal age-related changes of the GU system?

    a. Asymptomatic urinary tract infections
    b. Urinary incontinence
    c. Urinary retention
    d. Urgency, frequency, and nocturia

23. Because of the normal changes of aging, abnormalities often present differently in an older adult. What is the most common cause of delirium in an elderly patient?

    a. Drug intoxication
    b. Hypoxia
    c. Infection
    d. Hospitalization

24. Abnormal disease processes of the musculoskeletal system include:

    a. Bone demineralization
    b. Bony growths at joints
    c. Decreased strength and endurance
    d. Decreased muscle mass

25. One of the primary differences in clinical presentation of Alzheimer's dementia and vascular dementia is that:

    a. The symptoms of Alzheimer's dementia present before the sixth decade
    b. Depression is a common feature in early Alzheimer's disease
    c. Vascular dementia responds better to environmental interventions
    d. The symptoms of vascular dementia present incrementally

26. Aging results in a variety of normal, nonpathological changes in the body. Which of the following is a normal, age-related change in the structure or function of the ear?

    a. Decreased discrimination of pitch and acuity
    b. Increased sensitivity to low-pitched sounds
    c. Decreased hair growth in the canals
    d. Increased mobility of the tympanic membrane

27. Which of the following is not a true statement with respect to drug management of Alzheimer's dementia?

    a. Vitamin E has shown promising results in terms of slowing progression of neuronal degeneration
    b. Combination therapy with AChE inhibitors and NMDA receptor inhibitors is the standard of care
    c. Pharmacologic therapy can delay institutionalization
    d. Transdermal options are now available

28. Mrs. G. is an 86-year-old female who lives alone. She has been functionally independent until 2 days ago when her daughter found her to be disheveled, incontinent of urine, and "talking nonsense." When evaluating Mrs. G. to rule out causes of delirium, the nurse practitioner knows that which of the following is not typically a cause?

    a. Infection
    b. Polypharmacy
    c. Hyponatremia
    d. Depression

29. The drug of choice for pharmacologic therapy of depression in the elderly patient is an SSRI. Which SSRI is not indicated for this population?

    a. Sertraline
    b. Citalopram
    c. Fluoxetine
    d. Paroxetine

30. Which of the following is not a diagnostic feature of depression?

    a. Inability to concentrate
    b. Short-term memory impairment
    c. Mood swings
    d. Unintentional weight loss or gain

31. Some forms of Alzheimer's dementia have a clear genetic, familial component. A distinct feature of familial disease is that it:

    a. Is more rapidly progressive
    b. Presents before the age of 50
    c. Does not respond to traditional pharmacologic therapy
    d. Affects men disproportionately

32. It is important to remember that physiological changes in the elderly affect drug therapy. Which of the following statements is true?

    a. Metabolism of drugs usually occurs in the kidneys
    b. The liver increases in size in relation to the number and types of drugs used
    c. Gastric pH is decreased
    d. Decreased ability to excrete drugs is due to the decreased GFR

33. The U.S. Preventive Services Task Force made the following recommendation for routine screening of all individuals over 65 years old:

    a. Total cholesterol annually
    b. Prostatic specific antigen annually
    c. Complete skin exam annually
    d. Papanicolaou smear annually on all females

34. Polypharmacy contributes to a variety of symptoms in the older adult. Which of the following can exacerbate depression?

    a. H_2 receptor antagonists
    b. Beta adrenergic antagonists
    c. Benzodiazepines
    d. SNRIs

Answers

1.	**c**	18.	**c**
2.	**d**	19.	**a**
3.	**a**	20.	**b**
4.	**b**	21.	**b**
5.	**d**	22.	**d**
6.	**c**	23.	**c**
7.	**a**	24.	**a**
8.	**b**	25.	**d**
9.	**d**	26.	**a**
10.	**b**	27.	**a**
11.	**c**	28.	**d**
12.	**a**	29.	**c**
13.	**d**	30.	**c**
14.	**b**	31.	**b**
15.	**a**	32.	**d**
16.	**b**	33.	**c**
17.	**a**	34.	**b**

◘ BIBLIOGRAPHY

American Medical Association (AMA) and the National Transportation Safety Board (NTSB). (2003). *Physician guide to assessing and counseling older drivers.* Chicago: Author.

Cassel, C. K., Cohen, H. J., Larson, E. B., Meier, D. E., Resnick, N. M., & Rubenstein, L. Z. (Eds.). (2003). *Geriatric medicine* (4th ed.) New York: Springer.

Chobanian, A. V. (2004). Seventh Report of the Joint National Committee on Prevention, Detection, Evaluation, and Treatment of Hypertension. *Hypertension, 43*(1), 1–3.

Diegelman, N. M., Gilberston, A. D., Moore, J. L., Banou, E., & Meager, M. R. (2004). Validity of the Clock Drawing Test in predicting reports of driving problems in the elderly. *BioMed Central Geriatric, 4*(1), 10. Retrieved from www.pubmedcentral.nih /gov/articlerender.fcgi?tool=pubmed&pubmedid= 1511302

Duthie, E., & Katz, P. R. (2007). *Duthie: Practice of geriatrics* (4th ed.). Philadelphia: Saunders.

Fick, D. M., Cooper, J. W., Wade, W. E., Waller, J. L., MacLean, J. R., & Beers, M. H. Y. (2003). Updating BEERS criteria for potentially inappropriate medication use in the older adult. *Archives of Internal Medicine, 163*, 2716–2724.

Folstein, M. F., Folstein, S. E., & McHugh, P. R. (1975). Mini-mental state: A practical method for grading the cognitive state of patients for the clinician. *Journal of Psychiatric Research, 12*, 189–198.

Fulton, M., & Allen, E. (2005). Polypharmacy in the elderly: A literature review. *Journal of the American Academy of Nurse Practitioners, 17*(4), 123–132.

Gallo, J. J., Bogner, H. R., Fulmer, T., & Paverza, G. J. (2006). *Handbook of geriatric assessment* (4th ed.). Sudbury, MA: Jones & Bartlett.

Gore, V. F., & Mouzon, M. (2006). Polypharmacy in older adults: Front line strategies. *Advance for Nurse Practitioners, 14*(9), 49–52.

Hazzard, W. R., Blass, J. P., Ettinger, W. H., Halter, J. B., & Ouslander, J. G. (Eds.). (2003). *Principles of geriatric medicine and gerontology* (5th ed). New York: McGraw-Hill.

Katz, S. (1983). Assessing self-maintenance: Activities of daily living, mobility, and instrumental activities of daily living. *Journal of the American Geriatrics Association, 31*, 721–727.

National Highway Traffic Safety Administration (NHTSA) and American Medical Association (AMA). *Physician guide to assessing and counseling older drivers.* Retrieved from www.nhtsa.dot.gov/people/injury/olddrive /OlderDriversBook/pages/Chapter1.html#Anchor-Figur-42435

Pfeiffer, E. A. (1975). Short portable mental status questionnaire for the assessment of organic brain deficit in elderly persons. *Journal of the American Geriatric Society, 23*, 433–441.

Snyder, C. H. (2005). Dementia and driving: Autonomy versus safety. *Journal of the American Academy of Nurse Practitioners, 17*(10), 393–402.

Spirduso, W. W. (1995). *The physical dimensions of aging.* Champaign, IL: Human Kinetics Publishing.

Swanson, E. A., & Tripp-Reimer, T. (Eds.). (2002). *Advances in gerontological nursing: Issues for the 21st century, vol. 1.* New York: Springer.

U.S. Census Bureau. (2002). *Statistical briefs.* Economics and Statistical Administration, U.S. Department of Commerce.

United States Preventive Services Task Force (USPSTF). (2006). *The guide to clinical preventive services: Recommendations of the United States Preventive Services Task Force.* Retrieved from http://www.ahrq .gov/clinic/pocketgd.pdf

16

Advanced Practice, Role Development, Current Trends, and Health Policy

Leanne C. Busby

Mary A. Baroni

◻ INTRODUCTION

Advanced practice registered nurses (APRN) must remain informed regarding role development, current issues and trends related to their practice, as well as changes in healthcare policy, as each has an impact on the evolving practice environment. Although current information is presented, the reader is encouraged to contact local and state regulatory bodies for variations in practice requirements.

◻ ADVANCED PRACTICE NURSING

- Definition of Advanced Practice Registered Nurse (APRN)
  1. National Council of State Boards of Nursing (NCSBN)—an APRN is an individual who has "(a) completed a graduate-level educational program, (b) passed a national certification examination that matches the educational preparation, (c) acquired advanced clinical skills and knowledge, (d) practice built upon the competencies of an RN, (e) been educationally prepared to assume responsibility and accountability, (f) clinical experience of sufficient breadth and depth to reflect the intended license, and (g) obtained a license to practice as an APRN in one of the four roles (NCSBN, 2008). Practice as an advanced practice registered nurse means an expanded scope of nurs-

ing, with or without compensation or personal profit, and includes but is not limited to
  a. Assessing patients, synthesizing and analyzing data, and understanding and applying nursing principles at an advanced level
  b. Analyzing multiple sources of data, identifying alternative possibilities as to the nature of a healthcare problem, and selecting appropriate treatment
  c. Making independent decisions in solving complex patient care problems
  d. Developing a plan that establishes diagnoses, sets goals to meet identified healthcare needs, and prescribes a regimen of health care
  e. Performing acts of diagnosing, prescribing, administering, and dispensing therapeutic measures, including legend drugs and controlled substances, within the advanced practice registered nurse's focus of practice
  f. Managing patients' physical and psychosocial health-illness status
  g. Providing for the maintenance of safe and effective nursing care rendered directly or indirectly
  h. Promoting a safe and therapeutic environment
  i. Providing expert guidance and teaching
  j. Participating in patient and health systems management

k. Advocating for patients and communities by attaining and maintaining what is in the best interest of the patient or group

l. Evaluating responses to interventions, the effectiveness of the plan of care, and the health regimen

m. Communicating and working effectively with patients, families, and other members of the healthcare team

n. Utilizing research skills and acquiring and applying critical new knowledge and technologies to practice domain

o. Teaching the theory and practice of advanced practice nursing (NCSBN, 2008)

2. Advanced practice registered nurses (APRN) are educationally prepared to provide care to patients across the health wellness-illness continuum; the emphasis and how implemented within each of the four APRN roles varies. The four APRN roles are identified as (a) certified registered nurse anesthetists, (b) certified nurse midwives, (c) certified nurse practitioners, and (d) and clinical nurse specialist (NCSBN, 2008)

◻ ROLE DEVELOPMENT

- First nurse practitioner (NP) program established in 1964 prepared pediatric nurse practitioners (PNP) through collaborative efforts of Loretta C. Ford, EdD, RN, and Henry K. Silver, MD, at the University of Colorado
  1. PNP role development provided a model for other emerging NP specialties
  2. Original support of PNP role as "physician extender" to improve access concerns due to shortage of primary care providers (PCPs)
  3. Most early PNP education occurred within certificate and/or continuing education programs; e.g., Colorado program included 4 months didactic study followed by 18 months clinical practicum training
  4. Early research focused on quality of care, cost-effectiveness, productivity, clinical decision-making skills, and role satisfaction of the PNP
  5. National Association of Pediatric Nurse Practitioners (NAPNAP) organized in 1973 to establish PNP practice guidelines
  6. Early resistance to NP role as too much of a "medical model" from mainstream graduate nursing education that focused on "nursing model" of clinical nurse specialist (CNS) role development
  7. From 1980 to 1989 more physicians resulted in less need for NP
  8. From 1990 to 1998 increased emphasis on primary care resulted in decreased need for specialty care; NP seen as viable, cost-effective member of healthcare delivery team

- Majority of NP programs currently at the master's degree level within mainstream nursing education with increasing numbers moving toward the doctor of nursing practice (DNP) program
  1. By 1989, 85% federally funded NP programs were graduate level
  2. Distinction between NP and CNS roles in practice have blurred
  3. Blended NP/CNS programs focusing on advanced practice nursing (APN) emerged within graduate nursing education
  4. Advantages/disadvantages of blended NP/CNS role remains controversial
  5. Most current programs require 2 years of full-time or 3–4 years of part-time graduate study
  6. In October 2004 the American Association of Colleges of Nursing (AACN) endorsed the *Position Statement on the Practice Doctorate in Nursing*
  7. As of January 2012, 141 colleges and universities in the United States offered DNP programs; another 100 schools were in the planning stages
  8. A transition date of 2015 has been established for the implementation of the DNP as the entry-level degree for specialty nursing education

- Curriculum Guidelines and Content
  1. Association of Faculties of Pediatric Nurse Practitioner and Associate Programs (AFPNP/AP)—first published terminal competencies in 1981; later updated in 1996
  2. National Organization of Nurse Practitioner Faculties (NONPF)—published curriculum guidelines and standards for NP education in 1990; later updated in 1995 and again in 2000 as *Domains and Competencies of Nurse Practitioner Practice*
  3. Core graduate nursing content includes nursing theory and research, organizational/leadership theory, ethical/legal issues, multicultural care, economics, community-based care, managed care, and healthcare delivery systems
  4. Advanced practice core content includes advanced health assessment, pharmacology, physiology, advanced pathophysiology or other related sciences depending on the APRN specialty, clinical decision-making process, advanced nursing interventions/therapeutics, health promotion/disease prevention, community-based practice, role differentiation, and interpersonal and family theory
  5. APRN specialty content includes information that is unique to type of APRN role,

information that is unique to healthcare needs of respective specialty population, information that supports standards and competencies established by professional specialty organizations, clinical decision making applied to specialty practice, and faculty supervised clinical practice experience (NONPF, 1997)

6. NONPF competencies now available in specialty-specific form to include acute care nurse practitioner, psychiatric mental health nurse practitioner, and primary care in specialty areas, e.g., adult, family, gerontology, women's health, and pediatrics

• Conceptual Models for Advanced Practice Nursing
1. Benner's model of expert practice (1985)
2. Calkin's model of advanced nursing practice (1984)
3. Shuler's model of NP practice (1993; 1998)
   a. Holistic patient needs
   b. NP/patient interaction
   c. Self-care
   d. Health prevention
   e. Health promotion
   f. Wellness

▣ ADVANCED PRACTICE TRENDS AND ISSUES

• Components of Advanced Practice Registered Nursing Role
1. Coordinator of care
2. Patient advocate
3. Accountable for patient outcomes and cost-effectiveness
4. Direct caregiver
5. Educator
6. Administrator
7. Researcher
8. Consultant
9. Case manager
10. Change agent
11. Leader
12. Policy maker

• Standards and Scope of Practice
1. Standards of practice
   a. Described by American Nurses Association (ANA; 1998) as authoritative statements by which to measure quality of practice, service, or education
   b. Establishes minimum levels of acceptable performance
   c. Provides consumer with means to measure quality of care received (Hawkins & Thibodeau, 2002)
   d. Both generic and specific specialty standards exist
   e. Specialty groups have also developed standards, including National Association of Pediatric Nurse Practitioners (NAPNAP), Association for Women's Health, Obstetric, and Neonatal Nurses (AWHONN)—formerly NAACOG
   f. PNP relevant standards of practice
      (1) American Nurses Association (ANA) Maternal-Child Health (MCH) Standards—first published in 1983
      (2) NAPNAP Standards—first published in 1987
      (3) AWHONN Standards
   g. Can be used to provide legal expectations of practice but were not designed to define standards of practice for clinical or legal purposes
2. Scope of practice
   a. Based on what is legally allowable in each state under its nurse practice act
   b. Provides guidelines vs. specific mandates for nursing practice
   c. Is not mandated
   d. Varies widely from state to state (Hawkins & Thibodeau, 2002) and over time
   e. Often based on legal requirements within state and national standards
   f. NAPNAP first published Scope of Practice for PNPs in 1983 with updated statements published in 1990, 2000, and 2008
   g. Fluid and evolving (Hamric, Spross, & Hanson, 2000)
3. Nurse practice acts
   a. Authorizes boards of nursing in each state to establish statutory authority for licensure of registered nurse (RN)
   b. Authority includes use of title, authorization for scope of practice, and disciplinary grounds (Bosna, 1997)
   c. Evolves from statutory law, which after interpretation becomes regulatory language
   d. NCSBN website—(https://www.ncsbn.org) has full-text state practice acts for most states
4. Clinical practice guidelines or protocols
   a. Definition—"systematically developed statements to assist practitioner and patient about appropriate care for specific clinical outcomes" (IOM, 1990)
   b. Need/requirements for guidelines/protocol development
      (1) Variable requirements depending on individual state nurse practice act and standards of practice

(2) Protocol requirements may be met with recognized reference books and published clinical guidelines

c. Examples of practice guidelines for preventive care
   (1) Guidelines for Adolescent Preventive Services (AMA)
   (2) Guide to Clinical Preventive Services (USPSTF)

d. Examples of practice guidelines for illness management
   (1) Asthma (NIH, AAP)
   (2) Hearing screening (NIH, AAP)
   (3) HIV—Agency for Healthcare Research and Quality (AHRQ), formerly Agency for Health Care Policy and Research (AHCPR)
   (4) Otitis media with effusion (AHRQ)
   (5) Pain (AHRQ)
   (6) Sickle cell disease (AHRQ)
   (7) Hypertension (JNC VII)
   (8) Diabetes (ADA)
   (9) Dyslipidemia (ATP-III)

- Regulation of Advanced Nursing Practice
  1. Credentialing—regulatory mechanism(s) to ensure accountability for competent practice
     a. Mandates accountability/responsibility for competent practice
     b. Validation of required education, licensure, and certification
     c. Necessary to assure public of safe health care provided by qualified individuals
     d. Necessary to assure compliance with federal and state laws related to nursing practice
     e. Acknowledges APRN advanced scope of practice
     f. Should provide appropriate avenues for public or individual practice complaints
     g. Allows profession to be accountable to public and its members by enforcing professional standards for practice (Hickey, Ouimette, & Venegoni, 2000)
     h. Tension between certification bodies, state boards of nursing, and nursing education accrediting organizations regarding role and responsibility for credentialing intensified in the 1990s with the proliferation of NP programs
     i. National task force on quality nurse practitioner education convened in 1995 with broad-based representation
        (1) National Organization of Nurse Practitioner Faculties (NONPF)
        (2) American Academy of Nurse Practitioners (AANP)
        (3) American Association of Colleges of Nursing (AACN)
        (4) American Nurses Credentialing Center (ANCC)
        (5) National Association of Neonatal Nurses (NANN)
        (6) National Association of Nurse Practitioners in Women's Health (NPWH) (formerly the National Association of Nurse Practitioners in Reproductive Health)
        (7) National Association of Pediatric Nurse Practitioners (NAPNAP)
        (8) National Certification Board for Pediatric Nurse Practitioners and Nurses (NCBPNPN)—Pediatric Nursing Certification Board (PNCB) as of 2003
        (9) National Certification Corporation (NCC)
        (10) National League for Nursing (NLN)
        (11) National League for Nursing Accrediting Commission (NLNAC)
     j. Nurse practitioner credentialing remains within the domain of nongovernmental professional agencies with oversight of accreditation standards by the National Commission for Certifying Agencies (NCCA), http://www.credentialingexcellence.org/ProgramsandEvents/NCCAAccreditation/tabid/82/Default.aspx
     k. NP credentialing currently available through NCCA recognized certifying agencies
        (1) Pediatric Nursing Certification Board (PNCB)—formerly NCBPNPN 800 South Frederick Avenue, Suite 104 Gaithersburg, MD 20877-4250 (1-301-330-2921) (1-888-641-2767)
           (a) PNP
           (b) Pediatric acute care NP
        (2) American Nurses Credentialing Center (ANCC) 600 Maryland Avenue, SW Suite 100 West Washington, DC 20024-2572 (1-800-284-2378)
           (a) Adult nurse practitioners
           (b) Family nurse practitioners
           (c) Acute care nurse practitioner
           (d) Women's health nurse practitioner
           (e) Pediatric nurse practitioner
           (f) Gerontological nurse practitioner
           (g) Psychiatric mental health nurse practitioner
           (h) Major revisions to transition in 2013 and 2014 as a result of the blending of adult/gerontological primary care nurse practitioner

and acute care/gerontological nurse practitioner certification as required by the Consensus Model for Advanced Practice Registered Nurse (APRN) practice

   (3) American Academy of Nurse Practitioners (AANP)
Certification Administration
P.O. Box 12926
Austin, TX 78711
(1-512-442-4262)

    (a) Family nurse practitioners
    (b) Adult nurse practitioners
    (c) Gerontological nurse practitioner

   (4) American Association of Critical Care Nurses
101 Columbia
Aliso Viejo, CA 92656-4109
(1-949-362-2050)

    (a) Acute care nurse practitioner

2. Certification
  a. Definition—process by which nongovernmental agency or association confirms that an individual licensed professional has met certain predetermined standards as specified by that profession for specialty practice
  b. Purpose—to assure the public that an individual has mastered a body of knowledge and acquired skills in a particular specialty
  c. Required for licensure in most states and reimbursement available by most insurers

3. Prescriptive authority
  a. Some level of prescriptive authority for NP and certified nurse-midwives (CNM) since mid-1970s
  b. As of 2009, all states have approved and/or implemented some degree of prescriptive authority
  c. Required pharmacology education within graduate program and continuing education to maintain authority—specific requirements vary by state
  d. Scope of prescriptive authority varies by state; full scope includes ability to obtain federal DEA registration number

4. Multi-state Nurse Licensure Compact
  a. Since 1998, 24 states have passed legislation to recognize nursing RN licensure among participating states
  b. In 2000, Wisconsin became the first state to include advanced practice nurses within legislation on multi-state compacts
  c. NCSBN and NP stakeholders developed a position paper in 2000 to guide multi-state recognition of APRN licenses/authority to practice

5. Clinical privileges
  a. Possibility of hospital staff membership opened to nonphysician providers by Joint Commission on Accreditation of Healthcare Organizations (JCAHO) in 1983
  b. Current issue for APRN practice

- Practice Issues
1. Collaborative practice
  a. Definition—ANA's *Nursing: A Social Policy Statement* (2003) describes collaboration as "true partnership" in which all players have and value power, recognize and accept separate and combined areas of responsibility and activity, and share common goals
  b. Purpose—to enhance quality of care and improve patient outcomes through ongoing continuity and coordination of care (Hickey, Ouimette, & Venegoni, 2000)
  c. Interdisciplinary teams—examples of collaborative practice

2. Case management
  a. Definition—"case management is a collaborative process of assessment, planning, facilitation, and advocacy for options and services to meet an individual's health needs through communication and available resources to promote quality cost-effective outcomes" (Case Management Society of America, 2010)
  b. Purpose—to provide the means by which persons and firms offering services or products within or to the case management field may voluntarily coordinate their efforts to advance the practice in all respects
  c. Components of role
   (1) Planning care for cost-effectiveness and optimal outcomes
   (2) Procuring and coordinating care
   (3) Monitoring and evaluating outcomes
   (4) Performing physical assessments
   (5) Selecting laboratory and other tests
   (6) Prescribing medications
   (7) Requires that provider have strong communication skills and clinical expertise
   (8) Provides care along continuum, decreases fragmentation of services, enhances patient and family quality of life, and contains costs
  d. Key features associated with case management models
   (1) Standardized appropriate use of resources aimed at identified outcomes within appropriate time frames
   (2) Promotes collaborative practice among disciplines

(3) Promotes coordinated continuity of care over course of illness

(4) Promotes job satisfaction for providers

(5) Promotes patient and provider satisfaction with care delivery while minimizing cost to institution (Hickey, Ouimette, & Venegoni, 2000)

e. Populations appropriate for case management

(1) Those for whom course of treatment is costly and unpredictable

(2) Those who experience frequent or chronic readmission to hospital

(3) Those involved with multiple providers or multiple disciplines

3. Quality improvement (QI)

a. Definition—a formal approach to the analysis of performance and systematic efforts to improve it

b. Alternative terms—total quality management (TQM); continuous quality improvement (CQI); differs from quality assurance (QA) in being continuous rather than episodic process

c. Systematic, organized structures, processes, and expected outcomes focus on defining excellence and assuring accountability for quality of care

d. Provides framework for ongoing evaluation of practice through identification of norms, criteria, and standards that measure program effectiveness and minimize liability

e. QI mechanisms and strategies

(1) Peer review

(a) Recognize and reward nursing practice

(b) Leads to higher standards of practice

(c) Discourages practice beyond scope of legal authority

(d) Improves quality of care (Cherry & Jacob, 2002)

(e) Provides for accountability and responsibility

(2) Other methods of evaluation

(a) Audit—retrospective measurement of quality

(b) Interviews and questionnaires

(c) Patient satisfaction surveys or interviews

4. Risk management

a. Systems and activities designed to recognize and intervene to decrease risk of injury to patients and subsequent claims against healthcare providers; based on assumption that many injuries to patients are preventable

b. Evaluates sources of legal liability in practice such as

(1) Patients

(2) Procedures

(3) Quality of record keeping

c. Areas of liability risk

(1) Practitioner-patient relationship

(2) Communication and informed consent

(3) Clinical expertise

(4) Self-evaluation by professionals of need to stay current

(5) Documentation

(6) Consultation and referral

(7) Policies, procedures, and protocols

(8) Supervision of others

d. Includes educational activities that decrease risk in identified areas

5. Malpractice

a. Professional misconduct, unreasonable lack of skill; infidelity in professional or fiduciary duties; illegal, immoral conduct resulting in patient harm

b. Alleged professional failure to render services with degree of care, diligence, and precaution that another member of same profession in similar circumstances would render to prevent patient injury

c. Malpractice insurance

(1) Does not protect APRN from charges of practicing medicine without a license if APRN is practicing outside legal scope of practice for that state

(2) National Practitioner Data Bank collects information on adverse actions against healthcare practitioners, including nurses

(3) Types of coverage

(a) Occurrence coverage—covers malpractice event that occurred during policy period, regardless of date of discovery or when claim filed

(b) Claims made coverage—covers only claims filed during policy coverage period, regardless of when event occurred

(c) Tail coverage—covers malpractice event from the time that a claims made policy ends through the statute of limitations in the practitioner's state

6. Negligence—failure of individual to do what a reasonable person would do that results in injury to another

7. Reimbursement—whether working independently, sharing a joint practice with a physician, or practicing within a hospital, or managed care system, APRNs must be reimbursed

appropriately. Standards that determine private pay insurance mechanisms are often modeled after federal policies such as Medicaid and Medicare. However, even when the federal government establishes mandates that encourage direct payment of nonphysician healthcare providers, barriers to reimbursement are often encountered in state-level rules and regulations. (Hamric, Spross, & Hanson, 2000)

a. Medicaid
   (1) Authorized in 1965 as Title XIX of Social Security Act
   (2) Federal/state matching program with federal oversight
   (3) Financed through federal and state taxes, with between 50% and 83% of total Medicaid costs covered by federal government
   (4) Does not cover all people below federal poverty level, but state Medicaid programs are required by the federal government to cover certain categories such as
      (a) Recipients of Aid to Families with Dependent Children (AFDC)—states set own eligibility requirements for AFDC
      (b) People over 65, blind, or totally disabled who are eligible for cash assistance under federal Supplemental Security Income (SSI) program
      (c) Pregnant women (for pregnancy-related services only) and children under 6 with family incomes up to 133% of federal poverty level
      (d) Children born after September 1983 in families whose income is at or below federal poverty level
   (5) States can choose to cover "medically needy"
   (6) Coverage required for certain services
      (a) Hospital and physician services
      (b) Laboratory and radiographic services
      (c) Nursing home and home health-care services
      (d) Prenatal and preventive services
      (e) Medically necessary transportation
   (7) States can add services to list and can place certain limitations on federally mandated services
   (8) Although Medicaid recipients cannot be billed for services, states can impose nominal copayments or deductibles for certain services (Bodenheimer, 2002)

b. Medicare
   (1) Federally mandated program established in 1965, provides health insurance for aged and disabled individuals
   (2) Eligibility covers hospital service, physician services, and other medical services
   (3) Income level does not impact eligibility
   (4) Medicare Part A
      (a) Those 65 years of age and older who are eligible for Social Security are automatically enrolled, whether or not they are retired—persons are eligible for Social Security when they (or their spouses) have paid into Social Security system through employment for 40 quarters or more
      (b) Those who have paid into system for less than 40 quarters can enroll in Medicare Part A by paying monthly premium
      (c) Those who are under age 65 and are totally and permanently disabled may enroll in Medicare Part A after receiving Social Security disability benefits for 24 months
      (d) Those with chronic renal disease requiring dialysis or transplant may also be eligible for Part A without a 2-year waiting period
      (e) Services covered include some hospitalization costs; some skilled nursing facility costs, although custodial care is not covered; home health care—100% for skilled care; 80% of approved amount for medical equipment; and hospice care—100% for most services
      (f) Payment for hospitalization is based on projected costs of caring for patient with given problem—each Medicare patient admitted to a hospital is classified according to a diagnosis-related group (DRG); the hospital is then paid a predetermined amount for each patient admitted with the given DRG; if hospital costs are above payment rate, the hospital must absorb loss; if costs are below payment rate, hospital allowed to keep a percentage of excess
      (g) APRN not paid directly for services delivered in a hospital

(5) Medicare Part B—Supplementary Medical Insurance (SMI)

(a) Monthly premium is charged

(b) Some low-income people are eligible to have monthly premium paid by Medicaid

(c) Financed by general federal revenues and by Part B monthly premiums

(d) Covers all medically necessary services—80% of an approved amount after annual deductible; includes physician services, physical, occupational, and speech therapy; medical equipment and diagnostic tests and some preventive care such as Pap tests, mammograms; hepatitis B, pneumococcal, and influenza vaccines can be included in medical expenses

(6) Medicare Part C—Medicare Advantage Plans

(a) Like traditional PPO or HMO plans

(b) The plan pays all Part A and Part B costs

(c) May offer additional coverages, e.g., vision, hearing, dental, and wellness

(d) Most offer prescription coverage

(7) Medicare Part D—Prescription Drug Coverage

(a) Plan allows senior citizens to receive prescription drugs at reduced out-of-pocket costs for a monthly fee

(b) Allows some brand and generic drugs that are commonly prescribed to seniors to be covered; drugs have to fall into "commonly prescribed" categories

(c) Plan requires that first $250 per year be paid by the patient

(i) Patient pays 25% of drug costs from $251 to $2,250 in 1 year

(ii) Patient pays for cost of $2,251 to $5,100 in 1 year

(iii) Any costs > $5,100 paid completely by the plan

c. APRN—Medicaid/Medicare coverage

(1) Omnibus Budget Reconciliation Act (OBRA) 1989—mandated Medicaid reimbursement for certified pediatric and family nurse practitioners began July 1, 1990; providers required to practice within the scope of state law and do not have to be under supervision or associated with a physician or other provider

(a) Level of payment determined by states—reimbursement rates range from 70% to 100% of fee-for-service physician Medicaid rate (Pearson, 2010)

(b) Pediatric and family nurse practitioners may bill Medicaid directly after attaining provider number from state Medicaid agency

(c) States can elect to pass laws allowing them to extend Medicaid payment to other types of NP not identified in federal statutes

(2) Legislation (2005) has expanded direct Medicare reimbursement for APRN in all geographic locations

(a) APRN reimbursement at 85% of physician fee schedule when billing independently using APRN billing number; direct physician supervision not required

(b) When APRN is employed by physician, the physician practice may receive 100% of customary physician charge, according to "incident to" rules (Buppert, 2012)

(c) APRN must be RN currently licensed to practice in the state in which services are rendered; must meet requirements for NP practice in state in which services are rendered; must be currently certified as a primary care NP; must have successfully completed a formal advanced-practice educational program of at least 1 academic year that includes at least 4 months of classroom instruction and awards a degree, diploma, or certificate OR have successfully completed a formal advanced-practice educational program and have been performing in that expanded role for at least 12 months during the 18-month period immediately preceding February 8, 1978, the effective date for the provision of services of NP as reflected in the conditions for certification for rural health clinics

(d) NP covered services are limited to services an NP is legally authorized to perform under the state law in which the NP practices and must meet training, educational, and experience requirements prescribed by the Federal Secretary of Health and Human Services

(3) NP services covered under Part B if service would be considered physician's services if furnished by MD or doctor of osteopathy (DO); if NP is legally authorized to perform services in the state in which they are performed; if services are performed in collaboration with MD/DO (collaboration specified as a process whereby NP works with physician to deliver health care within scope of NP expertise with medical direction and appropriate supervision as provided for in jointly developed guidelines or other mechanisms defined by federal regulations and law of the state in which services are performed); and services are otherwise precluded from coverage because of one of the statutory exclusions

(4) "Incident to" refers to services provided as an integral, yet incidental, part of the physician's personal, professional services in the course of diagnosis or treatment of injury or illness—these services must occur under direct personal supervision of a physician, and the APRN must be an employee of the physician group; services must occur during the course of treatment where the physician performs an initial service and subsequent services in a manner that reflects the physician's active participation and management of the course of treatment—direct personal supervision does not mean that the physician must be in the same room as the APRN, however, the physician must be present in the office suite and available for assistance and direction while the APRN provides patient care (Buppert, 2005)

(5) When APRN performs "incident to" service in physician's office, billing must be submitted to Medicare by employing physician, under the physician's name, provider number, and CPT code—payment is made at full physician rate and is paid to physician or physician practice

(6) When APRN provides service in skilled nursing facility, or nursing facility located in urban area as defined by law, Medicare payment can be obtained—medicare reimbursement is also available for APRN services in skilled nursing facilities (SNF) in nonrural areas on a reasonable-charge basis; this amount may not exceed physician fee schedule amount for service, and payment is made to the APRN's employer

(7) Centers for Medicare and Medicaid Services (CMS)

(a) Formerly Health Care Financing & Administration (HCFA)

(b) Oversight of several federal programs including Medicare, Medicaid, State Children's Health Insurance Program (SCHIP), HIPAA, and clinical laboratory improvement amendments (CLIA)

(c) Website: http://www.cms.hhs.gov

d. Other third-party payors

(1) Private insurer reimbursement is contract specific per state insurance commission

(2) Triple Option Benefit Care Program (TRICARE), formerly Civilian Health and Medical Program of the Uniformed Services (CHAMPUS)

(a) Federal health plan for military personnel, including surviving dependents, families, and retirees

(b) APRN reimbursement for services

(3) Federal Employee Health Benefits Program (FEHBP)

(a) One of largest employer-sponsored group health insurance programs

(b) APRN recognized as designated healthcare provider

e. Methods of payment for advanced practice nurses

(1) Fee-for-service model

(a) Unit of payment by visit or procedure

(b) Can occur with utilization review in which case payor has right to authorize or deny payment of expensive medical interventions such as hospital admission, extra hospital days, and surgery

(2) Episodic model

(a) One sum is paid for all services delivered during a given illness

(b) DRG fee payment

(3) Capitation model, PPO, and HMO are covered in section on Managed Care in this chapter

- Professional Organizations
  1. Purpose and benefits
     a. Establish practice standards
     b. Collective voice to promote nursing and quality of care
     c. Monitor and influence policy and legislative initiatives
     d. Position papers on practice issues
     e. Disseminate information
  2. Examples
     a. American Nurses Association (ANA)
     b. National Association of Pediatric Nurse Practitioners (NAPNAP)
     c. National Conference of Gerontological Nurse Practitioners (NCGNP)
     d. National Organization of Nurse Practitioner Faculties (NONPF)
     e. American Academy of Nurse Practitioners (AANP)
     f. American College of Nurse Practitioners (ACNP)
     g. Nurse Practitioner Associates for Continuing Education (NPACE)
     h. National Association of School Nurses (NASN)
     i. Association of Women's Health, Obstetric, and Neonatal Nurses (AWHONN)
     j. National Association of Nurse Practitioners in Women's Health (NPWH) (formerly the National Association of Nurse Practitioners in Reproductive Health [NANPRH])

- Research in Advanced Practice
  1. Major trend is outcome studies
  2. Sources of federal funding
     a. Agency for Healthcare Research and Quality (AHRQ)
        (1) Formerly the Agency for Health Care Policy and Research (AHCPR)
        (2) Website: http://www.ahcpr.gov/
     b. National Institutes of Health (NIH)
        (1) Includes the National Institute for Nursing Research (NINR)
        (2) Website: http://www.nih.gov/
     c. Maternal and Child Health Bureau (MCHB)
        (1) Functions within Health Resources and Services Administration (HRSA)
        (2) Website: http://www.mchb.hrsa.gov/
  3. Sources of research findings
     a. Conferences
     b. Scholarly publications
     c. Distribution of summaries of research studies (Hawkins & Thibodeau, 2002)
  4. Use of research in practice setting
     a. Develop research-based clinical pathways
     b. Track clinical outcomes and variances
     c. Demonstrate quality and cost-effectiveness of care
     d. Give structure to demonstration projects
     e. Persuade lawmakers of NP value and contributions in today's healthcare system
     f. Improve quality and patient outcomes
  5. Benefit of research for patients
     a. Provides thorough understanding of patient situation
     b. Provides more accurate assessment of situations
     c. Increases effectiveness of interventions
     d. Increases provider sensitivity to patient situations
     e. Assists providers to more accurately determine need for and effectiveness of interventions
  6. Barriers to research utilization
     a. Time and cost of conducting research studies
     b. Resistance to change in work setting
     c. Lack of rewards for using research findings
     d. Lack of understanding or uncertainty regarding research outcomes
  7. Strategies to overcome barriers to research utilization
     a. Creation of organizational culture that values and uses research
     b. Creation of environment where questions are encouraged, critical thinking is appreciated, and nursing care is evaluated
     c. Support for research through time allocation and financial commitment

◻ HEALTH POLICY

- Policy Influences
  1. Healthy People 2020
     a. Released in 2010 by U.S. Department of Health and Human Services (DHHS)
     b. Builds on initiatives set in Healthy People 2010
     c. Purpose—designed to achieve four overarching goals
        (1) Attain high-quality, longer lives free of preventable disease, disability, injury, and premature death
        (2) Achieve health equity, eliminate disparities, and improve health of all groups
        (3) Create social and physical environments that promote good health for all
        (4) Promote quality of life, healthy development, and healthy behaviors across all life stages

2. Prevention guidelines—*Guide to Clinical Preventive Services* (U.S. Preventive Services Task Force, 2008) presents national clinical preventive services guidelines for practice and educational settings
   a. Age and gender specific
   b. Suggests targeted examinations, immunizations, and health counseling that should be part of periodic health visits
3. Nursing's Agenda for Health Care Reform (ANA, 1991; revised 2005 as ANA's Health Care Agenda)
   a. Supports creation of a healthcare system that assures access, quality, and services at affordable costs
   b. Supports ongoing primary care
   c. Calls for basic core of essential health services to be available to all, and for restructured healthcare system focusing on consumers and their health and healthcare delivery in familiar, convenient sites
   d. Proposes shift from focus on illness and cure to orientation on wellness and caring
   e. Supports provisions for long-term care and insurance reforms to assure improved access to coverage
   f. Calls for establishment of public/private sector review of resource allocations, cost-reduction plans, and fair and consistent reimbursement for all providers

- Utilization of Health Policy
  1. Shifting trend toward primary care and early preventive measures; supports need for APRN
  2. Four major factors influencing healthcare delivery services
     a. Payors—individual healthcare consumers, businesses that pay for health insurance for employees, and government through public programs and entitlement programs such as Medicare and Medicaid
     b. Insurers—take money from payors, assume risks, and pay providers
     c. Providers—includes hospitals, physicians, nurses, APRNs, physician assistants, pharmacies, home health agencies, and long-term care facilities
     d. Suppliers—pharmaceutical and medical supply industries
  3. Legislative strategies and political involvement
     a. Professional organizations monitor policy issues and keep membership informed—e.g., NAPNAP legislative newsletter
     b. Local networks of APRN develop practice guidelines and advocate for policies to enhance practice

- Types of Healthcare Delivery Systems
  1. Primary health care
     a. Definition—"primary care is the provision of integrated, accessible healthcare services by clinicians who are accountable for addressing a large majority of personal healthcare needs, developing a sustained partnership with patients, and practicing in the context of family and community"
     b. Activities and/or functions define boundaries of primary care, such as curing or alleviating common illnesses and disabilities
     c. Entry point to a system that includes access to secondary and tertiary care
     d. Attributes include care that is accessible, comprehensive, coordinated, continuous, and accountable
     e. Strategy for organizing healthcare system as a whole; gives priority and allocates resources to community-based rather than hospital-based care
     f. Categories of primary PCP and nature of care
        (1) Medical specialties—family medicine, general internal medicine, general pediatrics, obstetrics and gynecology
        (2) Other experts have included NP and physician assistants (PA) as PCP
     g. Many definitions stress self-responsibility for health
  2. Managed care
     a. Defined as any arrangement for health care in which an organization, such as an HMO, another type of doctor-hospital network, or an insurance company, acts as intermediate between the person seeking care and the physician (Houghton Mifflin Company, 2007)
        (1) Network connects consumers, sponsors, providers, and third-party payors
        (2) Initial managed care organization was Kaiser Health Plan (California) established in 1930s
     b. Objectives
        (1) Manage use and price of healthcare delivery system
        (2) Control type, level, and frequency of treatment
        (3) Restrict level of reimbursement for services
     c. Type of health insurance plan designed to control costs while assuring quality care
     d. Obligation to manage is shared among providers, consumers, and payers
        (1) Providers no longer dictate price of care delivery; must assume more financial

risk for population assigned to them for care

(2) Consumers have fewer choices of coverage and providers and greater financial responsibility

(3) Payors manage healthcare dollars through benefit design, selective contracting, and shifting financial risk to providers (Hickey, Ouimette, & Venegoni, 2000)

e. Types of managed care plans

(1) Health maintenance organizations (HMO)

(a) Most common type

(b) By 2009, enrollment at 64.5 million

(c) Offer preestablished benefit package—including preventive, inpatient, and outpatient care

(d) HMO contracts with providers to provide care to enrollees

(e) Providers at financial risk resulting in incentive to provide high-quality, cost-effective care

(f) Enrollees select a PCP who manages total care by authorizing specialty visits, hospitalization, and other services

(g) PCP may be MD, APRN, or PA providers; serving as "gatekeepers"

(2) Preferred provider organizations (PPO)

(a) Compromised managed care option that is alternative between indemnity and HMO insurance

(b) Uses financial incentives to influence consumer and provider behaviors

(c) Refers to variety of arrangements between insurers, providers, and third-party payers rather than standard plan

(d) Often owned by large insurance companies such as Prudential, Travelers, and Aetna

(e) Available primarily to employed commercial population

(3) Point of service plans (POS)

(a) Consumers decide whether to use a provider network or seek care outside the network

(b) If variation of HMO plan, PCP coordinates care for enrollees; if variation of PPO plan, enrollees may choose lower cost options outside of provider network

(c) Most rapidly growing type of managed care

(4) Integrated delivery systems

(a) Vertical integration of services across levels of care into seamless system with improved access for enrollees

(b) Capitated payment—financial risk shifts from payor to provider; unit of value is cost per member per month (PMPM); providers receive age- and sex-adjusted budget to cover services to maintain wellness of specific target population

(c) Emphasis on provision of appropriate but not unlimited care with financial benefit of keeping population healthy through systematic preventive services

f. Reimbursement under managed care

(1) Providers accept financial risk for care provided to specific population of enrollees

(2) Capitated payment

(a) Provider receives payment in advance

(b) Payment level reflects expected utilization by enrolled population for which provider is responsible

(3) Provider must control volume and cost

(4) Efficiency usually rewarded through bonus payments for operating within budget and meeting goals for quality and efficiency

g. Monitoring, evaluation, and accreditation in managed care

(1) Healthcare effectiveness data and information set (HEDIS)—provides quality measures and compares with benchmark standards and goals

(2) National Committee for Quality Assurance (NCQA)

(a) Major accreditation body for managed care organizations

(b) Standards in six critical areas are evaluated—quality management, utilization management, credentialing, preventive health services, medical records, members rights/responsibilities

h. Challenges and opportunities of managed care for APRN

(1) Need for balance between quality of care and costs inherent in diagnosis/management per patient visit

(a) Educational programs must incorporate managed-care content into curriculum

(b) APRN must combine strong clinical and financial skills to determine cost of providing care to target population

(c) Success in managed care environment requires systems-thinking skill to complement primary care skills; blended NP/CNS models may provide this necessary linkage with added focus on case management, utilization/resource management, quality improvement, and patient education/advocacy within systems of care

(2) APRN strategies for success within evolving managed care environment

(a) Determine strategies to increase efficiency without sacrificing quality of patient-provider interactions; e.g., group well-child visits

(b) Lobby for APN inclusion on provider panels

(c) Maintain partnerships with APRN educational programs for collaborative study and documentation of APRN effectiveness

◘ HEALTH INSURANCE PORTABILITY AND ACCOUNTABILITY ACT OF 1996 (HIPAA): PUBLIC LAW 104–191

- Purpose of HIPAA Provisions—improve efficiency and effectiveness of healthcare system by standardizing the electronic exchange of administrative and financial data

- Mandated Standards
  1. Specific transaction standards (claims, enrollment, etc.) including code sets
  2. Security and electronic signatures
  3. Privacy
  4. Unique identifiers, including allowed uses—for employers, health plans, and healthcare providers

- Privacy Rule—the privacy regulations control the use and disclosure of a patient's Protected Health Information (PHI) where the information could potentially reveal the identity of the patient. HIPAA regulates PHI by healthcare providers, health plans, and healthcare clearinghouses, i.e., entities that process or facilitate the processing of non-standard data elements of health information into standard elements or vice versa.

- Goals of Privacy Rule
  1. Provide strong federal protections for privacy rights
  2. Preserve quality health care

- Protected Health Information—all information
  1. Individually identifiable health information—health and demographic info; includes physical or mental health, the provision of or payment for health care; identifies the individual (includes deceased)
  2. Transmitted or maintained in any form or medium by a covered entity or its business associate

- Key Elements of Privacy Rule
  1. Covered entity—healthcare providers who transmit any health information electronically in connection with claims, billing, or payment transactions; health plans; healthcare clearinghouses
  2. Uses and disclosures of information
     a. Required
        (1) To individual when requested; to HHS
        (2) To investigate or determine compliance with Privacy Rule
     b. Permitted
        (1) Individual
        (2) Treatment, Payment, and Health Care Operations (TPO)
        (3) Opportunity to agree or object
        (4) Public policy
        (5) "Incident to"
        (6) Limited data set
        (7) Authorized

- Individual Rights
  1. Notice of privacy practices—must contain language in Privacy Rule describing uses and disclosures of PHI
  2. Individual rights and how to exercise them; provide information as follows
     a. Covered entity duties and contact name, title, or phone number to receive complaints with effective date
     b. Access—right to inspect and obtain a copy of PHI in a designated record set (DRS) in a timely manner
     c. Amendment—individual has right to have covered entity amend PHI; request may be denied by covered entity if record is accurate and complete
     d. Accounting—individual has right to receive an accounting of disclosures of PHI made in the 6 years or less prior to date requested
     e. Request restrictions—individual may request restrictions on uses and disclosures of PHI, but covered entity may disagree
     f. Confidential communication—provider must permit and accommodate reasonable requests to receive communications

of PHI by alternative means and at alternative locations

  g. Complaints to covered entity—a process must be established to document complaints and their disposition

  h. Complaints to secretary (HHS/OCR)—any person may file a written complaint if they believe a covered entity is not complying with the Privacy Rule

- De-identification of PHI
  1. Removal of certain identifiers so that the individual may no longer be identified
  2. Application of statistical method
  3. Stripping of listed identifiers such as names, geographic subdivisions, dates, SSNs

- Administrative requirements
  1. Implement policies and procedures regarding PHI that are designed to comply with the Privacy Rule
  2. Implement appropriate administrative, technical, and physical safeguards to protect the privacy of PHI
  3. Provide privacy training to entire workforce and develop and apply a system of sanctions for those who violate the Privacy Rule
  4. Designate a privacy official responsible for policies and procedures and for receiving complaints
  5. Compliance and enforcement—effective April 14, 2003
  6. Office for Civil Rights (OCR) enforces the Privacy Rule

- Complaint Process
  1. Informal review may resolve issue fully without formal investigation; if not, begin investigation
  2. Technical assistance

- Civil Monetary Penalties (CMPs)
  1. $100 per violation
  2. Capped at $25,000 for each calendar year for each identical requirement or prohibition that is violated
  3. Criminal penalties for wrongful disclosures
     a. Up to $50,000 and 1 year imprisonment
     b. Up to $100,000 and 5 years imprisonment if done under false pretenses
     c. Up to $250,000 and 10 years imprisonment if intent to sell, transfer, or use for commercial advantage, personal gain, or malicious harm
     d. Enforced by Department of Justice (DOJ)

- Employment Retirement Income Security Act (ERISA)
  1. Federal law that exempts self-funded health and other benefit plans (employer and union) from state jurisdiction

  2. Seven out of 10 U.S. employees are in self-insured plans
  3. Legal challenges are in process disputing the breadth of the ERISA exemptions

■ EVIDENCE-BASED PRACTICE

- Definition—the conscientious, judicious, and explicit use of current best evidence in making decisions about the care of individual patients incorporating both clinical expertise and patient values

- Major Clinical Categories of Primary Research and Their Preferred Study Designs
  1. Therapy—tests the effectiveness of a treatment; randomized, double-blinded, placebo-controlled
  2. Diagnosis and screening—measures the validity and reliability of a test or evaluates the effectiveness of a test in detecting disease at a presymptomatic stage: cross-sectional survey
  3. Causation or harm—assesses whether a substance is related to the development of an illness or condition: cohort or case-control
  4. Prognosis—determines the outcome of a disease: longitudinal cohort study
  5. Systematic review—a summary of the literature that uses explicit methods to perform a thorough literature search and critical appraisal of individual studies and that uses appropriate statistical techniques to combine these valid studies
  6. Meta-analysis—a systematic review that uses quantitative methods to summarize results

- Categories of strength of reviewed evidence from individual research and other sources
  1. Level I (A–D): Meta-analysis or multiple controlled studies
  2. Level II (A–D): Individual experimental study
  3. Level III (A–D): Quasi-experimental study
  4. Level IV (A–D): Nonexperimental study
  5. Level V (A–D): Case report or systematically obtained, verifiable quality or program evaluation data
  6. Level VI: Opinion of respected authorities; this level also includes regulatory or legal opinions

- Level I is the strongest rating per type of research, however quality for any level can range from A to D and reflects basic scientific credibility of the overall study; A indicates a very well-designed study, D indicates the study has a major flaw that raises serious questions about the believability of the findings

Note: The authors would like to thank Patricia Burkhardt, DrPH, CNM for her contributions to this chapter.

▫ QUESTIONS

Select the best answer.

1. The doctor of nursing practice:

   a. Will be the only graduate nursing degree accredited by the AACN after 2015
   b. Will be the entry-level degree for specialty nursing practice
   c. Is currently offered by > 200 colleges and universities
   d. Will replace the PhD in nursing by 2015

2. Which type of Medicare plan consists of a traditional PPO, HMO, or other managed care model?

   a. Part A
   b. Part B
   c. Part C
   d. Part D

3. Preventive health guidelines include references to:

   a. Immunizations, health screening, disease prophylaxis, education, and infection control
   b. Immunizations, counseling, health screening, disease prophylaxis, and education
   c. Health screening, disease prophylaxis, counseling, and CPR
   d. Health screening, disease prophylaxis, education, immunizations, and CPR

4. Nursing's Agenda for Health Care Reform:

   a. Is supportive of equal access, cost-effective, high-quality care
   b. Is a mandate to all nurses in the United States
   c. Is a summary of nursing research related to healthcare reform
   d. Is a report of the status of nursing in the 1990s

5. The nurse practitioner role was initially established to:

   a. Improve access to care and partially solve physician shortage
   b. Reduce the nursing shortage and improve access to care
   c. Improve working conditions of nurses while improving access to care
   d. Improve nursing's image through expansion of the role

6. Early nursing research focused on:

   a. The response of policy makers to the nursing shortage
   b. The effectiveness of the NP as a primary care giver
   c. An effort to demonstrate quality and cost-effectiveness of NPs
   d. The role of the NP as a physician extender

7. Which of the following is not a major factor influencing healthcare delivery services?

   a. Provider
   b. Payors
   c. Insurers
   d. Agencies

8. All definitions of primary health care include:

   a. The concept of universal access and accountability
   b. The concept of universal access and AIDS prevention
   c. The concept of universal access and a focus on self-responsibility for health
   d. The concept of universal access and a focus on reimbursement for services rendered

9. Standards of practice are:

   a. Authoritative statements used to measure quality
   b. Used to measure outcome but are not authoritative
   c. Designed for legal purposes
   d. Not designed for legal purposes and cannot be used to measure quality

10. Quality improvement activities include:

    a. Patient satisfaction surveys only
    b. Peer review, patient satisfaction surveys, chart audits
    c. Defining four practice domains
    d. Systems to decrease risk of injury to patients

11. Most risk management programs are based on the assumption that:

    a. Many injuries to patients are preventable
    b. Most legal liability is a result of poor documentation
    c. Most injuries to patients are not preventable
    d. Malpractice insurance is generally unnecessary

12. If an APRN practices beyond his/her scope:

    a. Malpractice insurance will protect him/her from a charge of practicing medicine without a license
    b. Malpractice insurance will not protect him/her from a charge of practicing medicine without a license
    c. He or she is legally accountable to the certifying body
    d. The collaborating physician is legally accountable to the certifying body

13. Standards of practice may be used to:

    a. Establish minimal levels of performance
    b. Establish reimbursement schemes for APRN
    c. Mandate nursing practice across the nation
    d. Mandate nursing practice in certain states

14. Scope of practice:

    a. Is identical across the states
    b. Is determined by the federal government
    c. Is mandated by the federal government
    d. Varies from state to state

15. Medicaid provides health insurance coverage to:

    a. Certain categories of people whose personal income falls below the federal poverty level
    b. Anyone whose personal income falls below the federal poverty level
    c. Newborns, pregnant women, and those over 65 whose personal income falls below the federal poverty level
    d. Those who are elderly

16. Medicaid reimbursement is available to an APRN:

    a. Practicing in federally designated areas
    b. At a rate that is between 70% and 100% of the physician rate
    c. Only if the APRN is in collaborative practice with a physician
    d. Practicing in nursing homes only

17. Medicare reimbursement for services:

    a. Is not dependent on the patient's income level
    b. Depends on the patient's income level
    c. Is not available to APRN under any circumstances
    d. Is only available to APRN who is in collaborative practice with a physician

18. Medicare Part A covers:

    a. Hospital, skilled nursing facility, and hospice care
    b. All medically necessary services
    c. Skilled nursing facility care only
    d. Hospice care only

19. Medicare Part B covers:

    a. All medically necessary services
    b. Inpatient hospital care
    c. Outpatient physician services only
    d. Skilled nursing facility and hospice care

20. To receive Medicare reimbursement, APRN must:

    a. Be nationally certified and maintain prescriptive privileges
    b. Maintain a current license in the state in which they are practicing
    c. Practice in a designated medically underserved area
    d. Practice with a physician

21. The term "incident to" refers to:

    a. The occasions when an APRN practices independently but occasionally consults with a physician
    b. The notion that the physician must be present in the office suite and immediately available to provide assistance in order for the APRN to bill for services rendered
    c. The notion that a physician must examine the patient along with the APRN if Medicare is to be billed for services rendered
    d. Medicaid only and is not pertinent to Medicare billing

22. "Incident to" billing is specific to:

    a. Medicare
    b. Medicaid
    c. Medicare and Medicaid
    d. Private insurance companies

23. TRICARE (formerly The Civilian Health and Medical Program of the Uniformed Services [CHAMPUS]):

    a. Is a federal health plan that covers health care for military personnel and their families and recognizes APRN as reimbursable provider
    b. Is a federal health plan that covers health care for military personnel and recognizes APRN as reimbursable provider
    c. Is a federal health plan that covers health care for military personnel and their families but does not recognize APRN as reimbursable provider
    d. Only covers hospital expenses of military personnel and their families

24. The knowledge base of the APRN is based on:

    a. Medical content
    b. Theoretical content only
    c. Scientific content and theory
    d. Theory and research

25. What has the role of the APRN traditionally focused on?

    a. The delivery of primary health care to all people
    b. The delivery of acute health care to all people
    c. Chronic care
    d. The medical model

26. The nurse practitioner role began:

    a. With the establishment of a pediatric nurse practitioner program in an effort to expand the role of the registered nurse in order to meet the needs of the children of the nation
    b. As a result of the new entitlement programs, Medicare and Medicaid
    c. When it was evident that medical schools across the United States could not prepare enough family practitioners to meet the nation's need
    d. As an experimental program at Duke University Medical Center

27. Legal authority for APRN practice is granted by:

    a. Federal law
    b. Regulations from the Department of Health and Human Services
    c. State law and regulations
    d. The board of medicine in most states

28. Direct reimbursement to APRN has resulted in:

    a. Increased access to cost-effective, quality primary care
    b. Increased malpractice claims against APRN
    c. Decreased consumer choice of healthcare providers
    d. Proliferation of APRN in independent practice

29. Malpractice insurance:

    a. Protects an APRN from charges of practicing medicine without a license when they are practicing outside the legal scope of practice
    b. Does not protect an APRN from charges of practicing medicine without a license when they are practicing outside the legal scope of practice
    c. Does not pay for legal defense if the APRN is practicing beyond the legal scope of practice
    d. Is important but should not be purchased if the facility in which the APRN is employed carries good coverage

30. Collaborative practice:

    a. Limits autonomy and is not reasonable in current managed care environment
    b. Will enhance quality of care and improve patient outcomes
    c. Will limit consumer choice of providers
    d. Excludes the concept of interdisciplinary teams

31. Case management:

    a. Balances quality and cost of patient care
    b. Has not been found to be cost-effective
    c. Decreases the autonomy of the APRN
    d. Is rarely used today

32. What is the major trend in health policy research today?

    a. Outcome studies
    b. Primary care studies
    c. Studies that compare practice strategies of MD and NP
    d. Studies that compare patient satisfaction with care delivered by MD versus NP

33. Current prescriptive authority for APRN:

    a. Varies among the states
    b. Is fairly consistent among the states
    c. Provides DEA numbers for APRN
    d. Allows APRN to move freely from state to state

34. Managed care is a term that describes:

    a. An established system of healthcare delivery that is mandated by the federal government
    b. A network of providers who contract to provide services for a specific group of enrollees
    c. A system that does not recognize APRN as a primary provider
    d. A network of hospitals and nursing homes that provide care to chronically ill people

35. Certification is:

    a. A procedure through which the government appraises and grants certification to the APRN
    b. Granted by the individual states
    c. Governed by each state's board of nursing
    d. A process in which a nongovernmental agency or group verifies that an APRN has met certain predetermined standards for specialty practice

36. Licensure:

    a. Is a federal process that is used to standardize healthcare facilities
    b. Is granted by a state government agency and grants permission to engage in the practice of a given profession
    c. Cannot be used to prohibit anyone from practicing a given profession
    d. Is a federal process that is used to standardize educational programs

37. Reimbursement under managed care:

    a. Requires that the provider accept the financial risk for the care provided to a specific population of enrolled patients
    b. Requires that the managed care organization accept the financial risk for the care provided to a specific population of enrolled patients
    c. Does not reward efficient care delivery
    d. Is not available to APRN

38. An integrated delivery system:

   a. Is one that delivers high-quality care but is often not cost-effective
   b. Delivers a vertical integration of services with capitated payment
   c. Does not include rationing of resources
   d. Does not include a capitated payment scheme

Answers

1. **b**	20. **b**
2. **c**	21. **b**
3. **b**	22. **a**
4. **a**	23. **a**
5. **a**	24. **c**
6. **c**	25. **a**
7. **d**	26. **a**
8. **a**	27. **c**
9. **a**	28. **a**
10. **b**	29. **b**
11. **a**	30. **b**
12. **b**	31. **a**
13. **a**	32. **a**
14. **d**	33. **a**
15. **a**	34. **b**
16. **b**	35. **d**
17. **a**	36. **b**
18. **a**	37. **a**
19. **a**	38. **b**

◘ BIBLIOGRAPHY

American Association of Colleges of Nursing. (1996). *The essentials of master's education for advanced practice nursing.* Washington, DC: AACN.

American Nurses Association. (1991). Nursing's agenda for healthcare reform. Washington, DC: American Nurses Publishing.

American Nurses Association. (2003). *Nursing's social policy statement* (2nd ed.). Washington, DC: American Nurses Publishing.

American Nurses Association. (2004). Scope of nursing practice: Advanced practice registered nurses. In *Nursing: Scope and standards of practice* (pp. 14–16). Washington, DC: Nursesbooks.org.

Association of Faculties of Pediatric Nurse Practitioner and Associate Programs. (1996). *Philosophy, conceptual model, terminal competencies for the education of pediatric nurse practitioners.* Cherry Hill, NJ: NAPNAP.

Bodenheimer, T. S. (2002). *Understanding health policy: A clinical approach* (3rd. ed.). New York: McGraw-Hill.

Bosna, J. (1997). Using nurse practitioner certification for state nursing regulation: An update. *The Nurse Practitioner: The American Journal of Primary Health Care, 22*(6), 213–216.

Bryant-Lukosious, D., DiCenzo, A., Brown, G., & Pinelli, J. (2004). Advance practice nursing roles: Development, implementation, & evaluation. *Journal of Advanced Nursing, 48*(5), 519–529.

Buppert, C. (2012). *Nurse Practitioners Business Practice and Legal Guide* (4th ed.). Burlington, MA: Jones & Bartlett Learning.

Cady, A. F. (2003). *The advanced practice nurse's legal handbook.* Philadelphia: Lippincott Williams & Wilkins.

Case Management Society of America. (2010). *CMSA's standards of practice for case management (revised 2010).* Little Rock, AR: Case Management Society of America.

Cherry, B., & Jacob, S. R. (2002). *Contemporary nursing: Issues, trends, and management* (2nd ed.). St. Louis: Mosby.

Department of Health and Human Services (DHHS). (2000). *Healthy people 2010 and leading health indicators.* Washington, DC: Government Printing Office.

Hamric, A. B., Spross, J. A., & Hanson, C. M. (2000). *Advanced practice nursing: An integrative approach* (2nd ed.). Philadelphia: W. B. Saunders.

Hawkins, J. W., & Thibodeau, J. A. (2002). *The advanced practice nurse: Current issues* (5th ed.). New York: Tiresias Press.

Health Care Financing Administration (HCFA). (1999). *Balanced Budget Act of 1997.* Baltimore, MD: HCFA. Retrieved from http://www.thecre.com/fedlaw/legal17/release.htm

Health Care Financing Administration (HCFA). (2012). *CY 2012 Physician Fee Schedule Final Rule Correction Notice.* Retrieved from https://www.cms.gov/PhysicianFeeSched/

Health Care Financing Administration (HCFA). (1999). *Medicare+Choice part C statutory requirement and regulatory implementation.* Baltimore, MD: HCFA.

Hickey, J. V., Ouimette, R. M., & Venegoni, S. L. (2000). *Advanced practice nursing: Changing roles and clinical applications* (2nd ed.). Philadelphia: J. B. Lippincott Williams & Wilkins.

Houghton Mifflin Company. (2007). *The American Heritage Medical Dictionary.* Boston, MA: Author.

Institute of Medicine. (1996). *20–20 vision: Health care in the 21st century. Primary care: America's health in a new era.* Washington, DC: National Academy Press.

IOM. (1990). *Clinical practice guidelines: Directions for a new program.* Washington, DC: National Academy Press.

Juran, M. (1999). *Juran's quality handbook* (5th ed.). New York: McGraw-Hill.

Mezey, M. D., & McGivern, D. O. (1998). *Nurses, nurse practitioners: Evolution to advanced practice* (3rd ed.). Philadelphia: W. B. Saunders.

NAPNAP. (1987). *Standards of practice for PNP/As.* Cherry Hill, NJ: Author.

NAPNAP. (1989). Risk management for pediatric nurse practitioners. Cherry Hill, NJ: Author.

NAPNAP. (2000). *Scope of practice.* Cherry Hill, NJ: Author.

National Council of State Boards of Nursing. (2008). *Consensus model for APRN regulation: Licensure, accreditation, certification, and education.* Retrieved from https://www.ncsbn.org/Consensus_Model_for_APRN_Regulation_July_2008.pdf

National Organization of Nurse Practitioner Faculties. (2008). *Criteria for evaluation of nurse practitioner programs: A report of the national task force on quality nurse practitioner education.* Washington, DC: Author.

Pearson, L. (2010). *The Pearson Report.* Retrieved from http://www.pearsonreport.com/overview

Shuler, P. A., & Davis, J. E. (1993). The Shuler nurse practitioner model: A theoretical framework for nurse practitioner clinicians, educators, and researchers, Part I. *Journal of the American Academy of Nurse Practitioners, 5*(1), 11–18.

Shuler, P. A., & Davis, J. E. (1993). The Shuler nurse practitioner model: Clinical application, Part 2. *Journal of the American Academy of Nurse Practitioners, 5*(2), 73–88.

Shuler, P. A., & Huebscher, R. (1998). Clarifying nurse practitioner's unique contributions: Application of the Shuler nurse practitioner practice model. *Journal of the American Academy of Nurse Practitioners, 10*(11), 491–499.

Snyder, M., & Mirr, M. P. (1999). *Advanced practice nursing: A guide to professional development* (2nd ed.). New York: Springer Publishing.

Social Security Act of 1965, Title XVIII—Health insurance for the aged and disabled. Retrieved from http://www.ssa.gov/OP_Home/ssact/title02/0226.htm

Trandel-Korenchuk, D. M., & Trandel-Korenchuk, K. M. (1998). *Nursing and the law* (5th ed.). Gaithersburg, MD: Aspen Publishers.

U.S. Department of Health and Human Services. (2010). *Healthy people 2020: National health promotion and disease prevention objectives.* Retrieved from http://www.healthypeople.gov/2020/topicsobjectives2020/default.aspx

U.S. Preventive Services Task Force. (2007). *The guide to clinical preventive services: Recommendations of the United States Preventive Services Task Force.* Retrieved from http://www.ahrq.gov/clinic/pocketgd.htm

Index

Pages followed by *t* or *f* denote tables or figures respectively.